Arthroscopic Management of the Knee

David J. Dandy FRCS

Consultant Orthopaedic Surgeon, Newmarket General Hospital and Addenbrooke's Hospital, Cambridge; Associate Lecturer, Faculty of Clinical Medicine, University of Cambridge.

SECOND EDITION

CHURCHILL LIVINGSTONE
EDINBURGH LONDON MELBOURNE AND NEW YORK 1987

CHURCHILL LIVINGSTONE
Medical Division of Longman Group UK Limited

Distributed in the United States of America by
Churchill Livingstone Inc., 1560 Broadway, New York,
N.Y. 10036, and by associated companies,
branches and representatives throughout
the world.

First edition entitled Arthroscopic Surgery of the Knee 1981
Second edition 1987

ISBN 0 443 02958 X

British Library Cataloguing in Publication Data
Dandy, David J.
    Arthroscopic management of the knee. – 2nd ed. –
    (Current problems in orthopaedics)
    1. Knee – Surgery
    2. Arthroscopy
    I. Title II. Dandy, David J. Arthroscopic surgery of the knee
    617′.582059   RD561

Library of Congress Cataloguing in Publication Data
Dandy, David J.
    Arthroscopic management of the knee. –
    (Current problems in orthopaedics)
    Rev. ed. of: Arthroscopic surgery of the knee. 1981.
    Includes bibliographies and index.
    1. Knee – Surgery.
    2. Arthroscopy.
    I. Dandy, David J. Anthroscopic surgery of the knee.
    II. Title.   III. Series. [DNLM: 1. Arthroscopy.
    2. Knee – Surgery. WE 870 D178a]
    RD561.D36 1986   617′.582   86-17609

Printed and bound in Great Britain by
William Clowes Limited, Beccles and London

Preface

Much has happened to arthroscopic surgery since *Arthroscopic Surgery of the Knee* first appeared five years ago. The manuscript for the first edition was prepared during 1979/80 and published in 1981, when arthroscopic surgery was a new technique regarded as a passing fad by many and a dangerous innovation by some; others regarded it with suspicion and disbelief. With this background, the aim of the first edition was to set out the operations that were then possible and to explain how they could be completed safely.

Since then, arthroscopic surgery has gained popularity at a rate little short of terrifying. In some countries, particularly the United States, where thousands of surgeons attend courses on arthroscopy every year, open meniscectomy is almost obsolete, and arthroscopy has been extended to the shoulder, elbow, ankle, wrist and the mid-carpal joints. In more conservative countries such as Great Britain, arthroscopy of the knee is already the most commonly performed orthopaedic operation in some centres, and there are very few orthopaedic centres where arthroscopic surgery is still unavailable. In areas such as Newmarket, where arthroscopic surgery has been established for several years, patients who were once astonished to find themselves back at work within a few days of meniscectomy now express amazement that friends and relatives in other areas are subjected to open surgery of the knee, with all its attendant incapacity and discomfort.

New equipment has been introduced at an alarming rate. Motorised instruments, a novelty at the time of the first edition, are now so well developed that some surgeons find themselves unable to operate without them. Television systems have developed beyond all expectations and have revolutionised both the teaching and the documentation of arthroscopic surgery, although television is no more essential for arthroscopy than it is for sigmoidoscopy. Electrodiathermy equipment is now available for intra-articular surgery, laser is under development, and there is an increasing body of opinion which believes that technological ingenuity may have outstripped common sense.

Operative techniques have followed the same pattern. Old techniques have been improved and new ones introduced to the extent that the only indications for arthrotomy are total joint replacement and ligament reconstruction. The conservative approach to the meniscus has progressed to the point where meniscal fragments are reattached rather than removed. The arthroscopic insertion of artificial ligaments, described in the first edition, but discontinued because the prosthetic materials were inadequate, has now been reintroduced and developed with new materials. Areas denuded of articular cartilage can be abraded in the optimistic expectation that they will heal, offering hope to patients for whom no treatment was previously available.

Such rapid development has led to many problems. Operations are done without the guidance of long-term studies to establish proper indications, and surgeons performing operations for the first time encounter new and unexpected complications. Arthroscopic surgery has forced a radical reappraisal of existing approaches to knee surgery, which has not endeared it to academic surgeons, to whom it seems that arthroscopic surgery has overturned long-established beliefs without any convincing evidence that the eventual long-term results justify the spectacular short-term benefits for the patient.

For all these reasons, the underlying philosophy of

this second edition is different from the first, which was essentially a 'how to do it' book describing operative techniques. Instead, the emphasis has been changed to show how arthroscopy and arthroscopic surgery contribute to the management of knee disorders as a whole, and the title has been changed accordingly. Little of substance has changed in the techniques and pathology, but some items – notably the lateral synovial shelf – have failed to stand the test of time. New chapters have been added on photography and television, the management of ligament instability, the unstable patella, and anterior knee pain. Other chapters have been split, as they became too long; the original chapter on meniscal surgery, for example, has now become three chapters. The decision was made to concentrate on disorders of the knee, rather than arthroscopy, because this bears a closer relationship to clinical practice; thus there is no reference to the arthroscopy of other joints.

The rapid expansion of arthroscopic surgery continues unabated, and it is inevitable that some parts of this manuscript will be out of date by the time the book appears on the shelves. The reader is asked to be tolerant of this unavoidable difficulty. Nevertheless, it is hoped that this edition will offer useful guidelines for the application of the arthroscope to the expanding field of knee surgery, and that arthroscopic surgery will not split off as a separate specialty, but become integrated into knee surgery as a whole.

Cambridge, 1987   D.J.D.

To Dr R W Jackson

Acknowledgements

I am indebted to Mrs C. Sheehan for transferring the manuscript of the first edition to disk and to Mrs S. French for secretarial assistance. The staff in the operating theatres and wards at Newmarket General Hospital, the Evelyn Hospital, Addenbrooke's Hospital, Cambridge, and the Hope Nursing Home have continued to encourage and support my arthroscopic endeavours, despite frequent and considerable tedium. My thanks are also due to Miss K. Sergeant, MCSP, whose skilful physiotherapy has contributed substantially to the success of the surgical procedures, and whose constructive and objective criticisms have proved invaluable.

For the illustrations, I am again indebted to Mrs M. Thorburn for the line diagrams and to many surgical instrument companies, but notably Chas F. Thackray Ltd, for supplying photographs of up-to-date equipment.

Finally, the work would not have been possible without the continued help and encouragement of my wife, Jane, and the tolerance of our children, James and Emma, who were deprived of access to the home computer for long periods while the project was in progress.

D.J.D.

Contents

The development of arthroscopy and arthroscopic surgery

ENDOSCOPY

The first report of endoscopy in clinical practice was presented by Phillip Bozzini to the Academy of Medicine in Vienna in 1806. In Bozzini's instrument, the 'lichtleiter', light from a beeswax candle passed down a polished silver tube which also served as a speculum (Fig. 1.1). This instrument was first used in the nasopharynx, but could also be used to examine the anal canal, rectum, vagina, bladder, urethra and the abscess cavities of osteomyelitis. The use of the instrument was painful, the illumination poor and the field of vision small (Bush et al 1974). Bozzini's audience in Vienna was unreceptive; his paper was greeted with derision and his instrument was considered to have no clinical importance – a reaction not unknown after the announcement of more recent advances in endoscopy. Bozzini returned from Vienna to his practice in Frankfurt, where he died three years later at the age of 36.

Pierre Ségalas presented a similar instrument to the Académie des Sciences in 1826, initiating an acrimonious dispute with Herteloupe (1827), who claimed that Ségalas had plagiarised his own idea, which used lampyrids (glow-worms) enclosed in a glass ampoule as a light source. Presumably the glow-worm must have emitted a constant light rather than an intermittent flash, and the abdomen of the female *Lampyris noctiluca*, which is 18 mm long and 5 mm wide, was probably used (Foster 1979). Little more was heard of endoscopy until 1853, when Desormeaux introduced an endoscope in which the light source was a spirit lamp burning a mixture of alcohol and turpentine called 'gazogene' (Fig. 1.2). The optical system included polished silver tubes,

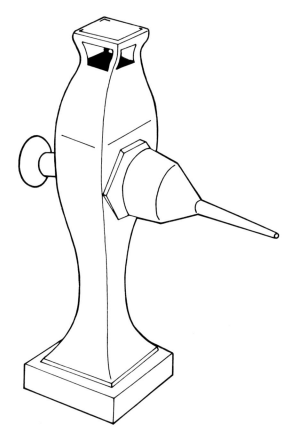

Fig. 1.1 The Bozzini endoscope. This instrument was covered with Morocco leather and the light source was a beeswax candle

mirrors and lenses. The operation must have been a trial for patient, surgeon and assistants alike: imagine a darkened room illuminated only by the lamp of the endoscope, which emitted as much heat as light, the smell of burning turpentine mixed perhaps with that of hot paint on a new instrument, and the apprehension of the unanaesthetised but stoical patient as the proboscis of this terrifying contraption entered his urethra. There are reports of burns to the surgeon's

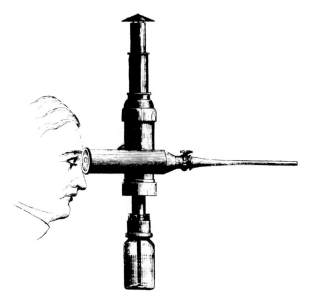

Fig. 1.2 The Desormeaux endoscope in use

face (Murphy 1972) and the patients probably suffered comparable injuries, although these are not mentioned.

Cumbersome and dangerous though the Desormeaux cystoscope may have been, it survived its critics and was improved by, among others, F.R. Cruise of Dublin who, in 1865, increased the brilliance of the flame by using a mixture of petrol and camphor and added a mahogany case to make handling easier and to protect the surgeon's hands from the heat of the lamp (Murphy 1972).

Other light sources included a burning magnesium filament introduced by J. Andrew in 1867, and Bruck's diaphanoscope. Bruck's innovation is worthy of mention not only because it was the forerunner of the electric lamp, but because it demonstrated the determination and enterprise of the endoscopic pioneers. Julius Bruck was a dentist from Breslau who, in 1867 developed a platinum filament that could be raised to white heat by electricity from a battery and cooled by a glass jacket through which water flowed (Fig. 1.3). Straying beyond the normal confines of dentistry, Bruck placed this crude electric light source in his patient's rectum so that the interior of the bladder could be observed by transmitted light, using a straight urethral speculum. A gynaecologist colleague of Bruck commented that if a lamp was placed in the vagina, he could make out the shape of the uterus and ovaries 'in a thin woman in a darkened room' (Wallace 1978).

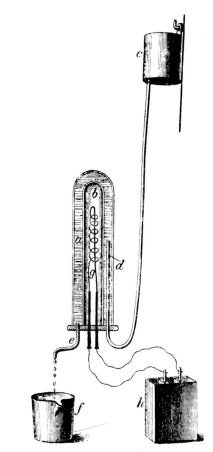

Fig. 1.3 Bruck's lamp (from E.H. Fenwick 1889)

Max Nitze (1848–1906) developed Bruck's lamp further, and in 1877 fitted a heated platinum filament shielded by a window of rock crystal and cooled by a continuous flow of water so that the light source itself was introduced into the bladder (Fenwick 1889). This instrument was improved with the help of Leiter, an instrument-maker of Vienna, and in 1879 the Nitze–Leiter cystoscope was produced (Fig. 1.4). The lighting and cooling systems of this instrument fell short of perfection, and the invention was ridiculed as a 'fire and water contraption' (Eikelaar 1975).

Joseph Swan, an Englishman, made a crude incandescent light in 1860, but it was Edison who produced the first effective electric lamp almost 20 years later, in 1879. The application of the incandescent bulb to endoscopy was quickly realised and was first used by David Newman of Glasgow in 1883. Leiter, in 1886, and Nitze, in 1887, used the same lamp to produce a cystoscope remarkably similar to those still in use today. Later improvements in-

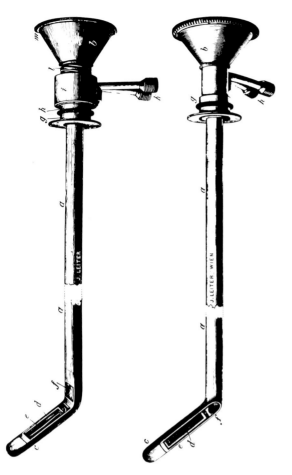

Fig. 1.4 The Nitze–Leiter cytoscope (1879). The electric filament (e) covered by a rock crystal window (d) illuminated the bladder, which could be observed through the lens (f) (from E.H. Fenwick 1889)

cluded the Amici prism, which for the first time produced an upright instead of an inverted image, and refinements in lens manufacture and design improved the quality of the image still further.

Optical design continued. Two recent innovations, both introduced by Professor H.H. Hopkins of Reading University, have done much to improve the reliability and versatility of endoscopy. These innovations are the rod lens system, which makes possible the construction of smaller telescopes that produce a better image with less light loss, and the glass fibre light guide used in all modern endoscopes. Less light is now required, the optical image is sharper and brighter, the instruments narrower, and the heat of the light source is kept well away from the patient. These developments, more than anything else, have been responsible for the rapid expansion of surgical endoscopy in the last decade.

DIAGNOSTIC ARTHROSCOPY

The first endoscopes were used for viewing the bladder, rectum or vagina and it was not until 1918 that Professor K. Takagi of Tokyo examined the interior of the knee with a cystoscope 7.3 mm in diameter (Watanabe et al 1979). The principal use of arthroscopy in Japan in those days lay in the management of tuberculosis of the knee, which could make squatting and kneeling impossible and led to serious social and physical incapacity. By 1920, Takagi had designed his own arthroscope, but its diameter, 7.3 mm, made it unsuitable for routine use. It was 1931 before a 3.5 mm instrument was developed and used routinely (Takagi 1982). The Takagi instruments evolved rapidly, and later included a focusable lens system, a 2.7 mm telescope for use in dogs, and an operating arthroscope. Takagi succeeded in taking both black and white still and 16 mm ciné photographs of the interior of the knee in 1932 (Takagi 1932, 1933), followed by colour photography in 1936 (Takagi 1939).

Independently of Takagi, Eugen Bircher of Aarau, in Switzerland, used the Jacobeaus laparo-thoracoscope to examine the knee, first distending the joint with oxygen or nitrogen by means of an artificial pneumothorax apparatus. Bircher reported the results of twenty 'arthro-endoscopies' in 1921, the first mention of arthroscopy in the world literature. The work of Takagi and Bircher stimulated much interest and it was not long before arthroscopy reached the English-speaking world. In 1925, Philip H. Kreuscher suggested to the Illinois Medical Society that arthroscopy might be helpful in the early diagnosis of meniscal lesions. The study of arthroscopy continued and advanced at the Hospital for Joint Diseases in New York, where Dr Michael Burman used an instrument with an outside diameter of 4 mm, designed by R. Wappler, to examine the elbow, ankle and shoulder as well as the knee (Burman 1931, Burman et al 1934, Burman & Mayer 1936, Mayer & Burman 1939). Burman's first paper (1931) described in detail the technique for distending the joint and the points of insertion that are still in use today. The second important paper by Burman and his colleagues (Burman et al 1934) described the clinical experience of more than 100 patients, and little new has been written about diagnostic arthroscopy since.

In Europe, the work of Bircher sometimes met the

same crushing scepticism that had greeted the work of Bozzini and Nitze in the previous century. In 1937, Hustinx, who had no experience of the instrument or its use, wrote:

> But what to think of the gonoscope which Bircher advocated at the Accident Congress held in Amsterdam in 1925? How can anyone venture to introduce a luminous object into the knee joint in an effort to look between the articular surfaces, which cannot be separated? Even at arthrotomy it is impossible to see the posterior horn of the meniscus if the knee joint is not sufficiently open. How then could one expect to see it in a closed joint? This is quite impossible. Moreover, this procedure is more dangerous than an exploratory arthrotomy. (Eikelaar 1975)

Despite such opposition, the work continued and arthroscopy was on the point of becoming an established technique when all work in Japan, North America and Europe was brought to an abrupt halt by the Second World War. Few articles about arthroscopy appeared during the war years but among them was the description by Wiberg (1941) of arthroscopy in disorders of the abnormal patellofemoral joint, included in a classic work remembered more for its anatomical analysis of the joint than its contribution to arthroscopy. Even when hostilities ended, several years passed before arthroscopy again progressed. In 1957, Dr Masaki Watanabe (Fig. 1.5), who had worked closely with Takagi, collaborated with Ikeuchi and Takeda to publish an *Atlas of Arthroscopy*, which included water-colour illustrations, and was followed in 1969 by a second edition that included endoscopic photographs, and a third edition in 1979. Of Watanabe's many contributions to arthroscopy, perhaps the greatest was his number 21 arthroscope (Fig. 1.6), which was introduced in 1959 (Watanabe & Takeda 1960) and became the instrument of choice for arthroscopists around the world for almost a decade.

In Europe and North America, interest in arthroscopy had been virtually extinguished by the Second World War. Although Dr I. Macnab of Toronto used a paediatric cystoscope to examine the interior of a knee in 1963 (Jackson 1979), general interest in arthroscopy was not rekindled until Dr R.W. Jackson returned to Toronto in December 1964, after working with Dr Watanabe. The teaching of Dr Jackson has since influenced many surgeons in

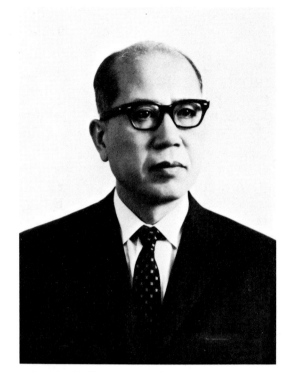

Fig. 1.5 Dr Masaki Watanabe

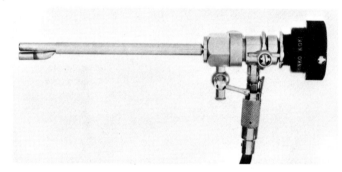

Fig. 1.6 The Watanabe 21 arthroscope. This instrument, with an off-set tungsten light bulb mounted on a separate light carrier, laid the foundations of modern arthroscopy (photograph courtesy of Colonel J. Carson, USAF)

America, Europe and Australasia, and has done more than anything else to establish arthroscopy as a routine procedure in the English-speaking world.

Instructional courses have also been influential. The first English-language course in arthroscopy was held in Philadelphia in 1972, where, in 1974, arthroscopy finally became established with the inauguration of the International Arthroscopy Association under the presidency of Dr Masaki Watanabe. The first instructional course in Europe was held in 1976 at Nijmegen, under the direction of

Professor T. Van Rens, followed by others in Scandinavia in 1977, and England in 1979.

ARTHROSCOPIC SURGERY

It has proved impossible to discover who first performed arthroscopic surgery, but the credit should probably go to Finkelstein and Mayer, who described synovial biopsy by the double puncture technique in 1931 (Finkelstein & Mayer 1931). The idea was published earlier, however, by E.S. Geist in 1926, when he wrote in a 'preliminary report' of the possibility of synovial biopsy through the arthroscope:

> We ought not only to be able to see through this tube inserted into the joint, but, like the genito-urinary surgeon, we ought to be able with suitable instruments to procure from the joint the necessary pathological material for microscopic study.
>
> As I conceive it, the performance of arthroscopy in the living ought not to be more distressing to the patient than a simple aspiration, provided local anaesthesia is employed.
>
> Further communications will follow.

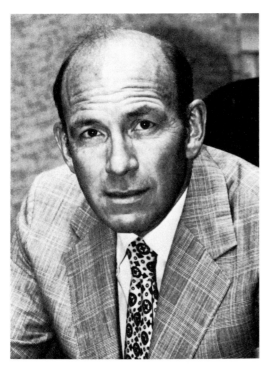

Fig. 1.7 Dr Richard L. O'Connor (1933–80) (courtesy of the *Journal of Bone and Joint Surgery*)

Sadly, there was no further communication until Lipson, Clemmons and Frymoyer described the successful results of arthroscopic synovial biopsy in 1967. The procedure has since become popular among those great surgical enthusiasts, the rheumatologists, often under local anaesthesia, just as Geist envisaged (Jayson & Dixon 1968).

Dr M. Watanabe became the first to perform an arthroscopic meniscectomy when he removed a posterior flap tear of the medial meniscus in 1962 (Carson 1979, O'Connor 1979, Ikeuchi 1979, Sprague 1982). Dr R.W. Jackson removed two loose bodies from the knee in 1966 (Jackson 1979) and a bucket-handle fragment of meniscus in 1970. Arthroscopic surgery was further developed by Dr R.L. O'Connor (Fig. 1.7), who made an enormous contribution before his death in 1980. Surprisingly, there do not seem to have been any reports of the clinical results of arthroscopic surgery until 1978 (Dandy 1978), although mention of arthroscopic surgery had been made earlier (Dandy & Jackson 1975).

EFFECT ON PRACTICE

Arthroscopic surgery has proved so successful that it has avoided much of the resistance that beset arthroscopy, but has instead been embraced with an almost indecent enthusiasm. In 1981, approximately 2000 surgeons attended instructional courses on arthroscopic surgery in North America alone, and the same reaction has been seen in many countries around the world. The results of arthroscopic surgery are so striking that the general public shares this enthusiasm as soon as it becomes aware of the technique, and patients with disorders of the knee quickly dominate the practice of any surgeon who offers arthroscopic surgery. Although few would consciously seek to be a 'one-operation' surgeon, this fate may be difficult to avoid. In some countries, there are now surgeons who confine their practice entirely to arthroscopic surgery of the knee and who are obliged to refer patients with ligamentous instability or osteoarthritis to a colleague. These points are worth considering before becoming too deeply involved in arthroscopic surgery, because however successful the results may be, the procedures themselves are technically exacting and often frustrating, and the operations are so different from the rest of orthopaedic surgery that many find them uncongenial. To give up a technique as successful as arthroscopic surgery is difficult, and it might be very reasonable to decide not to become involved before a graceful retreat becomes impossible.

Although the development of arthroscopic surgery as a separate specialty may well lead to a more rapid accumulation of research data, new techniques and experience, the need to refer so many common conditions to others for definitive treatment has obvious disadvantages. Other endoscopic specialties have avoided such a division: there are urologists, not cystoscopic surgeons; gynaecologists, not laparoscopic surgeons; and there are no bowel surgeons who perform only sigmoidoscopy and leave bowel resection to their colleagues. It is to be hoped that the specialty of pure arthroscopic surgery is a transient phenomenon that will vanish when every surgeon who operates upon the knee is a competent arthroscopist, but this may well take many years and perhaps even another generation of surgeons. By then, orthopaedic surgery may have become subdivided in much the same way as 'general' surgery is today. Hand surgery, joint replacement, scoliosis surgery, spinal surgery and children's orthopaedics are ready candidates for specialisation, and the development of arthroscopic surgery could provide the impetus for the evolution of knee surgery as a separate interest.

The speed and enthusiasm with which arthroscopic surgery has been accepted is an indication of its remarkable success, but should also sound a note of warning (Dandy 1983), not only because such an explosion of enthusiasm must inevitably be followed by reports of failures and complications, but also because new disorders and conditions are being found and treated without the benefit of long-term studies to establish the proper indications for operation.

Understandably, surgeons who have established a successful practice without the help of arthroscopy regard the technique with suspicion – sometimes almost as a form of witchcraft – and this has led to an unfortunate division among surgeons with a common interest in the knee. Because of this, all orthopaedic surgeons, whether arthroscopic or 'traditional', would be wise to maintain a healthy scepticism towards the sometimes extravagant claims made for arthroscopic surgery until arthroscopic surgery has 'shaken down' and found its true place in orthopaedic practice.

References

Bozzini P 1806 Lichtleiter, eine Erfindung zur Anschauung innerer Theile und Krankheiten nebst der Abbildung. In: Hufeland C W (ed) Journal der practischen Arzneykunde und Wundarzneykunst, Berlin 24: 107–124

Bruck, J 1867 Das Urethroskop und das Stamatoscop zur durch Leuchtung der Blase und der Zahne und ihrer Nachbartheile durch Galvanisches Gluhlicht. Maruschke und Berendt, Breslau

Burman M S 1931 Arthroscopy or direct visualization of joints. An experimental cadaver study. Journal of Bone and Joint Surgery 13: 669–695

Burman M S, Mayer L 1936 Arthroscopic examination of the knee joint. Archives of Surgery 32: 846–874

Burman M S, Finkelstein H, Mayer L 1934 Arthroscopy of the knee joint. Journal of Bone and Joint Surgery 16: 255–268

Bush R B, Leonhardt H, Bush I M, Landes R R 1974 Dr Bozzini's Lichtleiter. A translation of his original article (1806) Urology 3: 119–123

Carson R W 1979 Arthroscopic meniscectomy. Orthopedic Clinics of North America 10: 619–627

Dandy D J 1978 Early results of closed partial meniscectomy. British Medical Journal 1: 1099–1100

Dandy D J 1983 Arthroscopy of the knee: some problems. Journal of the Royal Society of Medicine 76: 448–450

Dandy D J, Jackson R W 1975 The impact of arthroscopy on the management of disorders of the knee. Journal of Bone and Joint Surgery 57B: 349–352

Desormeaux A J 1853 De L'endoscope. Bull Acad Med Académie des Sciences 1855

Eikelaar H R 1975 Arthroscopy of the knee – thesis for a doctorate in orthopaedic surgery at the University of Groningen, The Netherlands. Royal United Printers Hoitsema BV

Fenwick E H 1889 The electric illumination of the bladder and urethra. J & A Churchill, London

Finkelstein H, Mayer L 1931 The arthroscope. A new method of examining joints. Journal of Bone and Joint Surgery 13: 583–588

Foster W A 1979 Personal communication

Geist E S 1926 Arthroscopy: preliminary report. Journal-Lancet, Minneapolis 46: 306–307

Herteloupe C L S 1827 La lithotritie. Acad4émie des Sciences, Paris

Hustinx E J H 1937 Letsels van de menisci van het kniegewricht. Nederlands Tijdschrift voor Geneeskunde 81 Nr: 12 blz–1218

Ikeuchi H 1979 Meniscus surgery using the Watanabe arthroscope. Orthopedic Clinics of North America 10: 629–642

Jackson R W 1979 Personal communication

Jayson M I, Dixon A S 1968 Arthroscopy of the knee in rheumatic diseases. Annals of the Rheumatic Diseases 27: 503–511

Kreuscher P 1925 Semilunar cartilage disease, a plea for early recognition by means of the arthroscope and early treatment of this condition. Illinois Medical Journal 47: 290–292

Lipson R L, Clemmons J J, Frymoyer J W 1967 Arthroscopy: experience with percutaneous biopsy of intraarticular structures under direct vision. Arthritis and Rheumatism 10: 294

Mayer L, Burman M S 1939 Arthroscopy in the diagnosis of meniscal lesions of the knee joint. American Journal of Surgery 43: 501–511

Murphy L J T 1972 History of urology. C C Thomas, Springfield, Ill

O'Connor R L 1979 Personal communication

Ségalas P 1826 Académie des Sciences, Paris

Sprague N F 1982 Operative arthroscopy. Clinical Orthopaedics and Related Research 167: 4–5

Takagi K 1932 Journal of the Japanese Orthopaedic Association 7: 241

Takagi K 1933 Practical experience using Takagi's arthroscope. Journal of the Japanese Orthopaedic Association 8: 132

Takagi K 1939 The arthroscope. Journal of the Japanese Orthopaedic Association 14: 359–441

Takagi K 1982 The classic arthroscope. Kenji Takagi, Journal of the Japanese Orthopaedic Association 1939. Clinical Orthopaedics and Related Research 167: 6–8

Wallace D M 1978 In: Gow J G, Hopkins H H (eds) Handbook of urological endoscopy. Churchill Livingstone, Edinburgh

Watanabe M, Takeda S 1960 The number 21 arthroscope. Journal of the Japanese Orthopaedic Association 34: 1041

Watanabe M, Takeda S, Ikeuchi H 1957 Atlas of arthroscopy, 1st edn. Igaku Shoin, Tokyo

Watanabe M, Takeda S, Ikeuchi H 1979 Atlas of arthroscopy, 3rd edn. Igaku Shoin, Tokyo

Wiberg G 1941 Roentgenographic and anatomic studies of the femoro-patellar joint. Acta Orthopaedica Scandinavica 12: 319–410

2

Equipment

As in other fields of surgery, a wide choice of instruments is available. Each instrument company makes its own range, and each has its own good qualities. Every surgeon will want to choose his own instruments, but the following guidelines may help to make a decision.

ARTHROSCOPES

Standard arthroscopes

The work-horse of arthroscopic surgery is the 5 mm rod lens arthroscope with a 30° fore-oblique lens (Fig. 2.1). The 30° telescope can reach areas inaccessible to the 0° telescope, but anatomical landmarks within the joint must be used for navigation and a little experience is required before these can be recognised easily. Any surgeon considering arthroscopic surgery should be thoroughly familiar with arthroscopic anatomy and should be able to use the 30° arthroscope with confidence. For beginners – but only for beginners – the straightahead 0° telescope is recommended, because its field of vision lies directly in front of the telescope and

orientation is easy (Fig. 2.2). A 70° telescope is helpful in the postero-medial and postero-lateral compartments and is strongly recommended as an early addition to the basic set of instruments (Fig. 2.3).

The small-diameter arthroscope (Fig. 2.4), if used in conjunction with the multiple puncture technique

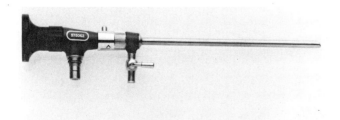

Fig. 2.1 A 5 mm 30° fore-oblique arthroscope (courtesy of Chas F. Thackray Ltd)

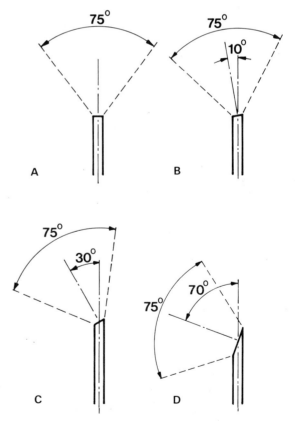

Fig. 2.2 The direction of vision of the arthroscope. (A) Straightahead arthroscope; (B) 10° fore-oblique (sometimes referred to as 170°); (C) 30° fore-oblique; (D) 70° fore-oblique

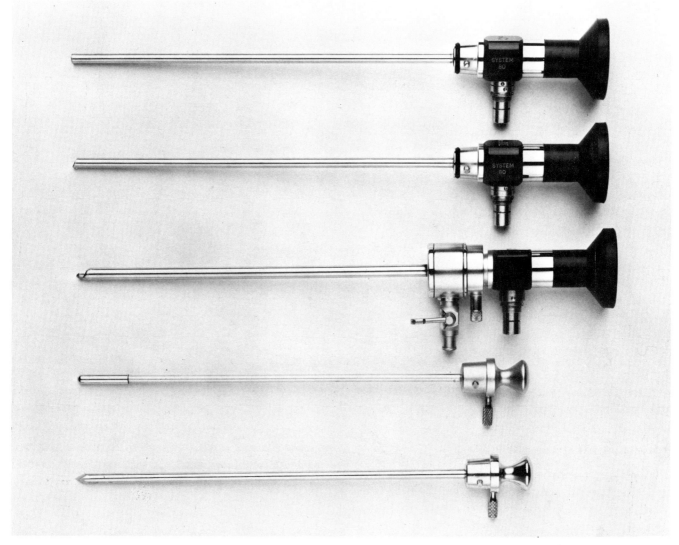

Fig. 2.3 A set of arthroscopes. From above downwards: 0° telescope, 30° telescope, 70° telescope in sheath, blunt obturator and sharp trocar

popularised by Johnson (Johnson 1977, Johnson & Becker 1976), is satisfactory for out-patient diagnosis under local anaesthesia, but the advantages of this instrument for routine use disappeared with the arrival of arthroscopic surgery. Small-diameter arthroscopes may find some application in the examination of the popliteus tunnel or other recesses, and in tight joints such as the wrist, but they are too small, too brittle, and have too narrow an angle of vision to be used routinely for arthroscopic surgery of the knee.

When selecting an arthroscope, do not choose a model which has a bridge (Fig. 2.5). The bridge was necessary in the original paediatric cystoscopes from which most arthroscopes evolved, because of the need for ureteric catheterisation and biopsy of the bladder wall, but it is not necessary for diagnostic arthroscopy and can easily be forgotten when the instrument is assembled. If the bridge is not inserted, several centimetres of unprotected telescope protrude from the sheath and arthroscopes have broken in the knee as a result; McGinty (1982) shows the radiographic appearance after such a mishap. The most effective insurance against this complication is to purchase an instrument which does not include a removable bridge. Check also that the saline ports are at the tip of the sheath. If the port is proximal to the tip, saline can run into the soft tissues and create serious problems by distending the fat-pad (Fig. 2.6).

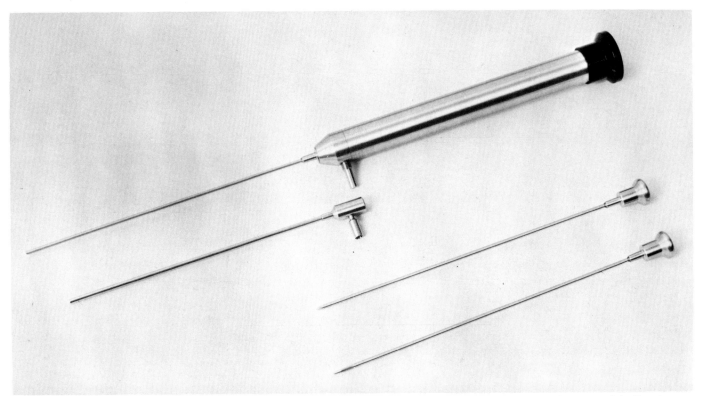

Fig. 2.4   The Dyonics Needlescope. From above downwards: needlescope, sheath, sharp trocar and blunt obturator (courtesy of the Dyonics Corporation)

Operating arthroscopes

An operating arthroscope is not a basic piece of equipment and is not necessary to perform arthroscopic surgery. Operating arthroscopes include a separate instrument channel parallel with the telescope, but moved away from the eyepiece by two 90° bends in the lens system (Fig. 2.7). Most use a

narrow telescope with a smaller field of vision than the diagnostic telescope, and the instrument is much thicker than a diagnostic arthroscope, because it

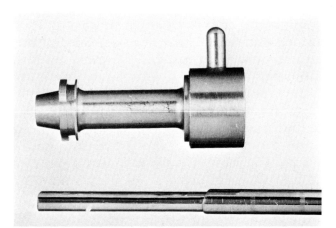

Fig. 2.5   The bridge from an early arthroscope. If the bridge (above) is omitted, a corresponding length of telescope is left protruding unprotected from the sheath

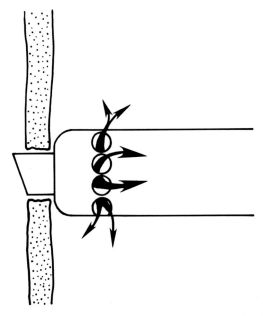

Fig. 2.6   If the saline ports are proximal to the telescope tip, they can lie outside the synovium (stippled) and distend the subcutaneous tissues

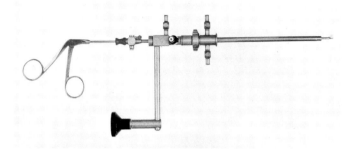

Fig. 2.7 The Wolf operating arthroscope with the scissors in the instrument channel

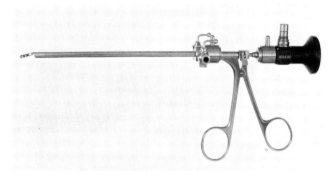

Fig. 2.9 The Storz diagnostic arthroscope with biopsy forceps inserted in place of the bridge

includes two irrigation channels as well as a glass-fibre light guide.

The instruments supplied with the operating arthroscopes include grasping forceps, basket forceps, and a selection of knives (Fig. 2.8). Meniscal tissue can be cut with the scissors as long as it is snipped in little bites, but both scissors and basket forceps quickly lose their cutting edge and need to be replaced after thirty or forty procedures.

A little practice is required before an operating arthroscope can be handled easily (Fig. 6.8). The main problems are difficulty in manipulating the instrument because of its bulk, the fragility of the 3 mm cutting instruments, the reduced field of vision

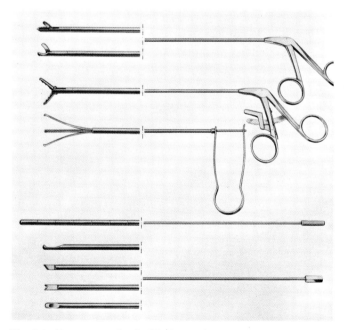

Fig. 2.8 Instruments for the Wolf operating arthroscope. From above downwards: basket forceps, scissors, grasping forceps, spring-loaded grasping forceps, probe and four knives

from the narrow telescope, which makes orientation difficult, and the fact that the instruments will only move parallel with the telescope. The problem of orientation can sometimes be overcome by identifying the target from a distance, touching it with the tip of an operating instrument passed through the instrument channel, and 'railroading' the arthroscope along the instrument.

Some arthroscopes started out in life as paediatric cystoscopes, and a few still have markings on the barrel at 1 cm intervals to show how far along the urethra they have passed. These instruments can be fitted with a diathermy lead for electrocoagulation of bladder polyps in place of a bridge and were the reason for the bridge that created so many difficulties in the early days (p. 9). With this type of instrument, biopsy forceps can be inserted by removing the telescope and bridge from the sheath and replacing them with a narrower telescope and forceps (Fig. 2.9). This instrument is excellent for working inside the bladder or the suprapatellar pouch, and is probably the arthroscope of choice for the rheumatologist taking synovial biopsy specimens. It is of little use, however, for other procedures, because the fixed position of the forceps at the end of the telescope only allows them to cut structures that can be brought flat against the end of the instrument (Fig. 2.10).

LIGHTING

Light sources

Apart from electronic flash generators, there are three principal sources of light: the tungsten filament, the mercury arc and xenon. A 150 watt

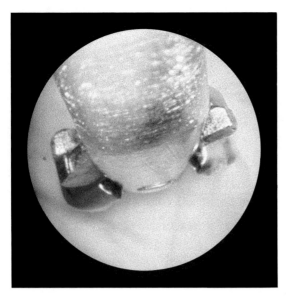

Fig. 2.10   The view down the Storz diagnostic arthroscope with the biopsy forceps in position

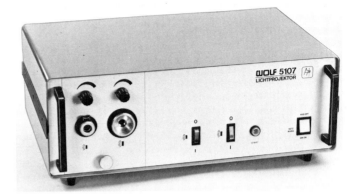

Fig. 2.11   A twin light source with a tungsten and mercury arc bulb (courtesy of Richard Wolf UK Ltd)

tungsten light, similar to that used in an ordinary slide projector, is the simplest and cheapest light source, but also the least brilliant. Tungsten light is not bright enough to use television cameras to their best advantage, and its yellow colour can interfere with television and photography.

Mercury arc lamps are bright enough for most television uses and for photography, but should not be used at full intensity unless coupled to a television camera, because their maximum intensity is too bright for the naked eye and can cause permanent retinal damage (Friedman & Kuwabara 1968, Calkins & Hochheimer 1979, 1980, Hochheimer et al 1979). Mercury arc lamps also have the disadvantage that they gradually become dimmer, and have a working life of 50–100 hours only. Xenon light sources, which are more intense than mercury arc lamps, were essential for early television cameras and for photography. They are very large, very costly, and are no longer needed for routine television or photography. Electronic flash units can also be interposed between the camera and the arthroscope, or can be built into the light source itself. These flash units are needed only for photographic work with slow films or dull arthroscopes (p. 28).

For most purposes, a simple 150 watt tungsten light is adequate, but a unit which includes a mercury arc lamp as well as a tungsten bulb (Fig. 2.11) is much more versatile and can be used for photography or television as well as routine work.

Light cables

The most commonly used light cable is a fibreglass bundle, the ends of the fibres sealed with an acrylic resin. The light from a fibre bundle can be manipulated optically as it leaves the cable, which can increase its efficiency, but the light transmission is diminished if the fibres are broken. The acrylic used to seal the end of the cable can cause a brownish discoloration that increases with time and repeated soaking in glutaraldehyde. Although satisfactory for routine use, an old or dirty light cable can spoil photographs or television.

A liquid light guide consisting of a fluid-filled flexible tube will carry more light than a fibreglass bundle, but the light cannot be directed as well after it has left the cable and it has a bluish tinge, which interferes with photography and television. Excellent photographs are produced with a 150 watt tungsten light source, however, because the blue tinge of the light cable compensates for the yellow of the tungsten light.

Light probes

Additional light sources consisting of a simple bundle of light fibres enclosed in a steel tube fitted with a light coupling can be slipped along an instrument cannula or passed through a separate incision (Fig. 2.12). However, because the direction of the light differs from the line of vision of the arthroscope, it will cast shadows. Light probes are therefore not as useful as they might seem, although they can be useful if inserted from the posterior approaches to transilluminate the cruciate ligaments and posterior structures.

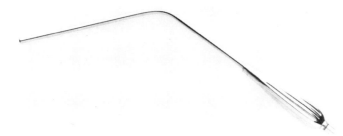

Fig. 2.12 A light probe (courtesy of Chas F. Thackray Ltd)

JOINT DISTENSION

Irrigation fluid and pH

The choice of irrigation fluid is not as simple as it might appear (Reagan et al 1983). Normal saline, although of the same osmolarity as blood, has a pH of 5.3, and is primarily intended for intravenous administration, where it can be rapidly diluted and exposed to the metabolic regulation of the kidneys, liver and lungs. Water has a pH closer to that of synovial fluid, but will cause lysis of red cells and oedema of the soft tissues, if it leaks into the calf through a capsular defect.

Other solutions are available with electrolyte and pH values closer to those of normal synovial fluid. Although clinical experience has not yet shown any evidence of complications or problems following the use of normal saline, the matter deserves careful thought and perhaps the development of an irrigation fluid with similar electrolytic and pH characteristics to those of normal synovial fluid.

Pumps

Hydrostatic pressure is sufficient to distend the knee, but some surgeons prefer a blood-pressure cuff to increase the pressure, or a pump (Fig. 2.13) to keep the knee at constant pressure and volume (Halperin et al 1978). The pressure within the knee can be set by adjusting the pump, and the flow can be controlled by foot pedal.

Although pumps offer good control of joint distension, they are expensive, and potentially dangerous if faulty (Henderson & Hopson 1982). If the capsule of the joint is ruptured, for example, the pressure within the joint cannot be increased, because the saline will flow into the calf and the pump may force large volumes of saline into the soft tissues. Saline can be introduced into the knee much

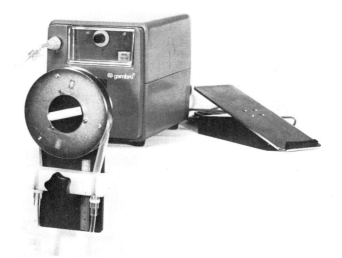

Fig. 2.13 A saline pump and foot pedal (courtesy of Gambro Ltd)

more safely by gravity, and this is strongly recommended for the beginner.

Irrigation needles

An 18 gauge disposable needle makes a good exit for the irrigation fluid, and can be discarded if it is blunt or bent, but it blocks easily and does not have a tap to control flow. A needle with side holes allows a more rapid flow of saline, and a tap can be used to shut off the outflow, if extra distension is needed (Fig. 2.14). Needles with a spring-loaded trocar minimise articular cartilage damage, but the more complicated the needle, the more expensive it will be to replace. Therefore a disposable 18 gauge needle has much to recommend it. The technique for setting up the irrigation system is described below (p. 38).

Suction probe

A simple smooth-ended sucker with straight sides is useful for removing articular cartilage debris and

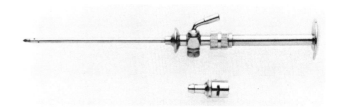

Fig. 2.14 An irrigation needle with stopcock and introducer (courtesy of Chas F. Thackray Ltd)

loose material. Jamming of the sucker can be kept to a minimum by restricting its use to small particles; meniscal fragments and loose bodies will not pass down the average sucker. Some surgeons prefer to use a powered shaver to remove debris from the joint at the end of the operation, but the reasons for such a preference are hard to find.

Plastic pouch

Plastic drapes designed to catch the outflow of saline in a central well which is fitted with a tap or tube connection at its lowest point are available, but their use is very much a matter of personal preference, and are most useful with a high rate of saline flow. Although ingenious, these drapes complicate the preparation of the patient and interfere slightly with manipulation of the knee. A further disadvantage is that the flow of saline from the exit needle projects beyond the lip of the pouch so that it misses the pouch, and the lip of the pouch itself obstructs access to the postero-medial and postero-lateral approaches to the joint.

Gas

Bircher (1921) used gas in his early arthro-endoscopies, and gas is still widely used in continental Europe (Henche 1979, Eriksson & Sebik 1982). Gas distension has the following advantages:

1. A wider angle of vision is possible, because the refractive index of glass to air is greater than that from glass to saline (Fig. 2.15). The wider angle is particularly useful in smaller joints such as the elbow and ankle.
2. Loose bodies fall to the bottom of the joint and do not bounce about under reduced gravity, as they do in saline.
3. Synovium does not float in front of the lens like seaweed in a fish tank (Fig. 2.16).
4. Articular cartilage defects and irregularities look much as they do at arthrotomy (Fig. 8.8).

Against these must be set the following disadvantages:

1. The shadows and highlights in the joint are more pronounced.
2. The shape of synovial fronds and flakes of cartilage cannot be assessed as well as with saline.
3. Gas escapes from the joint more easily than liquid and may cause surgical emphysema, which can be alarming.
4. Synovial fluid sticks to the lens, obscures vision, and can only be removed by withdrawing the telescope from its sheath.

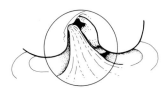

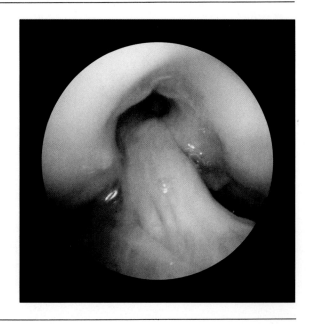

Fig. 2.15 The intercondylar notch in a knee distended with gas.
N.B. All arthroscopic photographs represent the right knee

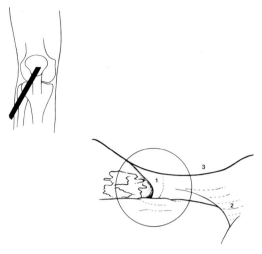

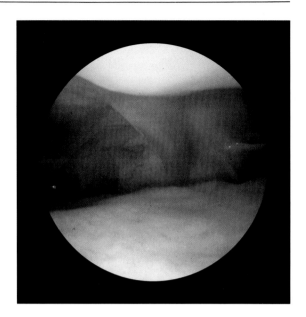

Fig. 2.16 The medial suprapatellar plica (1) and the medial synovial shelf (2) lying in different planes, in a knee distended by gas; the patella (3)

5. Synovial fluid sticks meniscal fragments together and can conceal their anatomy.
6. Gas distension needs expensive equipment.

The best pressure for distension with gas is 50–100 mm of mercury, which requires special equipment (Fig. 2.17). This is a higher pressure than that needed for laparoscopy, and the gas distension apparatus of the gynaecologist cannot be used for arthroscopy. Carbon dioxide, air, nitrogen or oxygen are all suitable, but carbon dioxide is probably the gas of choice. If lasers are ever used routinely, the selection of the appropriate gas will become critical (p. 25). Nitrogen, and thus air, takes several days to be absorbed and the knee can make an unpleasant squelching sound until all the gas has been resorbed, which can be socially embarrassing.

If the surgeon wishes to experiment with gas, he need not buy an expensive distension apparatus; a 20 ml syringe can be used to inflate the knee with air through the saline port. Although a proper gas distension apparatus gives a steady pressure, a syringe of air on the saline port gives a realistic impression of arthroscopy under gas and is much less expensive.

OTHER EQUIPMENT

Leg holders

A valgus strain in 30° of flexion and external rotation is essential to open up the back of the medial compartment, and a leg holder can make this easier. The simplest leg holder is a webbing sling placed around the thigh and fixed to the instrument rail on the opposite side of the table (Fig. 2.18). The sling is simple, inexpensive, and does not restrict movement of the leg when the postero-medial approach is used. A simple alternative is to place a vertical 'kidney' support against the lateral side of the thigh (Fig. 2.19), but the support is bulky, distorts the drapes and can interfere with the positioning of light cables and the irrigation system. On the other hand, the post does not hold the leg down on to the table or restrict movement of the thigh in any direction except laterally.

More complicated holders which clamp round the patient's thigh (Fig. 2.20) and are secured to the operating table are preferred by many, but these

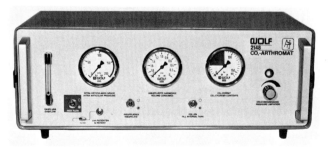

Fig. 2.17 A gas distension apparatus for arthroscopy (courtesy of Richard Wolf UK Ltd)

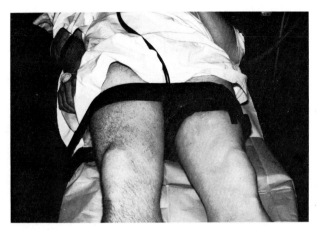

Fig. 2.18   A webbing strap attached to the operating table so that a valgus strain can be applied to the knee

devices interfere with free manipulation of the thigh and can actually make certain parts of the examination more difficult. Finally, there are leg holders that include an inflatable tourniquet – a logical, but cumbersome development of the fixed leg holder.

Although many surgeons find a leg holder indispensable for arthroscopy, it is the author's preference not to use a leg holder fulcrum for the following reasons:

1.   Equally good exposure can be obtained without one.
2.   The leg holder adds to the clutter of the operation.
3.   Applying the leg holder adds to the time taken for preparation and draping of the leg.
4.   The leg holder restricts the free movement of the thigh and makes manipulation of the knee more difficult.

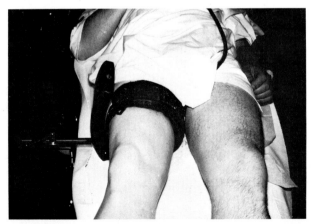

Fig. 2.19   The operating table fitment normally used to support patients lying on their side used instead to support the lateral side of the thigh so that a valgus force can be applied to the knee

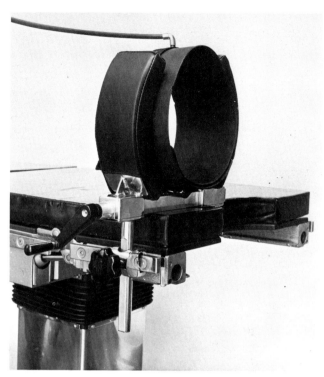

Fig. 2.20   An adjustable thigh holder for arthroscopic surgery (courtesy of Stille Ltd)

5.   The leg is held so firmly that a surgeon of average build can rupture the medial collateral ligament (Rosenberg & Wong 1982), fracture the femur, displace the lower femoral epiphysis, make partial ruptures of the anterior cruciate ligament complete, or displace undisplaced fractures.
6.   Having learned to perform arthroscopic surgery before leg holders were invented, the operation is easier without one.

Surgeons who consider using a leg holder are urged to have their own thigh fixed in the device and to invite the strongest resident available to open up the medial compartment of their knee.

Stool

A mobile stool makes arthroscopy easier. Wheeled stools are ideal, preferably four-wheeled rather than three, because they are more stable. If the operating theatre has a hard floor of terrazzo or similar material, a stool with brass feet is entirely satisfactory.

Dual viewing aids

Even though dual viewing teaching aids cannot be sterilised (p. 26), they familiarise the novice with the view down the arthroscope and help trainees to examine the knee correctly (Fig. 2.21). They also reduce the boredom of operating theatre staff, who have been known to tire of the uninterrupted view of the back of a surgeon's hat. Dual viewing aids may incorporate either a chain of surface polished mirrors and a lens system to produce a true optical picture (Fig. 2.22), or a flexible fibre-optic cable. Each system has its advantages and disadvantages, and the selection of a teaching aid is a matter of individual choice dependent on many factors, one of which is likely to be the cost. Whatever the cost, the acquisition of a dual viewing aid will increase the acceptability of arthroscopy and arthroscopic surgery to colleagues and operating theatre staff, and is a sound investment.

OPERATING INSTRUMENTS

Any instrument that can be passed through a 5–8 mm skin incision can be used for arthroscopic

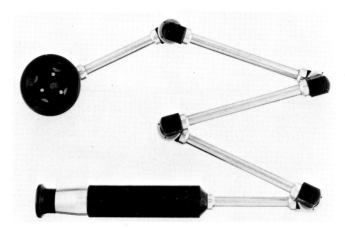

Fig. 2.22 The articulated dual viewing aid

surgery, provided that it is robust and has smooth edges that will not damage articular cartilage. It is quite possible to remove a locked bucket-handle fragment of meniscus using only a pair of pituitary rongeurs, but specially designed instruments extend the range of operations and make them simpler.

Instruments for laparoscopy and other endoscopic procedures can be used, but the special requirements of cutting tough meniscal tissue inside the narrow potential space of the knee rather than soft tissue in a cavern such as the bladder or abdomen make laparoscopic instruments unsuitable for arthroscopic surgery. The instruments need not be complicated; the author's first few hundred arthroscopic operations were done with the basic instruments shown in Figures 2.23 and 2.24.

The instruments should be without sharp edges or corners and run smoothly over articular cartilage without causing damage (Fig. 2.25); the jaws must be strong enough to cut and grasp meniscal tissue without bending or breaking, yet be small enough to be opened in the intercondylar notch, requirements which are difficult to reconcile.

The shape of the handles deserves thought. Bow handles (Fig. 2.26) are light and convenient, but the thumb can be caught in the bow if the instrument is used upside down, and firm pressure of the thumb against the side of the bow can damage the cutaneous nerve of the thumb at the level of the proximal phalanx (Fig. 2.27), a lesion which takes between two and twelve weeks to resolve. Although altered sensibility of the skin along the edge of the thumb is only a minor inconvenience, it is nevertheless worth avoiding by the use of handles that are specifically

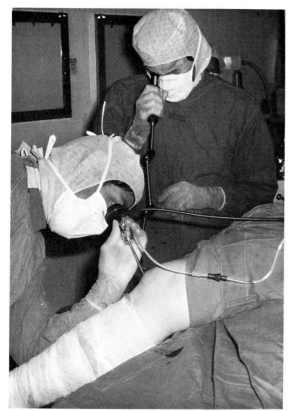

Fig. 2.21 The articulated dual viewing aid in use

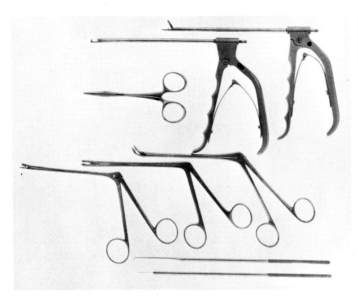

Fig. 2.23 A set of basic instruments used for the double puncture technique in the early days of arthroscopic surgery. From above downwards: arthroscopic scissors, guillotine, artery forceps with screw joint, Northfield's curved pituitary rongeurs, Cushing's straight rongeurs with 4 mm bite, punch forceps, hook and knife

designed for gripping (Fig. 2.28) and do not include a metal ring for the thumb.

Finally, it is helpful if the instruments, which are all superficially similar, can be identified quickly and easily by the scrub nurse or assistant in a darkened operating theatre by a mark or number on the handle of the instrument.

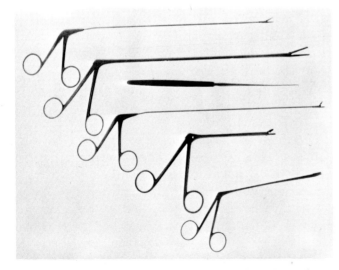

Fig. 2.24 Fine instruments used as additions to the basic set of instruments in the early days of arthroscopic surgery. Microlaryngeal forceps, sigmoidoscopic grasping forceps, modified Gillies' skin hook, microlaryngeal cup forceps, punch scissors and flat nasal scissors

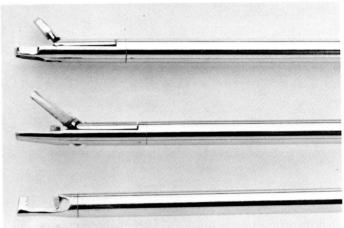

Fig. 2.25 Tips of arthroscopic instruments. From above downwards: punch forceps, scissors and guillotine

Basic instruments

The basic set of operating instruments will vary from one surgeon to the next, but most surgeons will find their basic instruments in the following list:

1. 30° telescope
2. blunt hook
3. large and small basket forceps, also known as punch forceps
4. straight rongeurs
5. a retractable or rigid knife
6. sideways-cutting basket forceps
7. curved or angled rongeurs
8. a guillotine
9. grasping forceps

Some surgeons declare themselves unable to operate without a video system, powered instruments or an irrigation pump, but none of these is essential and all are expensive.

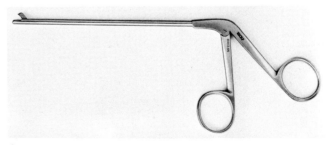

Fig. 2.26 Punch forceps with bow handles (courtesy of Richard Wolf UK Ltd)

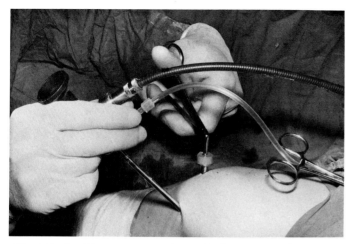

Fig. 2.27 Double puncture technique. The forceps are held wrongly with the surgeon's thumb passed completely through the bow of the handle

Probing hook

The probing hook should have a smooth rounded tip, with the angled segment approximately 3 or 4 mm long and 1 or 2 mm wide (Fig. 2.29). Markings to indicate size are not particularly helpful, but do little harm unless they are cut into the hook, which produces a point of weakness and can lead to fracture. The shaft of the instrument should be robust, but not so hard that it fractures under stress. It is better to have a hook which will bend slightly than a hard and brittle hook that will fracture inside the joint.

The handle of the instrument should not be heavy enough to pull the hook out of the knee so that it falls

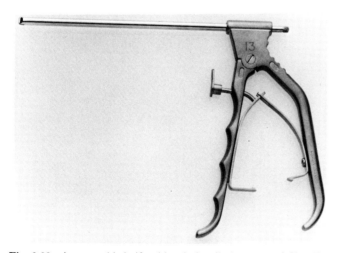

Fig. 2.28 A retractable knife with grip handle (courtesy of Chas F. Thackray Ltd)

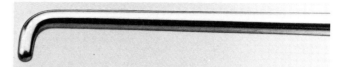

Fig. 2.29 The tip of a probing hook

to the floor, if left unsupported in the knee. Some hooks have a cylindrical handle (Fig. 2.30) that fits the operating instrument cannula so that the cannula can be withdrawn over the hook without first removing the hook, and this can be helpful. A small ball-ended probe is also valuable for assessing the hardness of articular cartilage, but is not effective for manipulating meniscal fragments.

Trocar and cannula

A cannula can be used as a second channel for irrigation, if there is excessive bleeding or a turbid effusion (Fig. 2.31). It can also be used as an additional inflow channel when powered instruments are used, or left in the knee to maintain the portal for instruments, if they need to be inserted repeatedly. This can be particularly helpful in obese patients and those with osteoarthritis, in whom the channel can be difficult to find.

Scissors

Two patterns of scissors are generally available, hook and straight. Both patterns are useful, and are used in different situations. Hook scissors (Fig. 2.32) cut at their tip, but need a large space for the jaws to open and are more suitable for cutting synovium in the suprapatellar pouch or tissue at the front of the joint than the posterior attachment of the meniscus, where there is little room to open the jaws. Straight scissors with narrow tips can be used as shears to cut the meniscus at the back of the intercondylar notch, but they will not cut fine structures such as synovium with their tips.

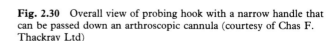

Fig. 2.30 Overall view of probing hook with a narrow handle that can be passed down an arthroscopic cannula (courtesy of Chas F. Thackray Ltd)

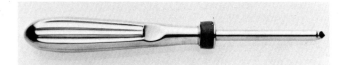

Fig. 2.31 Trocar and cannula (courtesy of Chas F. Thackray Ltd)

Punch or basket forceps

A pair of forceps which punches out a segment of tissue like a ticket punch is invaluable for trimming meniscus or excising synovium, and can be used as an alternative to scissors (Fig. 2.33). In the early days, the basket forceps used for bowel or bladder biopsy were often used, but the wire basket which retained the fragment was a disadvantage because it held the tough meniscal tissue in the jaw of the instrument and attempts to close the jaws often broke the hinge pin. To overcome this problem the basket was omitted from the design, but the instrument is still known as the 'basket' forceps rather than punch forceps. The instrument will cut better if the upper jaw is hollowed or hooked at its tip, rather than flat. Both large (4 mm) and small (2.5–3 mm) instruments are required.

Rotatory instruments

The hinge pin in the jaw of the cutting mechanism is the weakest point of most instruments. This pin can

(a)

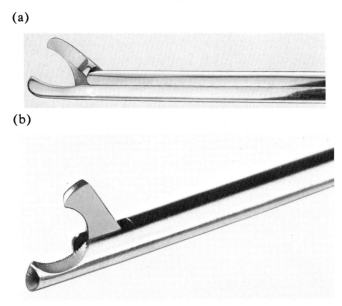

(b)

Fig. 2.32 Hook scissors: (A) with rounded blades (courtesy of Chas F. Thackray Ltd); (B) with serrated blades (courtesy of Richard Wolf UK Ltd)

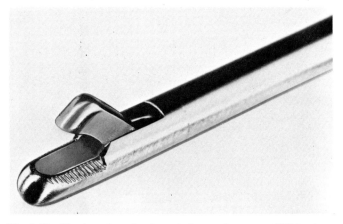

Fig. 2.33 The jaw of a pair of punch forceps (courtesy of Richard Wolf UK Ltd)

be eliminated if the up-and-down hinge mechanism is replaced by a rotatory action so that the upper and lower jaws of the instrument meet each other in an arc instead of a flat plane. The rotatory action also allows the instrument to cut sideways, but not directly ahead (Fig. 2.34). Elimination of the hinge pin as a point of weakness does not eliminate fractures, but shifts the point of failure to another part of the instrument. Rotatory side-cutting forceps (Fig. 2.35) are among the most useful and versatile instruments available.

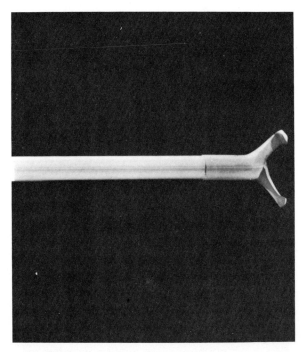

Fig. 2.34 Side-cutting hooked rotary scissors (courtesy of Acufex Microsurgical Inc)

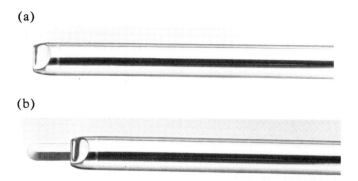

Fig. 2.36 A retractable knife: (A) with blade retracted; (B) with blade extended (courtesy of Chas F. Thackray Ltd)

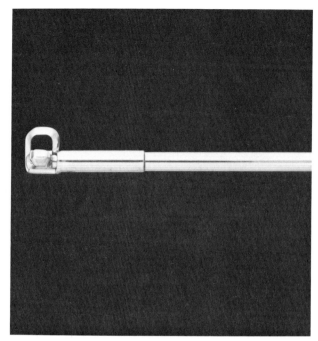

Fig. 2.35 Side-cutting rotary punch forceps (courtesy of Acufex Microsurgical Inc)

Knives

Knives are basic surgical instruments, but in arthroscopic surgery their value is limited. A knife works best if the tissue is held still or under tension, but this is not always possible in the knee, and the blade must be kept very sharp to cut the tough meniscus. Fixed blades need frequent resharpening, and replaceable or disposable blades are often brittle and have a bulky attachment to their handle, which limits their mobility. In the early models, replaceable blades often fell out of the jaws of the handle and remained in the knee as a foreign body, but this problem has now been overcome.

Retractable blades are, in general, preferable to a simple knife (Fig. 2.36). If the knife is inserted with the blade retracted, there is less chance of damaging the articular cartilage, and the shaft of the instrument can be used as a probe. When the knife tip is in position, the blade can be exposed and the meniscus cut with the minimum of damage to other structures.

Straight, curved and backward-cutting blades are available and each has its place. A curved knife (Fig. 2.37) is useful in the posterior third of the meniscus, and a backward-cutting knife is often helpful in the middle third. Backward-cutting knives have a tendency to 'self steer', which sometimes makes the line of cut unpredictable, and the tip of some backward-

cutting knives is so sharp that it can damage the underlying articular cartilage.

Grasping forceps

Artery forceps, Kocher's forceps or any other pattern of grasping instrument can be used for arthroscopic surgery, but if the jaws are to be opened widely, the hinge must be at the level of the skin incision. A selection of instruments with different length jaws is nevertheless a useful addition to the basic set. Instruments that have sliding shafts instead of a cross action hinge can be used anywhere in the joint, and most arthroscopic graspers follow

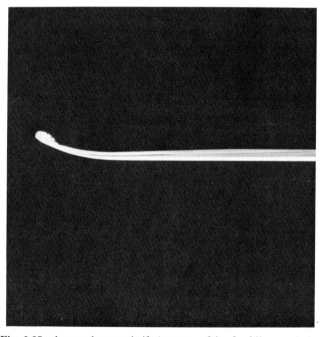

Fig. 2.37 A curved rosette knife (courtesy of Acufex Microsurgical Inc)

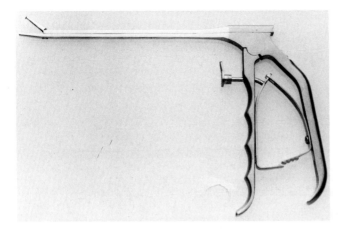

Fig. 2.38   Grasping forceps (courtesy of Chas F. Thackray Ltd)

this pattern (Fig. 2.38). If none is available, Anderson's tendon tunnelling forceps, which are standard orthopaedic instruments, can be used, but the jaws do not open widely enough to hold a large loose body. Curved graspers are helpful in the suprapatellar pouch and the gutters, and a curved pituitary rongeur is very effective if no toothed grasping forceps are available.

Size of instrument

In general, 5 mm arthroscopic instruments are ideal for most purposes and, provided they are inserted correctly and handled properly, will reach all areas of the joint except for the posterior thirds of the menisci. Although 2 or 3 mm instruments will reach further back, they are more fragile and must be used very gently. As a general rule, the largest and stoutest instrument that will reach the lesion should be used, and fine instruments should be reserved for tight corners. The areas where fine instruments must

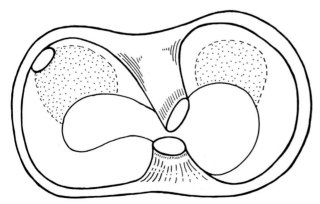

Fig. 2.39   The area of the knee where fine (3 mm) instruments are required; 5 mm instruments will reach the areas that are not stippled

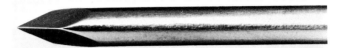

Fig. 2.40   The tip of a trocar-pointed Kirschner wire

be used are indicated in Figure 2.39. Apart from breakage, fine instruments blunt quickly and need to be replaced more often than thicker instruments, but they are an essential item in the basic set of instruments.

Drills

If a hole is to be drilled in bone, a simple 1.5 mm Kirschner wire or bone awl is more versatile than a standard twist bit. If a twist bit is not inserted exactly at right angles to the surface of the bone, it will not only skid and wander across the joint surface, but the groove in its side will catch the soft tissue, unless it is passed through a cannula. A trocar-pointed Kirschner wire (Fig. 2.40) or an awl with a trocar point does not have this disadvantage, and an awl with a pointed tip and counter-helical groove (Fig. 2.41) is particularly useful.

Retrievers

Fracture of instruments in the knee, though unusual, is disturbing. A 'golden retriever' has been devised that consists of a suction probe made of a yellow non-magnetic metal with a powerful magnet at its tip. In theory, the suction draws the metallic fragments towards the tip of the instrument, where they are held by the magnet. In practice, however, the magnets are of less value than might be supposed, because the attractive force of the magnet operates in straight lines that cross the natural highways of the knee, and the fragment must retrace its course if it is to be extracted. A curved metal strip with a magnet at its tip, which will reach to the recesses beneath the meniscus, where fragments often settle, is more effective (Fig. 2.42), and should

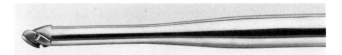

Fig. 2.41   The tip of a hand burr with counter-helical groove (courtesy of Chas F. Thackray Ltd)

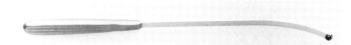

Fig. 2.42 A flexible metal strip with magnetic tip for retrieving broken metallic fragments (courtesy of Chas F. Thackray Ltd)

be kept available in every operating theatre where arthroscopic surgery is practised.

POWERED INSTRUMENTS

Powered instruments have a place in arthroscopic surgery, but they are by no means an essential or basic piece of equipment and should not be purchased until the surgeon is thoroughly competent with simple hand instruments. Powered instruments are not passports to arthroscopic expertise and will do little that cannot be done just as neatly with a hand instrument. A set of powered instruments, including shaver heads and burrs, is shown in (Fig. 2.43).

A good steady flow of saline is essential to remove debris and ensure a clear field of view and a high flow system (p. 38) must be used with any powered instrument.

Shavers

The original powered instrument was the patellar shaver designed by Dr Lanny Johnson and made by the Dyonics Corporation. The instrument consists of a hollow tube containing a cylindrical blade that revolves slowly and cuts tissue drawn into a small window by gentle suction (Johnson 1981). The blade is driven by a small battery-powered motor controlled by a foot-pedal. The shaver is most effective in removing flakes of articular cartilage from the patella and femoral condyles and can produce a very pleasing arthroscopic appearance (Fig. 8.17). Different cutting ends, including 3 mm shaving heads and a variety of end cutting instruments, can be used for synovectomy and 'contouring' the irregular surfaces of damaged menisci. The shaver is also an effective, albeit expensive, vacuum-cleaner for removing debris. Other shavers, powered by air or electricity, are readily available from most surgical companies.

Burrs

Powered burrs will smooth rough areas of bone and roughen smooth areas. The instruments themselves are safe, but can be dangerous in the wrong hands and should be used cautiously; in at least one patient,

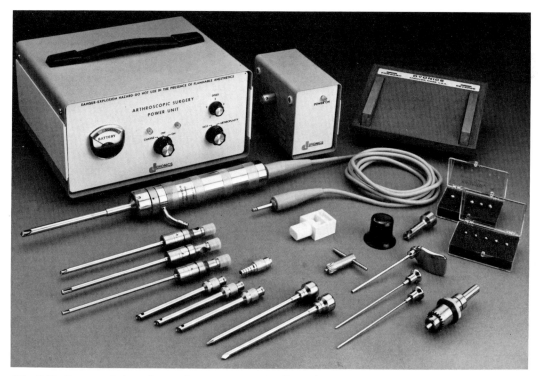

Fig. 2.43 Power tools for arthroscopic surgery including (from above) power unit, hand piece with large burr, small burr, large and small meniscal cutters, sheath, obturator and trocar (courtesy of the Dyonics Corporation)

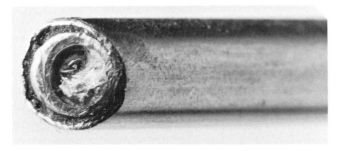

Fig. 2.44 The tip of an arthroscope damaged by contact with a power burr

the popliteal artery and vein have been divided by a burr inserted from the postero-medial approach. The lens of the arthroscope is particularly vulnerable (Fig. 2.44) and should be kept well away from the burr to avoid damage.

Electrocautery

The electrocautery or 'diathermy' used in conventional surgery must be modified for use in the knee, because the meniscus is largely avascular and has a high impedance. The surgical technique must also be modified because the 'live' electrode will cut with the gentlest touch. The equipment consists of an electrode plate for the patient, a stylus, and an assortment of cutting electrodes (Figs. 2.45–2.47).

The advantages of electrosurgery in the knee are twofold:

1. Bleeding points can be coagulated, which is particularly helpful during a subcutaneous lateral release.

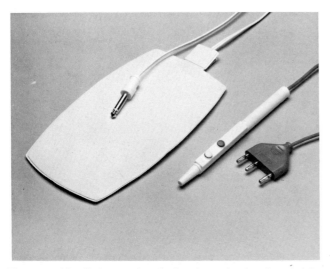

Fig. 2.45 The diathermy plate, lead, stylus and connecting plug for electrocautery (courtesy of Concept Inc)

2. Inaccessible areas of meniscus, notably the posterior third and the posterior menisco-synovial junction, can be cut with precision.

The list of disadvantages is longer, but perhaps less important.

1. Sterile water, glycine, sorbitol, mannitol or gas must be used to distend the knee, because normal saline conducts electricity too well. Glycine corrodes surgical instruments, particularly cutting edges, and the disadvantages of sterile water are listed above (p. 13); sorbitol or mannitol are expensive for routine use.

2. If gas is used to distend the knee, the joint fills with smoke. There is no smoke in a fluid-filled knee, but the stream of bubbles from the tip of the electrode obscures vision while the electrode is cutting.

3. Accidental damage to articular cartilage can easily occur. A standard knife blade can be rested on articular cartilage without causing damage, but this does not apply to an electrode.

4. The equipment interferes with television, causing the picture to disappear when the current flows, unless the camera is heavily shielded, which adds to its bulk. Low-light-sensitive cameras are affected particularly by this problem.

5. The equipment is expensive, complex, and potentially dangerous, if not properly maintained. The patient electrode must be correctly applied, and the strength of the current must be varied according to the tissue being cut and the distension medium used. Although these are small points and the technical details are easily learned, they complicate an otherwise simple operation.

Laser

The idea of lining up troublesome or inaccessible fragments of meniscus in a gun sight and vaporising them with laser, rather than struggling to reach them with conventional steel cutting instruments, is attractive, but the practical problems are considerable. Moreover, laser will cut meniscus as well as articular cartilage or soft tissue, and there is no reason to suppose that it will prove any less dangerous than other cutting instruments.

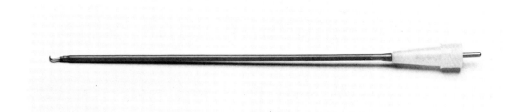

Fig. 2.46 An insulated electrode with hook tip for electrosurgery (courtesy of Concept Inc)

Three types of laser have been examined. The Argon laser, which is towards the green end of the spectrum, is not effective against white tissue such as meniscus and has insufficient power for practical use. The Neodymium Yag (Yttrium Aluminium Garnet) laser produces a red beam that will cut meniscus, but the cutting is slow and the meniscus becomes charred. To make a cut 1 cm long takes approximately 4.5 minutes. The Neodymium Yag laser has the advantage that it can be passed along a glass-fibre bundle and is not absorbed by a glass lens system, but it is absorbed by saline and the joint must therefore be distended with gas. An alternative is the carbon dioxide laser, which will cut meniscus easily,

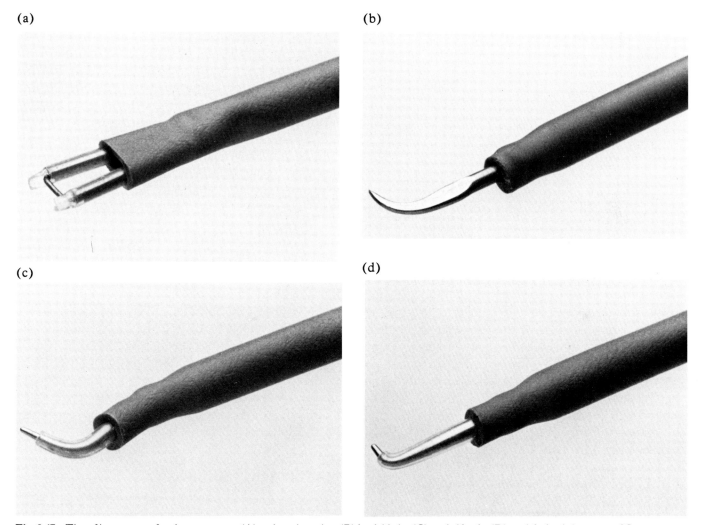

Fig. 2.47 Tips of instruments for electrosurgery: (A) end cutting wire; (B) hook blade; (C) angled hook; (D) straight hook (courtesy of Concept Inc)

but has the great disadvantage that because it is absorbed by glass or saline, the beam must be passed along a line of surface polished mirrors and focused by lenses made of zinc selenite.

Laser superheats the target tissue, which vaporises and passes directly from the solid to the gaseous state. The heat released is so great that a fire can be started inside the knee and the joint must therefore be distended with a gas that does not support combustion, which excludes air, oxygen and nitrous oxide. Carbon dioxide absorbs the power of the laser slightly, and nitrogen is commonly used.

Whipple et al (1983, 1984a) found that rabbit or human cadaveric meniscus can be cut using 0.2–0.5 second blasts of carbon dioxide laser at a 35 watt energy level. At this level, the depth of cut is easily controlled; 63% of the energy is absorbed within 10 μ of the surface and 99% within 50 μ of the surface, which means in effect that the meniscus will not cut deeper than 50 μ. The cut surface of the meniscus is blackened, burnt tissue tends to spatter onto articular cartilage, and the ash produced causes a low-grade synovitis in rabbits (Whipple et al 1984b).

STERILISATION AND CARE OF INSTRUMENTS

Sterilisation

Metal parts of the arthroscope, such as the sheath and the obturator, can be sterilised in a steam autoclave like any other instrument, but the sterilisation of the optical equipment – telescopes, light guides, dual viewing aids and television cameras – presents considerable problems. A high-pressure steam autoclave will damage the cement used to secure the components of the lens system in most arthroscopes, although some manufacturers claim their instruments will withstand such treatment. In practice, the users of these arthroscopes often find that the lens system becomes less clear and slightly yellow with repeated autoclaving, perhaps because the autoclaves are operating at excess pressures or temperatures. In the United Kingdom, hospital autoclaves are checked every three months to ensure that the pressures and temperatures are correct, but faults can develop between the checks and super-heating can occur, with sad consequences for the telescope. In many instances, the problems of autoclaving arthroscopes and optical equipment can

be more fairly attributed to a defect in the sterilising equipment than in the telescope.

Ethylene oxide will sterilise an arthroscope completely in one hour at 56°C, but the telescope must be absolutely dry before it is placed in the gas and must be free of both dirt and salt crystals, neither of which can be penetrated by ethylene oxide. In the United Kingdom, steam and formaldehyde are often preferred to ethylene oxide, but this policy may change with time.

Immersion of the telescope and light guide in glutaraldehyde for ten or twenty minutes is the almost universal clinical practice. True sterilisation (that is, the killing of all spores and viruses), requires 24 hours continual immersion, which means that each telescope and light guide can be used only once each day, making it necessary either to restrict the number of arthroscopies performed or to purchase an unreasonably large number of telescopes.

Glutaraldehyde has other disadvantages. It is essential to rinse all traces of glutaraldehyde off the instrument before it is used, to avoid irritation not only of the synovium and soft tissues, but also the surgeon's eye; if glutaraldehyde remains on the eyepiece of the instrument, it will cause an uncomfortable, but transient conjunctivitis. Prolonged immersion of telescopes and light guides in glutaraldehyde may also cause yellowing of the resin used to bind the glass fibres in the light guides of the telescope and the light leads, and a thin film may form over the tip of the arthroscope and cause discoloration.

The sterilisation of dual viewing aids presents additional problems because they incorporate surface polished mirrors, which will not stand even one immersion in any fluid. Dual viewing aids incorporating a fibre-optic bundle can sometimes be sterilised, but users are strongly urged to consult the manufacturer's instructions before the instrument is immersed in any liquid. Sterilisation of television cameras is also possible. Small solid-state cameras can be soaked between cases, and total sterility can be maintained by using such a camera and operating off the screen.

Sterilisation or disinfection?

The difference between disinfection and true sterilisation has often led to difficulty with infection-control officers and hospital administrators, which is well illustrated by the correspondence in the *Journal of Bone and Joint Surgery* between Johnson (1982) and Roth (1982). In some countries (but not in the United Kingdom, which is blessed with wise and sensible hospital administrators), hospital authorities have both insisted on the total sterilisation of the telescope between each use, and refused to purchase enough telescopes to allow an arthroscopic service to be established. Practising surgeons have come to regard such problems as another example of an obstructive bureaucracy designed to eliminate progress and prolong the suffering of patients. In fairness, however, it must be said that the risk of transmitting viral diseases on an arthroscope that is disinfected and not sterilised must remain a theoretical risk, even though early fears that the disinfected arthroscope might be a health hazard comparable with the tattooist's needle have not been justified. A practical compromise between the bacteriological ideal and disinfection might perhaps be a glutaraldehyde soak between each operation and a gas sterilisation of the instruments at the end of each operating day – 'soak between cases and gas between days'.

Care of instruments

Telescopes are very brittle and should always be handled as if they were made of the finest crystal – as indeed they are. The lens system will shatter if the telescope is dropped, and a very slight bend in the telescope is enough to put the lens system out of alignment. Accidental bending can occur if something is rested on top of the telescope, or if it is withdrawn from the sheath while still attached to the light cable. The light cable should always be disconnected before the telescope is moved in or out of its sheath, and special care must be taken to ensure that the telescope is moved only in the line of the sheath.

The telescope will also be damaged if it is picked up by the tip rather than the eyepiece, and nurses must not slap the telescope into the surgeon's hand as if it were a bone lever. The telescope should be held by the eyepiece only and never with Cheatle's or other instrument-holding forceps applied to its barrel. Damage can also occur during cleaning and storage. The telescope should be washed separately from the other instruments, and should be stored in a foam-lined box or carrying case.

The push/pull rod and other moving parts become stiff and rusty, if they are not kept properly clean and lubricated, and instruments should be kept clean and free of organic material. If the instrument can be dismantled for cleaning, this should be done regularly because dirt – even sterile dirt – interferes with the hinges and leads to corrosion and eventually to fracture.

The irrigation stopcocks, which are in frequent contact with saline, become stiff unless washed in water after use to remove saline. If the stopcock has become jammed either through disuse or poor maintenance, do not attempt to force it or the handle will break off; a light tap with the heavy end of the obturator will usually be sufficient to free it.

References

Bircher E 1921 Die Arthroendoskopie. Zentralblatt fur Chirurgie 48: 1460–1461

Calkins J L, Hochheimer B F 1979 Retinal light exposure from operating microscopes. Archives of Ophthalmology 97: 2363–2367

Calkins J L, Hochheimer B F 1980 Retinal light exposure from ophthalmoscopes, slit lamps, and overhead surgical lamps. An analysis of potential hazards. Investigative Ophthalmology and Visual Science 19: 1009–1015

Eriksson E, Sebik A 1982 Arthroscopy and arthroscopic surgery in a gas versus a fluid medium. Orthopedic Clinics of North America 13: 293–298

Friedman E, Kuwabara T 1968 The retinal pigment epithelium IV. The damaging effects of radiant energy. Archives of Ophthalmology 80: 265–269

Halperin N, Axer A, Hirschberg E, Agas M 1978 Arthroscopy of the knee under local anaesthesia and controlled pressure. Clinical Orthopaedics and Related Research 134: 176–179

Henche H R 1979 Arthroscopy of the knee joint. Springer–Verlag, New York

Henderson C E, Hopson C N 1982 Pneumoscrotum as a complication of arthroscopy. Journal of Bone and Joint Surgery 64A: 1238–1239

Hochheimer B F, D'Anna S A, Calkins J L 1979 Retinal damage from light. American Journal of Ophthalmology 88: 1039–1044

Johnson L L 1977 The comprehensive examination of the knee. C V Mosby, St Louis, Mo

Johnson L L 1981 Diagnostic and surgical arthroscopy of the knee and other joints, 2nd edn. C V Mosby, St Louis, Mo

Johnson L L et al 1982 Two per cent glutaraldehyde: a disinfectant in arthroscopy and arthroscopic surgery. Journal of Bone and Joint Surgery 64A: 237–239

Johnson L L 1982 Correspondence. Journal of Bone and Joint Surgery 64A: 954

Johnson L L, Becker R L 1976 Arthroscopy, technique, and the role of the assistant. Orthopaedic Review 5: 31–43

McGinty J B 1982 Arthroscopic removal of loose bodies. Orthopedic Clinics of North America 13: 313–328

Reagan B F, McInerny V K, Treadwell B V, Zarins B, Mankin H 1983 Irrigation solution for arthroscopy. A metabolic study. Journal of Bone and Joint Surgery 65A: 629–631

Rosenberg T D, Wong H C 1982 Arthroscopic surgery in a free-standing outpatient surgery centre. Orthopedic Clinics of North America 13: 277–282

Roth R A 1982 Correspondence. Journal of Bone and Joint Surgery 64A: 954

Whipple T L, Caspari R B, Meyers J F 1983 Laser energy in arthroscopic meniscectomy. Orthopaedics 6: 1165–1169

Whipple T L, Caspari R B, Meyers J F 1984a Synovial response to laser induced carbon ash residue. Lasers in Surgery and Medicine 3: 291–295

Whipple T L, Caspari R B, Meyers J F 1984b Laser subtotal meniscectomy in rabbits. Lasers in Surgery and Medicine 3: 297–304

3

Photography and television

PHOTOGRAPHY

Photography is important for teaching and research, but presents technical difficulties not found in other types of photography (Eriksson 1979).

Camera adaptors

Adaptors that fit in the lens mount will link most 35 mm reflex cameras to any arthroscope (Fig. 3.1). Most adaptors are made without an iris diaphragm and therefore have a large aperture that cannot be reduced. A large aperture will admit the maximum possible amount of light, but the depth of field is small and the lens must therefore be focused accurately.

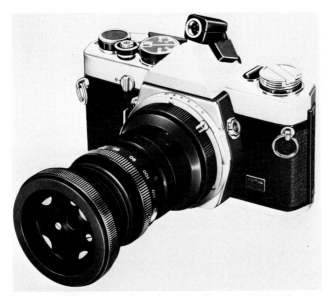

Fig. 3.1 Camera with endoscopic adaptor (courtesy of Karl Storz Ltd)

It is helpful if the adaptor includes a zoom lens so that the picture size can be adjusted to fill the full height of the frame, which not only produces the ideal picture size, but also standardises the area of light-sensitive screen exposed to light and makes incorrect exposure less likely.

Light sources

Illumination is a problem, particularly in the suprapatellar pouch, where there is a large cavity and little reflected light. A mercury arc lamp provides ample illumination for most purposes, but a standard 150 watt light source can also be used successfully, although the exposure time may be uncomfortably long.

Flash units built into the light source are available and can be set at one of three levels of illumination. Adequate exposure cannot be guaranteed, and an exposure at each setting will be needed if this method is used. At present no 'dedicated' flash system is available with automatic exposure control based on the light reflected from the film, but these systems are widely used in conventional photography and it is only a matter of time before the technology is applied to endoscopy.

Exposure

Exposure based on guesswork is often disappointing and wasteful of film, and some form of metering is invaluable. If a camera with a built-in automatic exposure meter is used, problems arise from the fact that the image is circular and does not cover the entire surface of the light-sensitive screen. If the camera mechanism determines the exposure time on the assumption that the light is equally distributed across the screen, overexposure will occur and experience with the individual camera/arthroscope combination is needed to determine the correct setting. Most cameras can be adjusted to underexpose by one stop, which will usually correct the error. Alternatively, the film-speed adjustment can be set at twice the correct speed, thus halving the exposure time and compensating for the error. If the camera has a compensation control, it may be set at -1.

Focusing

Most adaptors include a focusing mechanism, essential with the small depth of focus that accompanies a large aperture. The focusing screen may need to be changed, because the screen for normal photography requires more light than is available endoscopically. Most dealers will be able to supply the appropriate screen for endoscopic photography, but a professional photographic supplier may be needed to give specialist advice.

Film

Because light is at a premium in endoscopic photography it is preferable to use a fast film, even though the colour quality and definition may be less satisfactory. Most processing laboratories can 'force' the film so that the film speed is effectively doubled or even quadrupled, but this results in increased contrast, graininess and loss of quality. For transparencies, Ektachrome 400 will produce satisfactory results with xenon or a mercury arc, but with tungsten light the colour temperatures will be incorrect. A slow film can be used with a flash unit, but the problems of incorrect· exposure already described mean that much film will be wasted.

Transparencies, although ideal for teaching, are unsatisfactory for record purposes because they cannot easily be stored in the patient's notes. A Polaroid camera back, available for most cameras, gives very satisfactory (but expensive) prints that are more easily filed than transparencies.

Colour temperature

The colour of the light reaching the interior of the knee depends upon the same factors as those described for endoscopic television (p. 33), and is often so distorted that even the use of daylight film with a tungsten light source does not produce the terrible result that might be expected. Film for tungsten light, however, produces a very blue picture if used with xenon, quartz halogen or mercury arc light sources. If the colour is unsatisfactory, it can be corrected when copying the slides, if appropriate filters are used; copying, however, always results in some loss of quality.

Record keeping

A practical problem of endoscopic photography is the accumulation of unlabelled slides. Matching the slide to the patient can be difficult and accurate records are essential. The longer the interval between taking the photograph and writing the patient's name upon the transparency, the greater will be the difficulty in recalling which patient belongs to which slide. One method of avoiding this difficulty is to record the name of each patient photographed with the date and the number of exposures in a special book kept in the operating theatre. Provided that the slides are kept in the correct order, correlation of the slide with the patient is then simple.

An alternative is to use a camera back (Recordataback) (Fig. 3.2) that imprints letters or numbers on the film so that the date or a code can be simply recorded on the picture itself. Provided that a record is kept to correlate the code number with the patient, the number is changed between each patient and the device is reliable, this system is entirely satisfactory.

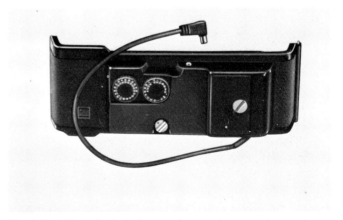

Fig. 3.2 A Recordataback for recording numbers on arthroscopic photographs (courtesy of Karl Storz Ltd)

Orientation

Orientation of the picture is a problem when taking circular photographs and is best achieved by ensuring that the camera body is parallel with the tibial plateau. If the slide is accidentally taken in a different orientation, it can be corrected by making a copy of the slide.

Slide copying

Slide copiers which fit into the lens mount of the camera are readily available, simple, inexpensive and allow both orientation and colour to be corrected or the picture reversed. It is now becoming almost conventional for publications to illustrate the right knee only, which means that photographs of the left knee must be reversed, if they are to be published. The quality of copies obtained from these devices is fair, but better quality is achieved by using a much more complex and expensive copier such as an Illumitran, which can also correct excessive contrast by pre-fogging the film.

A practical photographic system

Most of the photographs in this book were made using an Olympus OM2N camera body, fitted with a Storz endoscopic adaptor and a 1.12 focusing screen. The film generally used was Ektachrome 400, developed normally and without forcing, but with the automatic exposure-compensation dial set at -1 to allow for the incomplete distribution of light on the light-sensitive screen, and the zoom lens on the endoscopic adaptor set so that the picture fills the full height of the frame. The best results are achieved using a mercury arc or xenon light source; 150 watt tungsten light with a liquid light cable will give good results in the smaller and brighter parts of the knee, such as the tibio-femoral compartments, but is less satisfactory in the suprapatellar pouch. This system works well in practice and gives consistent results. The very best photographs, however, are produced using a slower film such as Kodachrome 64 with electronic flash, but the waste of film and the lack of consistently good results makes this technique a 'hit and miss' affair; therefore for everyday use the system described above is preferred. When dedicated off-the-film flash metering becomes available for arthroscopic use, it will probably become the system of choice.

TELEVISION

Although the technical developments of television move so quickly that anything written is out of date before it appears in print, some general principles are unlikely to change.

Why use television?

Television is no more essential for arthroscopy than it is for cystoscopy, sigmoidoscopy, bronchoscopy or any other endoscopic procedure. Nevertheless it does make it possible to record the operation, allows assistants to see what is happening inside the knee and is therefore essential in any teaching centre. Secondly, being able to watch the operation allows the operating theatre staff to take a more active part in the procedure, but it must be said that a television set-up is a needlessly expensive device for alleviating boredom. Thirdly, television allows the surgeon to operate in the upright posture instead of sitting curled up in a ball, a grotesque position that is not only uncomfortable and likely to aggravate degenerative changes in the surgeon's neck and back, but also makes it impossible to converse intelligibly or maintain complete sterility. Finally, operating off the television screen eliminates any risk of retinal damage from exposure to excessive light levels.

Television cameras

The early cameras were too heavy to be attached to the telescope and needed a powerful light source; when lightweight cameras were developed, they lacked sensitivity and had to be coupled directly to the arthroscope to minimise light loss. Cameras incorporating a vacuum tube have now been reduced to a tube approximately 1.5 cm thick and 10 cm long, about half the size of the cameras shown in Figures 3.3 and 3.4. In some cameras, the vacuum tube is replaced by a solid-state chip, making the camera slightly smaller than the coupling unit of a dual viewing aid (Fig. 3.5). Chip cameras can be designed to fit the hand (Fig. 3.6), and it is very likely that the camera will soon be incorporated into the telescope itself.

Chip cameras, and some tube cameras, can be sterilised by soaking (Fig. 3.7) (p. 26), making a completely sterile operation possible. They do,

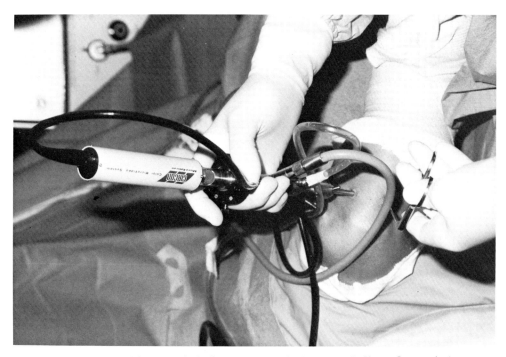

Fig. 3.3 A soakable camera including a vacuum tube (courtesy of Circon Corporation)

however, need more light than a tube camera, and produce a grainy picture if there is inadequate light.

There are different colour systems in different countries, and an American camera therefore may not work with a European monitor or recorder. The American system, NTSC (which stands for National Television Standards Committee as well as Never The Same Colour), is perhaps gaining the ascendency, but many monitors will still accept only a PAL signal. It is therefore essential to check that all the items in a proposed television system are compatible, and to see it working, before buying anything.

Light levels

When endoscopic television was first attempted, the greatest single problem was introducing enough light to obtain a picture. This problem has been largely overcome by the introduction of more sensitive cameras, brighter light sources, liquid light guides, and optical design, which minimise loss both in the light guides and the arthroscope itself. Light loss is greater if a beam splitter or dual viewing aid is used, because light is directed away from the television camera to the surgeon's eye, and some light is lost in the prism and other elements of the optical system of the aid. To overcome this and keep light loss to a minimum, the cameras can be coupled directly to the arthroscope, but the surgeon must then operate 'off the screen'.

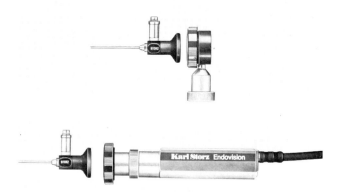

Fig. 3.4 A vacuum tube camera with straight and right-angled adaptors (courtesy of Karl Storz Ltd)

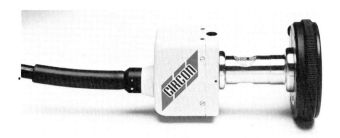

Fig. 3.5 A soakable solid-state 'chip' camera with arthroscope adaptor (courtesy of Circon Corporation)

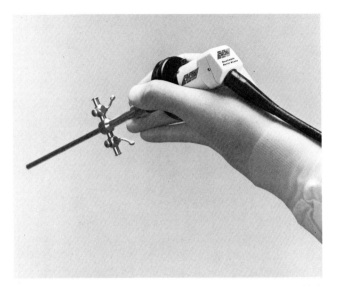

Fig. 3.6 A soakable solid-state 'chip' camera with adaptor moulded to fit the hand and wrist (courtesy of Circon Corporation)

Adjustment of light level

Because the knee includes a dark cavern with non-reflecting walls – the suprapatellar pouch – as well as many small white-walled crevices, a television camera must be able to work over a great range of light levels. If the light is sufficient for the suprapatellar pouch, it may be too bright for the menisci, and will produce a ghost-image or 'lag' when the camera is moved. The brightest areas will also tend to appear brighter than they really are, to produce 'blooming', and, if excessive light levels are maintained, the camera may be permanently damaged.

All television systems include some mechanism for regulating light level automatically, but because the range is so great it can overload the compensating

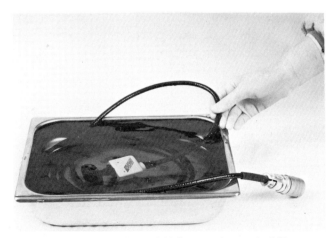

Fig. 3.7 Soaking a solid-state 'chip' camera (courtesy of Circon Corporation)

mechanism of the camera and some therefore include an iris diaphragm either on the camera or the coupling unit. In the early days, many of these devices were unsatisfactory. At least one lens coupling included an iris that worked admirably in air, but lay in the wrong focal plane when attached to an arthroscope immersed in saline, with the result that closing the iris made the picture become smaller, but no darker. Some cameras included a motor-driven iris, which operated so slowly that it prolonged the examination. A simple way of regulating the light is to loosen the light guide from the arthroscope, but a more elegant solution is for an optical wedge to be interposed between the light source and the light cable and controlled automatically by the light level at the face plate of the camera.

Picture size

The size of the image on the screen depends upon the optical characteristics of the eyepiece, the size of the light-sensitive faceplate in the camera, and the focal length of the lens in the coupling unit. If the image is small – occupying less than one-third of the height of the monitor screen – the picture will be difficult to see, but brighter than the same image spread over the whole of the screen. In simple terms, there may be enough light for a small picture, but not enough for a large one. Many early cameras would work only if the picture was small, and some have not been modified since.

If an articulated viewing aid is used, the image will move about the screen and may rotate off the screen altogether if the picture is large. It is often better to accept a smaller image that stays within the limits of the screen than a picture that occupies the entire height of the screen, but keeps disappearing off its edge. A large image also has the disadvantage that it must be viewed from further away than a smaller picture.

Focusing

The focusing mechanism of the television camera is usually sealed to avoid accidental disturbance, but most coupling units include an optical focusing mechanism. As in conventional photography, the depth of field depends upon the size of the aperture, but because light is scarce the small aperture necessary for a good depth of field may be unobtainable. Some coupling units developed for use in air have an unsatisfactory range of focus for arthroscopy, and in some the aperture and focusing rings become jammed together in use. To avoid these difficulties, it is again urged that the entire system – arthroscope, light cable, light source, camera and monitor – be used together before purchasing single items separately.

Colour balance

The balance between red and blue is as important for endoscopic photography as for clinical photography, and is affected by many things. The colour temperature of the light source is variable, xenon having a colour temperature of 5000°C and tungsten a temperature of 3500°C. The light can be tinged with yellow or brown as it passes through the glass-fibre light guide – particularly if the guide is old and the resin used to secure the fibres has become discoloured – but if a liquid light guide is used, the transmitted light will be towards the blue end of the spectrum. The type of tube in the television camera also affects the colour.

Many camera control units are now equipped with a control to compensate for difference in colour temperature, but they cannot compensate for discoloured light cables. The television monitor also influences the colour and quality of the picture, some producing a sharp, brightly coloured picture, whereas others have softer and more muted tones. Finally, the colour controls of the monitor must be correctly adjusted, and it is advisable to check the setting of the controls on the monitor with colour bars or a test card before criticising the television camera or the optical equipment.

Video recorders

When selecting a video recorder, it is better to buy one based on the Umatic system rather than VHS or Betamax. The Umatic system is accepted internationally for academic purposes, and there are security advantages in having a system that cannot be used for home video.

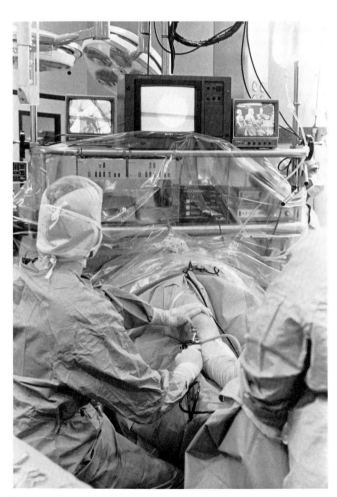

Fig. 3.8 Operating 'off the screen'. The arthroscopic view is displayed on a television mounted on a gantry over the patient

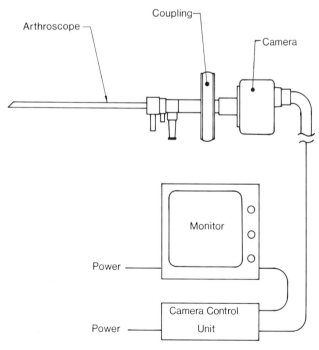

Fig. 3.9 The simplest arrangement for arthroscopic television. The arthroscope is linked directly to the camera, camera control unit and monitor

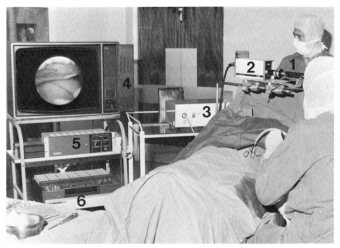

Fig. 3.10 Displaying the arthroscopic view on a television monitor (4). The arthroscope is connected by an articulated dual viewing aid (1) to a television camera (2). A high-intensity light source (3) is required. Camera control unit (5), video-cassette recorder (6). This was very early equipment. Note the large camera (2) and camera control unit (5)

Owning a video recorder is a mixed blessing. Although a video recorder will record operations for research, teaching or record purposes, it leads to the accumulation of a vast stack of unedited tape. Unedited video tapes are interesting only to their maker, and a social menace in the hands of an undisciplined enthusiast. To record an operation is simple, but to edit the recording so that it can be shown to others without embarrassment requires an expensive and well-equipped editing studio, and editing is both time consuming and hugely expensive.

Other accessories

A timing device that displays the time and date on the picture gives an unambiguous reference point that makes editing much quicker and simpler. A moving marker to indicate interesting features is also helpful, and comparatively inexpensive.

SETTING UP A TELEVISION SYSTEM

Operating 'off the screen'

Television can either be used with a dual viewing aid so that the surgeon looks down the arthroscope while observers watch the television monitor, or the surgeon can watch the screen and not look down the arthroscope at all (Fig. 3.8). To operate 'off the screen' makes orientation more difficult, but this becomes simpler with practice. A special problem is rotatory instability of the picture, which can be overcome by remembering that the picture is always the same way up as the camera; if the camera has its top uppermost, the picture will also be correct,

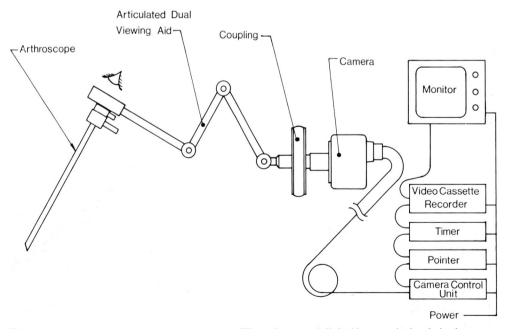

Fig. 3.11 An even more complicated arrangement. The arthroscope is linked by an articulated viewing aid to the camera and the system includes a video-cassette recorder, timer, pointer and camera control unit

unless a dual viewing aid with a rotating element has been interposed between the camera and the arthroscope.

The television camera converts an optical image into an electric signal which passes by cable to a camera control unit, which may either be incorporated into the monitor or exist as a separate unit, where it is modified and converted before reaching the television monitor. The monitor is just like an ordinary domestic television set, except that it is not adapted to receive a radio frequency signal.

Set-up 1

The simplest arrangement is shown in Figure 3.9. A lightweight television camera is coupled directly to the arthroscope and the image is displayed on the television monitor, but with this system the surgeon must operate directly off the screen. With an 'old-fashioned' camera, a powerful mercury arc or xenon light source must be used, but with a more sensitive camera and a good light cable, a simple 150 watt tungsten light source is sufficient.

Set-up 2

If the camera is linked by an articulated viewing aid to the arthroscope, a larger television camera can be mounted either beside the operating table or on a gantry attached to the instrument rail at the side of the operating table (Fig. 3.10).

Set-up 3

Timing devices and pointers can be placed between the camera control unit and the monitor (Fig. 3.11) and the signal is fed via a video recorder into the monitor. This is the standard arrangement for use with a video recorder.

In the future, a solid-state television camera may be incorporated into the eyepiece of the arthroscope. If the camera control unit were placed in the base of the monitor, the system would be simplified still further.

Reference

Eriksson E 1979 Problems in recording arthroscopy. Orthopedic Clinics of North America 10: 735–744

4

Technique of operation

The greatest danger of arthroscopy is the inexperienced enthusiast who believes that buying a set of expensive instruments exempts him from the need to learn how to use an arthroscope correctly and who does not understand that it is better to 'open it rather than wreck it' (McLean 1983). The havoc wrought by such individuals is terrifying and it cannot be emphasised too strongly that arthroscopic surgery should only be attempted by competent arthroscopists. To recognise an abnormality at arthroscopy and examine it more thoroughly at arthrotomy is easy, but to define the anatomy of a lesion precisely enough to insert operating instruments at the correct site demands confidence of a different order.

Arthroscopy is a dynamic examination and there is more to a full arthroscopic examination than admiring the view as if it were a series of still photographs. The movement of the intra-articular structures can be assessed as the knee is flexed and extended with rotatory and lateral stresses. The menisci can be lifted with percutaneous needles to inspect their under-surface, and a hook can be used to manipulate suspicious structures, assess the stability of the posterior third of the meniscus and palpate softened articular cartilage. To omit these additional techniques and rely solely on the view down the arthroscope is to conduct a partial arthroscopy, with results that can only be disappointing (Gillies & Seligson 1979).

INDICATIONS FOR ARTHROSCOPY

Arthroscopy is indicated before any arthrotomy for internal derangement of the knee, in the assessment of complex knee problems such as ligament injuries or persistent symptoms following meniscectomy, in the investigation of supposed hysterics or malingerers, and in the diagnosis of acute injuries. These are wide indications, but the patient's account of his symptoms and their onset can provide as much information as clinical examination, radiography and arthroscopy combined. Arthroscopy does not replace the clinical history as the single most useful weapon in the investigation of any knee disorder, and is neither a substitute for clinical acumen nor a short cut to the correct diagnosis. The findings of arthroscopy cannot be considered in isolation, and are useful only if they are correlated with the patient's symptoms and the findings of clinical and radiological examination. If these three principles are not followed, disaster is bound to follow (Joyce & Mankin 1983).

CONTRA-INDICATIONS

There are very few contra-indications to arthroscopy, and it often happens that one person's contra-indication for diagnostic arthroscopy is another person's indication for arthroscopic surgery. For example, a complete diagnostic arthroscopy is impossible unless the knee flexes to 90°, but restriction of flexion is often an indication for arthroscopic mobilisation of the joint (p. 74). Routine diagnostic arthroscopy of an infected joint is unwise, but septic arthritis can be treated by arthroscopic lavage, provided that it is part of the treatment regime.

Arthroscopy through areas of infected or abraded skin is always inadvisable and may be followed by infection of the synovial cavity, presumably by direct inoculation of the joint space with bacteria carried into the joint on the tip of the arthroscope. Operation through unsound skin is therefore contra-indicated, unless special precautions, such as prophylactic antibiotics, are taken to avoid spread of the infection.

ANAESTHESIA

General anaesthesia has many advantages (Rosenberg & Wong 1982). The injured knee is painful and manipulation of the joint is an unnecessary discomfort for the patient and a hindrance to the surgeon. General anaesthesia also avoids the need for repeated infiltration of the skin when extra incisions are made. Moreover, many arthroscopic procedures are best done under tourniquet control, and the use of a tourniquet on the unanaesthetised patient for more than a few minutes is unkind.

Perhaps the greatest advantage of general anaesthesia is that it renders the patient oblivious to events in the operating theatre. It is by no means unusual for a planned operation to change imperceptibly into an ad hoc adventure requiring the sterilisation of additional instruments and the rejection of those already prepared. On these occasions, the confidence of the patient and the credibility of the surgeon are more likely to survive the operation if the patient is asleep.

Local anaesthesia

Local anaesthesia is successful, provided that the surgeon is experienced and confident in his arthroscopic technique. Many techniques for local anaesthesia have been described (Johnson 1977, Klein & Schultz 1979, Halperin et al 1978, McGinty & Matza 1978, Pevey 1978), but the following is simple and effective. The skin is infiltrated with lignocaine 1%, containing adrenaline (epinephrine) 1 in 200 000 along the medial joint-line, the antero-lateral joint-line, and the supero-lateral corner of the patella, using a total of approximately 10 ml (100 mg of lignocaine) of solution. The injection should be placed deeply enough to infiltrate the capsule as well as the subcutaneous fat – this is important.

The synovial cavity is then distended with 10 ml of 0.25% bupivacaine containing adrenaline 1 in 200 000, and the solution left in the knee while the surgeon scrubs and the limb is prepared. Time is important: at least ten minutes should elapse between injection and incision. The joint is then distended with saline in the usual way, but a further 10 ml of 0.25% bupivacaine is left in the joint at the conclusion of the procedure.

If local anaesthetic is used, it is better to operate without a tourniquet to avoid pain; a high rate of saline flow should therefore be used to maintain a clear field. Adrenaline may also help to minimise bleeding, but is not essential and can be omitted if there is any anxiety about the patient's myocardium.

Spinal anaesthesia

Both epidural and spinal anaesthesia are suitable for arthroscopic surgery, and will allow a tourniquet to be used if necessary. As with any regional block, anaesthesia may be less than complete or uncomfortably short, and the surgeon must be prepared either to operate under local anaesthesia and without a tourniquet or to abandon the procedure if difficulties arise. A further disadvantage is that because the patient is awake, it is unwise to try and learn arthroscopic surgery or attempt new techniques under either spinal or local anaesthesia.

Any standard technique for epidural or spinal anaesthesia is acceptable, but the following gives a well-localised area of anaesthesia from the second lumbar to the first sacral roots, lasting about one hour. Five ml of 2% lignocaine is diluted in 5 ml of 10% dextrose to produce 10 ml of a heavy solution of 1% lignocaine in 5% dextrose. Between 5 and 10 ml of solution (50–100 mg of lignocaine) is injected into the spinal theca in the usual way using a No. 25 gauge spinal needle, with the patient lying on the side of operation so that the solution reaches the appropriate nerve roots. Younger patients generally require a slightly higher dose than older patients. The patient is then turned on the back, a tourniquet applied and inflated, and the operation completed without unnecessary delay. This technique has been used on thirty patients as day cases without serious difficulty.

PREPARATION

Examination under anaesthesia

Examination under anaesthesia is important, particularly if a ligament injury is suspected, and should

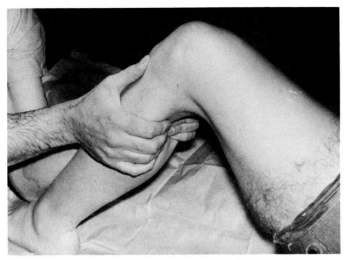

Fig. 4.1 Examination of the knee under general anaesthesia

always precede arthroscopy (Fig. 4.1). The patient should be fully relaxed; a quick tussle with the leg in the anaesthetic room immediately after induction is useless, but time spent on a careful examination of ligamentous stability with the patient fully relaxed is time well invested.

Tourniquet

Elevation of the leg and inflation of a tourniquet controls bleeding without losing the subtleties of synovial vascularity. Exsanguination is unnecessary and blanches the synovium to such an extent that even the menisco-synovial junction may be difficult to identify.

Some surgeons prefer not to inflate the tourniquet routinely, but it is sensible to apply it to the thigh in case bleeding is a problem. If inflation becomes necessary, the arthroscope should be withdrawn and

the leg elevated for at least a minute. If this is not done or the tourniquet is inflated with the knee flexed over the edge of the table, venous congestion of the leg is common and venous thrombosis may follow. At the end of the procedure, the tourniquet should be released and the joint irrigated thoroughly before a dressing is applied, although many people apply the bandage before releasing the tourniquet.

Irrigation – flow and pressure

Fluid should enter through the sheath and leave through a needle in the suprapatellar pouch to maintain a steady flow of saline away from the lens and keep the field of view clear. If the flow is towards the sheath, and therefore the telescope, blood and debris will be washed towards the lens instead of away from it, obscuring vision.

Although draining the fluid down a plastic tube into a bucket reduces spillage, the tube adds to the pipes and light cables already needed, and the weight of the tube can tilt the needle so that its tip lies against the synovium and blocks, or its weight may pull the needle out of the joint altogether. A drainage tube is only really necessary when a high rate of flow is used, and suction apparatus may then be more appropriate.

Controlling the rate of flow and pressure of saline within the knee is critical, and depends largely on the relative sizes of the outflow and inflow channels (Fig. 4.2). To keep the knee distended, either the outflow channel must be narrower than the inflow channel, or the saline must flow into the knee under pressure, because if saline can run out of the joint faster than it can run in, the joint will stay empty. If the outflow needle is blocked, the knee will remain distended,

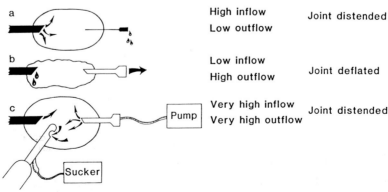

High inflow Low outflow	Joint distended
Low inflow High outflow	Joint deflated
Very high inflow Very high outflow	Joint distended

Fig. 4.2 Balancing inflow and outflow to maintain joint distension

but no saline will flow through the knee, however much pressure is applied to the saline reservoir. If, on the other hand, the outflow channel is larger than the inflow channel, much saline will flow, but the knee will remain deflated and examination will be impossible. In simple terms, if there is more saline running out of the joint than into it, arthroscopy is impossible.

A high rate of flow has advantages and disadvantages. If there is bleeding, for example, a high flow rate will help clear the field of view. A high flow rate is also necessary when powered instruments are used, because they have a large exit channel to which suction is applied and unless a correspondingly high inflow of saline is maintained, the joint will deflate. The principal disadvantage of a high rate of flow is distension of the soft tissues with saline, if the tip of the sheath accidentally slips out of the synovial cavity into the extra-synovial layers, or the saline leaks around the sheath into the subcutaneous tissue. With a high rate of flow the tissues will become engorged more quickly than with a slow rate of flow, but whether the flow is high or low, the saline should always be turned off whenever the tip of the sheath is outside the synovial cavity. A second disadvantage is that unless the saline is kept at body temperature, a high rate of flow will produce a marked drop in temperature around the knee. If cold saline is used or the operation is prolonged, the tissues become cold to the touch and the subsynovial fat solidifies and takes on a firm and waxy appearance. Although such localised hypothermia does not appear to have any ill effects, little is known of the effects of low temperatures on articular tissues and the hazard is best avoided.

For all these reasons, continuous irrigation of the joint under low pressure and with a low flow rate has many advantages. No. 18 gauge needles, often used in spinal anaesthesia, are readily available as exit needles and, with the infusion bag 1 m above the knee, ensure a steady flow of fluid through the joint without the synovial cavity collapsing.

Skin preparation and draping

Arthroscopy has no place as an unsterile 'office procedure' and should only be performed in a fully-equipped operating theatre. The leg should be shaved before operation to avoid hairs being driven into the joint on the tip of the trocar, and the skin should be prepared as if an arthrotomy were to be performed. Because it is virtually impossible to avoid the surgeon's mask, eyelashes or hood touching either his gloves or the patient's leg during the examination, the procedure ceases to be truly sterile as soon as the eye is brought to the eyepiece. Some semblance of sterility can be maintained by insisting that all instruments should be held by the handle or eyepiece only and that nobody should touch the barrel of the arthroscope or any instrument that might enter the joint, but true sterility can be guaranteed only by using a sterile television camera.

The leg should be draped in such a way that the knee can be manipulated freely without the towels, irrigating tube or light cable falling to the floor. The towels around the calf and the foot should be applied firmly so that they do not come adrift when the knee is manipulated, and should not be bulky or irregular. There are many ways to satisfy these simple requirements and every surgeon will have his own technique, but it may be helpful to describe one routine that has proved effective.

The patient is anaesthetised in the anaesthetic room, and when fully relaxed is placed on the operating table and the knee carefully examined. The leg is elevated, and a pneumatic tourniquet applied and inflated by a technician or assistant while the surgeon scrubs. A diathermy plate is applied only if an arthrotomy may be necessary. With the leg still elevated, a waterproof sheet is placed across the table and under the leg, and the skin prepared from the middle of the calf to the level of the tourniquet with an antiseptic solution such as 0.5% chlorhexidine in 70% alcohol (Fig. 4.3). The first sterile waterproof sheet is replaced with a second and covered with a sterile linen sheet. A small square towel is folded into a triangle, wrapped around the thigh at the junction of its lower and middle thirds, and secured with two towel clips which do not enter the skin. The leg is lowered into a second small towel, which is laid under the leg, wrapped around the calf and foot, and secured throughout its length with a 10 cm cotton bandage tied with the knot on the inner side of the calf or ankle. This part of the draping must be done neatly and correctly. If the towel is crumpled untidily around the calf or secured loosely with some feeble material such as tubular gauze, the drapes will slide down to the ankle at the most inconvenient and difficult stage of the procedure.

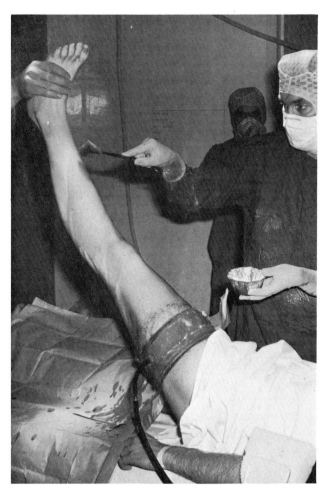

Fig. 4.3 Preparation of the leg with antiseptic solution after application of a tourniquet

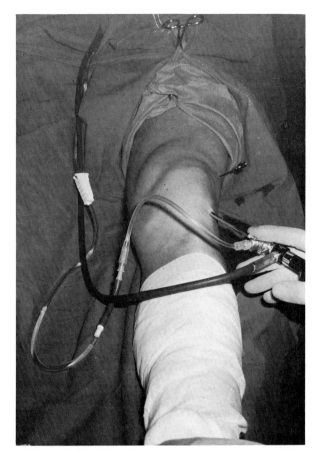

Fig. 4.4 The draped leg with the irrigation tube, light cable, drainage needle and arthroscope in position

A large abdominal sheet with a central hole is then passed over the leg and secured with a towel clip. The sterile light cable and irrigation tube are laid over the abdomen, held with a clip in a fold of towel at the level of the groin, and covered with another sheet. A good length of cable and tube should be left free to allow easy manipulation of the arthroscope without tension (Fig. 4.4).

Positioning of the infusion set, light source, instrument trolley and assistant is important (Fig. 4.5). The assistant should stand next to the surgeon, towards the patient's head. The drip set and light source should be at the patient's head, preferably on the side away from the surgeon, with the instrument trolley on the opposite side and not at the foot of the table, where the surgeon is certain to back into it during the procedure. If a television is used, space must be found for the monitor, camera control unit and other equipment. The layout in Figure 4.6 and

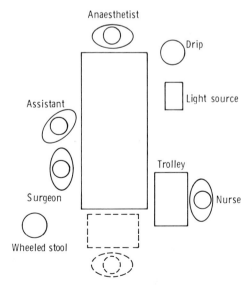

Fig. 4.5 Theatre layout. For arthroscopic surgery the instrument trolley can be brought to the position indicated by a broken line at the end of the operating table

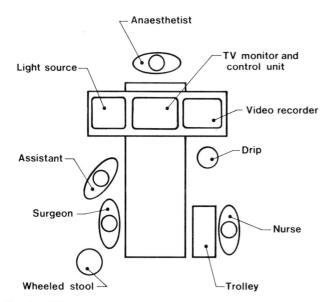

Fig. 4.6 Theatre layout including television

allows the monitor to be seen easily without making the patient inaccessible.

THE ANTERO-LATERAL APPROACH

Of the many possible points of insertion of the arthroscope (Whipple & Bassett 1978), the antero-lateral insertion described by Dr R.W. Jackson and based on the technique of Dr M. Watanabe (Jackson & Abe 1972, Jackson & Dandy 1976) is the most useful for routine initial examination of the knee. Although it is essential to be familiar with all the insertions, an established routine approach for the initial examination is important and the antero-lateral approach serves this purpose well. The central approach is a satisfactory alternative.

Insertion of the arthroscope

The point of insertion for the antero-lateral approach lies 2 mm above the anterior horn of the lateral meniscus and as close to the patellar tendon as possible (Fig. 4.7). This point can be identified by flexing the knee to 90° and pushing the thumbnail into the small depression just lateral to the patellar tendon. A 5 mm incision extending down through the joint capsule is then made with a small No. 15 blade immediately above the thumbnail (Fig. 4.8). With the blunt obturator locked into the sheath, the trocar is directed upwards, medially and backwards

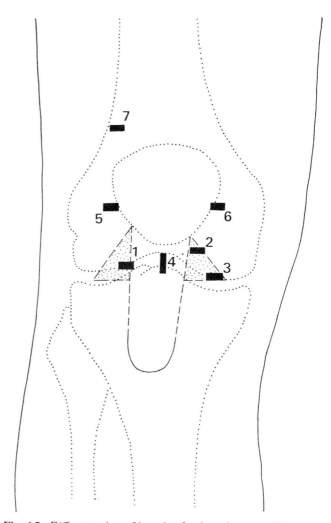

Fig. 4.7 Different points of insertion for the arthroscope: (1) antero-lateral approach (anywhere in the stippled area); (2) and (3) antero-medial approach (anywhere in the stippled area) – insertion (2) is suitable for the back of the intercondylar notch, insertion (3) for the medial gutter; (4) central approach; (5) lateral mid-patellar approach; (6) medial mid-patellar approach; (7) lateral mid-patellar approach

towards the intercondylar notch (Fig. 4.9). The sharp trocar can be used, but may damage the articular surface, however carefully it is handled.

The patella is then lifted on the sheath and the instrument passed into the suprapatellar pouch as the knee is straightened. It is important to make certain that no 'assistant' is holding the patient's leg during this manoeuvre, because any interference with the smooth movement of the instrument can cause unnecessary trauma to the articular cartilage and even damage the instrument.

As an alternative to putting the arthroscope into a dry knee, the joint can first be distended with saline by running a little irrigation fluid into a sterile

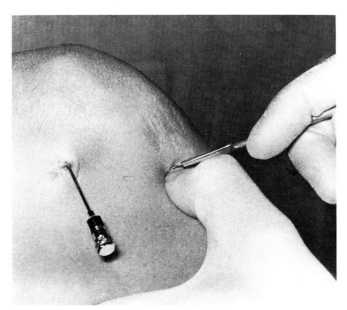

Fig. 4.8 Incising the skin before inserting the arthroscope from the antero-lateral approach

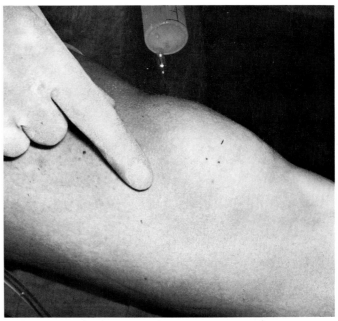

Fig. 4.10 Irrigation fluid running down in the medial gutter, confirming that the needle tip is correctly placed in the synovial cavity

container, drawing it up into a 20 of 50 ml syringe, and injecting the saline into the suprapatellar pouch through a No. 18 gauge needle, which is left to act as an exit needle. To inject the saline into the subsynovial layers instead of the synovial cavity is surprisingly easy, but attention to the following points should avoid this. First, insert the needle at the supero-lateral angle of the patella and feel its under-surface with the side of the needle, before injecting any saline. Next, inject a few millilitres of saline and watch carefully to be sure that the fluid runs down into the medial gutter (Fig. 4.10). If in

doubt, detach the syringe to see if fluid runs back along the needle. When it is certain that the needle is well in the joint, hold it still and inject a further 20–50 ml.

Assembling the arthroscope

With the sheath in the suprapatellar pouch, the obturator can be withdrawn and the joint washings examined. Yellow or bloodstained fluid is evidence of an intra-articular disorder and flakes of articular cartilage in the washings indicate generalised osteoarthrosis or synovial chondromatosis. The joint is then irrigated thoroughly until completely clear fluid is obtained, or visibility within the joint will be poor.

The instrument is assembled by placing the telescope in the sheath and attaching the light cable and irrigation inflow tube. If the arthroscope includes a bridge, it must be inserted correctly and locked into position.

Suprapatellar pouch

Because of the irregular shape of the lower end of the femur and the convolutions of the synovial cavity, arthroscopy involves manipulation of the leg around the arthroscope as well as manipulation of the arthroscope around the joint.

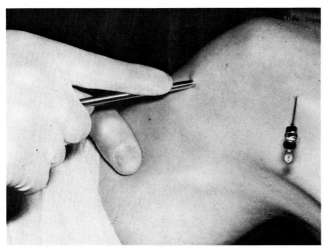

Fig. 4.9 Inserting the arthroscopic trocar

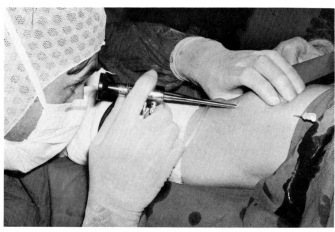

Fig. 4.11 Examining the under-surface of the patella

The examination begins at the apex of the suprapatellar pouch (Fig. 4.11), which is most easily examined with the table raised so that the knee is at the level of the surgeon's umbilicus. The first structure to be identified is the insertion of the articularis genu muscle onto the synovium. The next structure to be identified should be the medial suprapatellar plica (alias the plica synovialis suprapatellaris and plica medialis suprapatellaris) (Figs. 4.12, 4.13), which lies on the medial side of the joint and can conceal loose bodies or other interesting pathology (Fig. 7.1). If there is generalised synovitis, the changes are often less marked in the synovium hidden behind the plica than in the rest of the joint. If there is a complete suprapatellar membrane dividing the pouch into two separate compartments, the free margin of the plica will be absent and it may seem that the medial suprapatellar plica is missing altogether (Fig. 13.3). To be certain that there is not a complete membrane, look for the insertion of

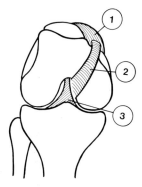

Fig. 4.12 The synovial folds in the knee: (1) medial suprapatellar plica, (2) medial synovial shelf, (3) infrapatellar fold or ligamentum mucosum

articularis genu; if the muscle is visible, the apex of the knee has been reached and a complete membrane cannot be present.

At this stage, the synovium can be examined. If the synovium is inflamed, special note should be made of the shape of the villi, which will appear fatter and rounder in acute synovitis than in a chronic synovitis, in which they are finer and filiform.

Patello-femoral joint

The surface of the patella is examined next by withdrawing the arthroscope slightly and turning the lens upwards. By moving the patella across the tip of the telescope, the whole of its surface can be examined and any suspicious areas probed with the irrigation needle (Fig. 8.7). The relationship of the patella to its groove is also important, but can be assessed more easily from the lateral suprapatellar approach (p. 53) than the antero-lateral (Fig. 4.14).

Medial synovial shelf

The telescope should then be aimed medially and slightly upwards towards the medial synovial shelf (alias the plica synovialis medio patellaris, plica alaris elongata, Iino's band (Iino 1939), Aoki's ledge, meniscus of the patella, medial patellar plica), which runs in the coronal plane and ends in the fat-pad below the inferior pole of the patella (Fig. 4.12). The shelf, which was first reported by Mayeda (1918), was not widely recognised until arthroscopy became a routine procedure, and examination of the distended synovial cavity under magnification from within led to the recognition of folds not noticeable in an empty joint opened widely either post-mortem or at operation. The medial synovial shelf should not be confused with the medial suprapatellar plica, which lies entirely above the patella (Fig. 2.16).

The medial synovial shelf is a normal structure that is more obvious in some patients than others, and is absent altogether in approximately 40–60% of patients (Sakakibara 1976, Patel 1978, Jackson et al 1982). Histological study of the shelf shows it to consist of fibrous tissue covered by synovium (Fig. 4.15). The shelf is usually seen as a white crescent (Fig. 4.16), but may be thickened and inflamed if the rest of the joint is affected by synovitis or if there has been localised trauma to the shelf itself. The white

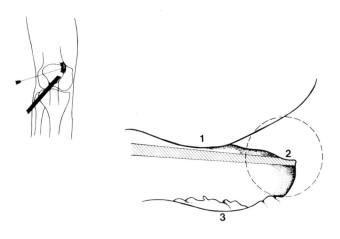

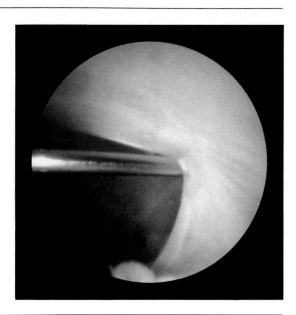

Fig. 4.13 The medial suprapatellar plica (1) manipulated with the irrigation needle; patella (2), femur (3)

crescentic appearance of a thickened shelf is similar to a meniscus, and the shelf is sometimes aptly referred to as the 'meniscus of the patella'.

The shelf sweeps across the medial femoral condyle during flexion of the knee and comes into contact with the area of femoral condyle that strikes the anterior horn of the meniscus in full extension. If the 'impingement lesion' (p. 45) is present (see Figs. 4.20, 4.21), the shelf sweeps across it in approximately 45° of flexion, which corresponds with the click and the position in which the knee is most painful. The 'impingement lesion' and the

groove in the medial femoral condyle described by Patel (1978) may be one and the same.

A fold of synovium may also be seen on the lateral side of the patella, but the lateral 'shelf' is neither as clean nor as sharp as its medial counterpart (Fig. 4.17) and probably has no clinical importance.

Medial compartment

The medial compartment is entered by turning the telescope downwards to identify the edge of the medial femoral condyle and rolling the tip around

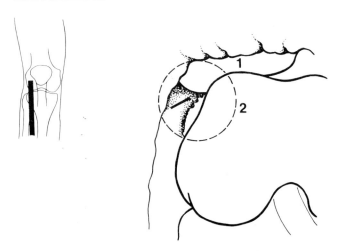

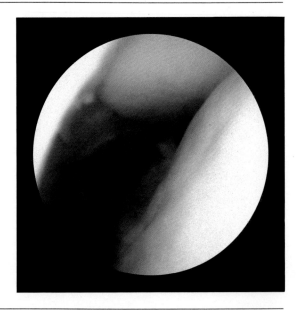

Fig. 4.14 Lateral tracking of the patella with the lateral edge of the patella (1) overhanging the edge of the lateral femoral condyle (2), seen from the lateral gutter

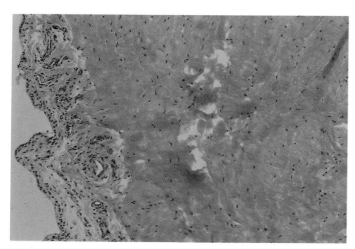

Fig. 4.15 Histological appearance of the medial synovial shelf. There is much collagen, covered by synovium

the condyle while the knee is flexed. The menisco-synovial junction can then be identified and inspected for peripheral tears and localised synovitis, before moving on to the meniscus itself. The edge of the medial meniscus can almost always be seen throughout its length by applying a firm valgus and external rotation strain with the knee in 30° of flexion (Fig. 4.18), which sometimes displaces concealed meniscal flaps into the joint space (Figs. 10.28, 10.29). Visual inspection does not always provide complete information about the meniscus, however, and probing with a percutaneous needle or hook is

essential, if a tear is suspected. The anterior horn of the meniscus is best seen with a 70° telescope (Fig. 4.19).

Before leaving the medial compartment, the articular surface of the femoral condyle should be examined for irregularities and for the 'impingement lesion' that is often seen at the point of contact of the medial femoral condyle and the anterior horn of the medial meniscus in full extension (Figs. 4.20, 4.21). This lesion is usually asymptomatic and appears as an area of heaped up tissue immediately above a slightly depressed area of irregular articular cartilage, and may catch on the synovial shelf (p. 183).

The intercondylar notch

Because structures in the notch are very close to the lens, they appear unnaturally white and excessively magnified, which can lead to difficulties of interpretation. A small synovial frond, for example, can look like a meniscal fragment, if it is directly in front of the lens. Synovitis, fronds of synovium, meniscal fragments, a prominent tibial spine and osteophytes add to the problems.

The anterior cruciate ligament is a convenient landmark and can be identified by slipping the arthroscope laterally out of the medial compartment and withdrawing it slightly. Care must be taken not to withdraw the arthroscope so far that its tip enters

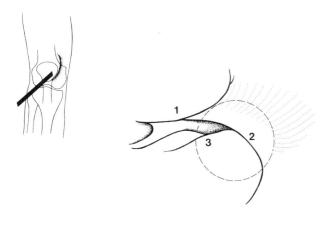

Fig. 4.16 The medial synovial shelf (2), patella (1), medial femoral condyle (3)

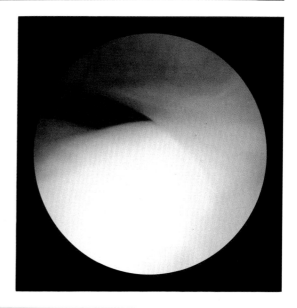

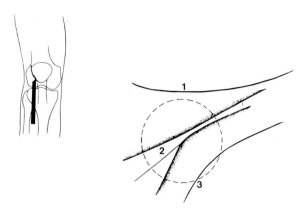

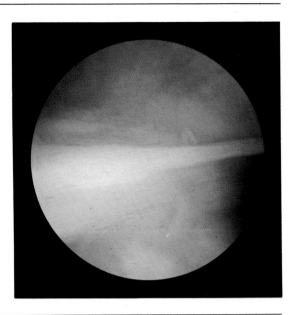

Fig. 4.17 The lateral synovial shelf (2), patella (1), lateral femoral condyle (3)

the subsynovial fat-pad, because, if this is done, saline will distend the subsynovial tissues. Once the anterior cruciate has been identified (Fig. 2.15), its fibres should be followed upwards and backwards to the insertion on the lateral femoral condyle. The small fat-pad overlying the attachment of the posterior

cruciate ligament to the medial femoral condyle, and towards the classical site of osteochondritis dissecans, should also be inspected.

The lateral compartment

To enter the lateral compartment, the joint space is opened with a varus strain in approximately 30° of flexion by applying the surgeon's thigh to the outer side of the patient's ankle and using the edge of the table as a fulcrum (Fig. 4.22). Difficulty in passing the arthroscope across the notch may be caused by the infrapatellar fold (alias the ligamentum muco-sum, plica synovialis infrapatellaris, inferior patellar plica, or inferior synovial fold), which is the anatomical vestige of the septum which divided the knee into separate medial and lateral compartments.

This method of examining the lateral compart-ment of the knee differs slightly from that in which the patient's foot is put on the operating table in such a way that the knee falls outwards, with the hip abducted and flexed (Jackson & Dandy 1976) (Fig. 4.23). Although a good view of the lateral compart-ment can be obtained with the knee in this position, manipulation of instruments within the joint is difficult, the position of the leg is harder to control precisely, and loose bodies tend to fall into the recess beneath the posterior horn (Fig. 4.24) of the lateral meniscus or the postero-lateral compartment, from which retrieval may be difficult (Figs. 7.2, 7.3).

Fig. 4.18 Applying a valgus stress in external rotation to open up the medial compartment

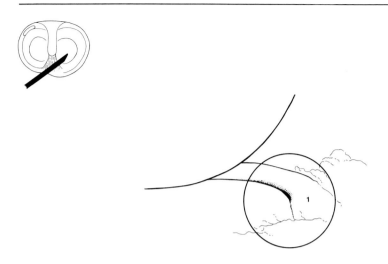

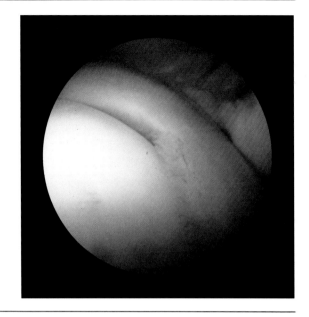

Fig. 4.19 The anterior horn of the medial meniscus seen with a 70° arthroscope inserted from the antero-lateral approach

When the meniscus has been inspected, the articular surface of the lateral condyle should be examined by scanning its surface with the tip of the telescope as the knee is flexed and extended. The telescope is then guided into the lateral gutter and the popliteus tendon brought into view (Fig. 4.25). Although pathology in this area is unusual, loose bodies may lurk around the popliteus tendon and localised synovitis is sometimes seen. Defects in the inferior menisco-synovial junction opposite the popliteus tunnel are not uncommon and are probably of no serious significance; they are emphatically not an indication for total lateral meniscectomy. Before leaving the lateral gutter, the arthroscope should be turned upwards to assess the relationship of the lateral edge of the patella and the underlying femur. Between a third and a quarter of the patellar surface usually overhangs the lateral condyle (Fig. 4.14).

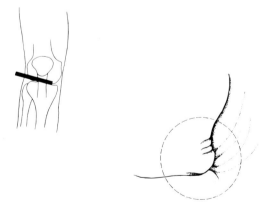

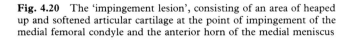

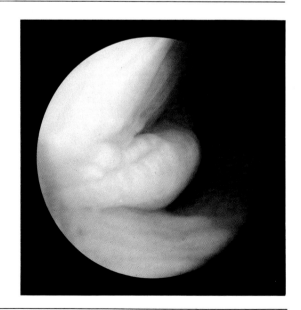

Fig. 4.20 The 'impingement lesion', consisting of an area of heaped up and softened articular cartilage at the point of impingement of the medial femoral condyle and the anterior horn of the medial meniscus

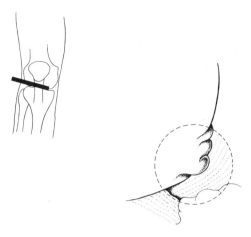

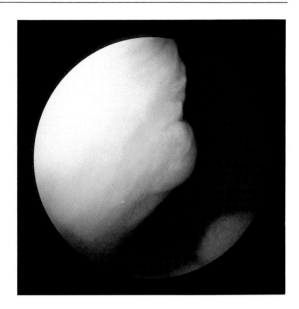

Fig. 4.21 The 'impingement lesion' seen with the knee slightly flexed and the lesion raised above the anterior horn of the medial meniscus

The median ridge can be brought into view in patients with abnormal ligament laxity, and the medial facet in those with dislocation, but in patients with excessive lateral pressure syndrome the patella will feel tight and less mobile than normal. The lateral suprapatellar approach is also helpful in assessing the patello-femoral joint. Finally, if there is a possibility that a loose body is lying under the posterior horn of the lateral meniscus, the arthroscope should be passed beneath the meniscus.

If the telescope cannot be brought into the lateral compartment through the intercondylar notch, per-

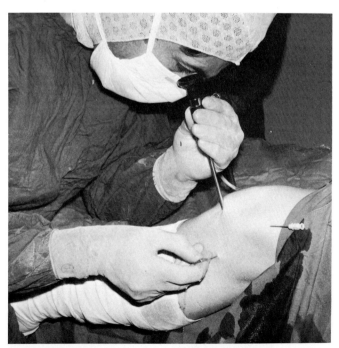

Fig. 4.22 Applying a varus stress to the knee using the edge of the table as a fulcrum, while manipulating the lateral meniscus with a percutaneous needle

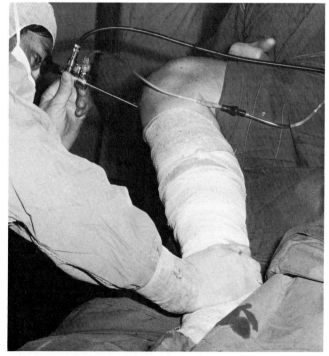

Fig. 4.23 Examining the lateral compartment with the patient's foot on the table. The most dependent part of the joint is the postero-lateral corner

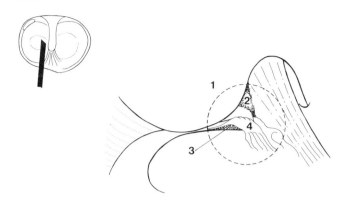

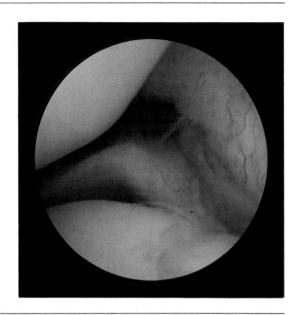

Fig. 4.24   The posterior horn of the meniscus seen from the antero-lateral approach. The opening (2) below the lateral femoral condyle (1) and above the lateral meniscus (4) leads to the postero-lateral compartment. The opening (3) beneath the lateral meniscus leads to a recess in which loose bodies and foreign bodies may become lodged

haps because of a locked bucket-handle fragment or a loose body in the notch, it can often be passed down from the suprapatellar pouch via the lateral gutter. If this is also impossible, it is better to stop struggling and insert the arthroscope from the antero-medial approach.

Posterior compartments

The postero-medial compartment of the knee is entered by passing the telescope between the medial

femoral condyle and the anterior cruciate ligament (Fig. 4.26). This can be achieved from the antero-lateral approach in most knees if the leg is held in external rotation and the knee flexed to approximately 30°, provided that there are no osteophytes and the tibial spine is of normal size. The posterior attachment of the medial meniscus can be seen clearly as the telescope enters the compartment and its posterior surface can be examined in more detail with the 70° telescope. A ruptured posterior cruciate ligament may be seen in the lateral wall of the

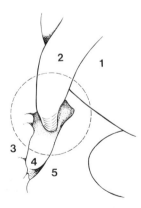

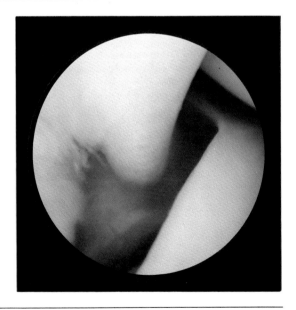

Fig. 4.25   The popliteus tendon (2) entering its tunnel (4) with the knee in slight flexion; femur (1), synovium of lateral gutter (3), lateral meniscus (5)

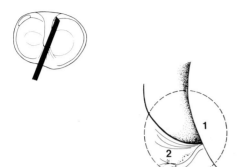

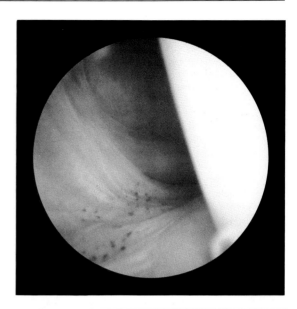

Fig. 4.26 Postero-medial compartment of the knee from the antero-lateral approach. The speckled appearance of the synovium (2) is sometimes seen and is probably a normal variant; medial femoral condyle (1), medial meniscus (3)

compartment (Fig. 4.27) and loose bodies or debris often settle on the floor of the compartment (Fig. 10.23).

The postero-lateral compartment can be entered from the antero-lateral approach in almost every patient by passing the telescope between the lateral femoral condyle and the anterior cruciate ligament. The back of the lateral femoral condyle and the lateral meniscus can then be examined, if necessary with the 70° telescope. Finally, the arthroscope should be brought back to the suprapatellar pouch.

OTHER APPROACHES

The central approach

The central approach directly through the patellar tendon (Gillquist & Hagberg 1976) is a practical alternative to the antero-lateral insertion for the routine initial examination, and offers easy access to the posterior compartments. With the knee flexed to 60°, a short skin incision is made in the midline of the knee – which is just lateral to the midline of the tendon and not in its centre – 1 cm below the lower

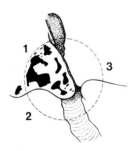

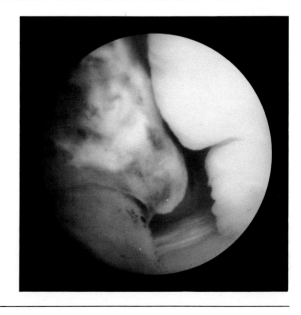

Fig. 4.27 A ruptured posterior cruciate ligament seen with a 70° arthroscope inserted from the antero-lateral approach and passed through the intercondylar notch. The ruptured end of the posterior cruciate ligament (1) is seen lying above the posterior margin of the tibia (2), and anterior to the posterior capsule (3)

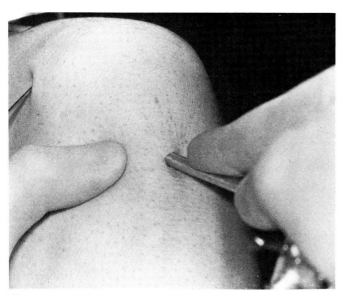

Fig. 4.28 Inserting the trocar of the arthroscope from the central approach

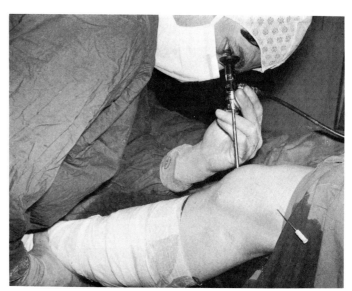

Fig. 4.29 Examining the lateral compartment from the antero-medial approach

pole of the patella and down to the patellar tendon, but not into it (Fig. 4.7). The trocar is then directed backwards and slightly upwards through the tendon (Fig. 4.28), the tip of the instrument tilted, the knee straightened, and the arthroscope brought into the suprapatellar pouch in the usual way. The mobility of the arthroscope is restricted very slightly by the patellar tendon and examination of the suprapatellar pouch, particularly the medial shelf, is not as easy from this approach as from the antero-lateral.

The medial compartment can be examined very thoroughly and it is easier to enter the postero-medial compartment from this approach than from the antero-lateral (Gillquist et al 1979). The inter-condylar notch and lateral compartment can also be examined as well from this approach as from the antero-lateral, but the lateral gutter, including the popliteus tendon, is less accessible.

One minor disadvantage of the central approach is that operating instruments inserted through second and third channels from the antero-medial or antero-lateral routes lie very close to the arthroscope. Apart from the undesirability of three wounds so close together, the arthroscope and instruments tend to clash and make manipulation difficult. A second disadvantage is that the fibres of the patellar tendon close together so neatly that it is difficult to find the original passage if the arthroscope is withdrawn, and repeated insertion of instruments is potentially more harmful through the patellar tendon than through

the capsule. Despite the simplicity and proven safety of this approach, some surgeons have seen granulo-mata of the tendon, and if every beginner learns arthroscopy from the central approach and uses it for routine examination, problems are likely to follow. Nevertheless, the central approach has the great virtue of allowing two operating instruments to be brought to bear on a lesion, and this can be invaluable in a difficult situation.

Antero-medial approach

The antero-medial approach has no place as the routine initial insertion for diagnostic arthroscopy. Although the medial side of the patella, medial gutter, postero-medial compartment and anterior horn of the lateral meniscus can be seen better from the medial approach than the lateral, the medial synovial shelf, lateral gutter and anterior part of the medial meniscus are more difficult.

Apart from the limitations of the field of vision, manipulation of an arthroscope from the medial side of the knee makes it necessary for the arthroscopist to adopt some curious postures, unless a television is available (Fig. 4.29). Despite this criticism, a thorough understanding of the antero-medial ap-proach is essential because it is the usual route for operating instruments, and transposition of the instruments and arthroscope during arthroscopic meniscectomy is often necessary.

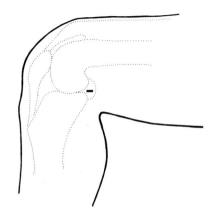

Fig. 4.30 The point of insertion of the arthroscope from the postero-medial approach

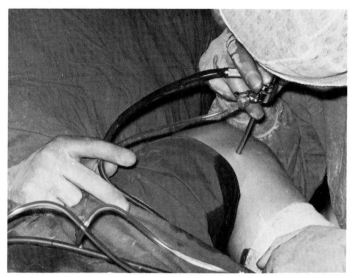

Fig. 4.31 Examining the postero-medial compartment from the postero-medial approach

The exact point of insertion is determined by the lesion to be dealt with and will be described later (p. 127). In general, the point of insertion will lie in an area approximately 1 cm above the anterior horn of the medial meniscus and 1.5 cm medial to the patellar tendon (Fig. 4.7). If the point of insertion lies about 1 cm above the medial meniscus, the posterior attachment of the meniscus, the intercondylar notch and lateral meniscus can all be seen easily. The posterior third of the medial meniscus is best seen if the insertion is a little lower, and the middle third or medial gutter if the arthroscope is inserted 1 cm medial to the edge of the patellar tendon.

Postero-medial insertions

The postero-medial compartment, including the posterior aspect of the medial meniscus, the posterior cruciate ligament and the inferior recess, can be seen well from the postero-medial approach. Although the anterior margin and inferior surface of the posterior horn can be seen from the antero-lateral approach and the posterior surface from the postero-medial approach, it is still possible for small splits in the substance of the meniscus itself to escape detection from any approach.

The point of insertion for the postero-medial approach lies in the triangle above the tibial plateau and behind the posterior edge of the medial femoral condyle when the knee is flexed to 90°, directly over the pouch of loose capsule and synovium that appears when the knee is flexed (Fig. 4.30). The point of insertion must be defined exactly, for if an

instrument is placed too far anteriorly, it will damage articular cartilage, and if placed too far posteriorly, it will be outside the capsule and endanger the popliteal vessels. The point of insertion is found by distending the joint fully with saline with the knee extended, flexing it to 90°, and inserting a needle at the proposed site of insertion. If there is a free flow of saline from the needle, it must be in the joint and the arthroscope can be inserted safely at that point. The arthroscope can then be inserted through the usual 5 mm horizontal skin incision, aiming slightly upwards and forwards (Fig. 4.31).

The postero-medial compartment is best seen from this approach with the knee flexed to 90°, the outer edge of the foot lying on the operating table, and the hip in abduction. The cruciate ligaments block entry to the lateral compartment, making it impossible for instruments, or loose bodies, to pass directly from the postero-medial to the postero-lateral compartment (Fig. 4.32). A small defect is sometimes seen in front of the cruciate 'mesentery', but is not large enough to admit the arthroscope, unless the posterior cruciate ligament is ruptured.

Rotating the arthroscope brings the posterior capsule and its femoral reflection into view, but the synovium in this area is usually featureless, apart from the striations of the posterior oblique ligament. Openings leading to popliteal cysts are disappointingly rare, but can sometimes be identified medial to the medial tendon of the gastrocnemius.

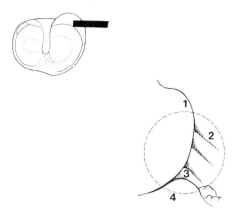

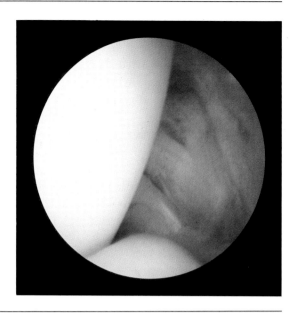

Fig. 4.32 A normal postero-medial compartment from the postero-medial approach; medial femoral condyle (1), posterior capsule (2), posterior cruciate ligament (3), medial meniscus (4)

Lateral suprapatellar approach

The lateral suprapatellar approach is helpful in the evaluation of the synovial folds, the patella and its alignment, as well as the fat-pad (Fig. 4.33). Procedures involving the patella or fat-pad are often easier with the arthroscope in the suprapatellar pouch and the instruments inserted from the antero-medial or antero-lateral route (Fig. 6.17).

The suprapatellar approach is easier in a lax knee than in a patient with a tight patella or a deep intercondylar groove and a correspondingly sharp angle between the patellar facets. The most convenient point for the insertion is 1 cm proximal and posterior to the supero-lateral angle of the patella.

From this route the upper pole of the patella, fat-pad, medial synovial shelf and the patello-femoral joint can be seen from above, the relationship of the shelf and femoral condyle observed, and the stability of the patello-femoral joint assessed (p. 43). The arthroscope can also be directed downwards into the lateral gutter, which gives an excellent view of the popliteus tendon and its tunnel.

Medial and lateral mid-patellar incisions

Insertions at the mid-patellar level, popularised by Patel (1982), are useful when examining the anterior horns of the menisci, the transverse ligament, the fat-pad and the tibial insertion of the anterior cruciate ligament. The front of the intercondylar notch can be seen with the 30° telescope and the entrances to the postero-medial and postero-lateral compartments with the 70° telescope. The mid-

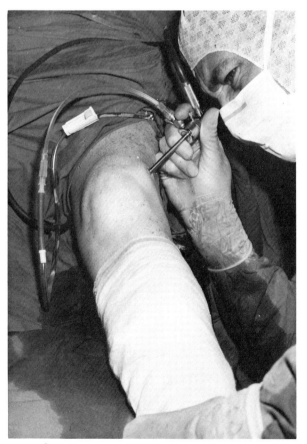

Fig. 4.33 Examining the knee from the suprapatellar approach

patellar approaches are especially useful if the anterior part of the knee is obscured by oedema or extra-synovial saline, because the arthroscope can be directed downwards towards the fat-pad instead of passing directly above or through it. Although some surgeons use the mid-patellar approach routinely, most prefer to reserve it for times when it is difficult or particularly important to inspect the anterior part of the joint.

Patel (1982) described an incision opposite the widest point of the patella, but most surgeons find that the soft tissues in this area restrict the mobility of the arthroscope considerably. This difficulty is overcome if the incision is made about 5 mm from the border of the patella, midway between its upper and lower poles. The incision then lies just below the widest point of the patella, which is a little above its midpoint and about 1.5 cm above and lateral to the antero-lateral approach (Fig. 4.34). A better name for this approach might be the 'high antero-lateral approach'.

The mid-patellar approaches have some disadvantages. The incision passes through an area with little subcutaneous tissue, and leakage of saline into the extra-synovial tissue leads to the rapid formation of an extra-synovial 'salinoma', as it does after a lateral suprapatellar approach. Secondly, the patella limits mobility of the arthroscope, making it difficult to see

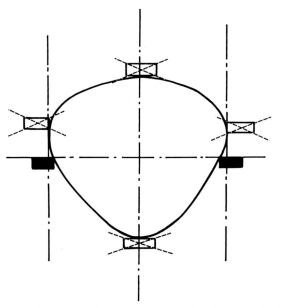

Fig. 4.34 The mid-patellar approach. The point of insertion is at the middle of the height of the patella, not its widest point

all of the suprapatellar pouch or the back of the opposite compartment. Thirdly, because the arthroscope points distally and the operating instruments proximally, it is difficult to control leg, instruments and arthroscope simultaneously without the help of an assistant or television, which is almost essential when these approaches are used.

Postero-lateral approach

The postero-lateral approach is useful when removing loose bodies and meniscal fragments from the postero-lateral compartment, but is seldom needed for diagnosis. If the postero-lateral approach is used, the lateral side of the posterior cruciate ligament can be clearly seen. The posterior aspect of the lateral meniscus and the superior menisco-synovial junction can also be seen, but no better than with the arthroscope passed through the intercondylar notch from the antero-lateral approach. The popliteus tendon lies so close to the point of insertion that it is only visible with a 70° telescope from this approach.

The 'window' for the postero-lateral insertion is approximately 1 cm in diameter (Fig. 4.35), and much smaller than that for the postero-medial approach. Special care must be taken to identify the exact point of insertion of the instruments. If the 30° arthroscope can be passed into the postero-lateral compartment through the intercondylar notch and the lens turned laterally with the knee flexed to 90°, the patch of transilluminated skin indicates the point of insertion, which can then be confirmed with a hypodermic needle. If there is a free flow of saline from the needle and it moves freely inside the compartment, the needle marks the correct point of insertion. The point of insertion can also be found by holding the knee at a right angle, identifying the lateral joint-line, the head of the fibula and the lateral femoral condyle, and passing a needle just behind the condyle to check that fluid flows. The needle can then be withdrawn without altering the position of the knee and a short incision made in the line of the fibres of the ilio-tibial tract. The incision is extended deeply and slightly forwards to enter the postero-lateral compartment. The knee must not be flexed or extended after the skin incision has been made or the ilio-tibial tract will move in relation to the capsule and the incisions in the tract and capsule will not coincide.

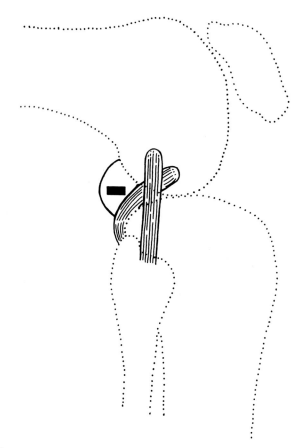

Fig. 4.35 The 'window' for the postero-lateral insertion of the arthroscope

Alternative approaches

The medial suprapatellar approach is sometimes helpful in the release of synovial adhesions or ankylosis, and the lateral submeniscal approach (Fig. 10.12) can be invaluable (p. 158). The central suprapatellar approach through the quadriceps tendon has no advantage over other approaches.

PROBING NEEDLES AND HOOKS

The use of a percutaneous needle and blunt hook is an essential part of a complete arthroscopic examination of the knee, and an important phase in the learning of arthroscopy and arthroscopic surgery. The roles of the joint-line needle and probing hook in the examination of the joint are described here, and their place in the learning of arthroscopic surgery is discussed in Chapter 15. It is essential to be thoroughly familiar with the use of these instruments before attempting arthroscopic surgery.

Percutaneous needles

The use of percutaneous needles to assess the meniscus is simple in principle, but slightly more difficult in practice. A No. 21 gauge hypodermic needle placed beneath the meniscus will sweep out flaps or lift the meniscus so that its under-surface can be inspected (Fig. 4.36); it can also be put directly into the substance of the meniscus itself to check its stability (Figs. 10.5, 10.6, 11.2, 11.4).

The point of insertion of the needle is found by pointing the arthroscope at the desired point of entry and passing the needle just below the area of transilluminated skin. The first placement of the needle may be a few millimetres off target, but the second attempt should be exact; random percutaneous stabbing of the meniscus is not to be encouraged. The irrigation needle in the suprapatellar pouch can also be used to explore the patella, the medial synovial fold or the synovial shelf, and needles at other sites can be used to examine chondral lesions (Fig. 8.6).

Probing hook

If the clinical history indicates that a meniscus lesion is possible, the examination is incomplete unless a probing hook is used (Fig. 10.7). To test the inferior menisco-synovial junction, the hook should be slipped under the meniscus and moved to the doubtful area with its tip trailing. The hook is then turned upwards so that it engages the under-surface of the meniscus, which can then be pulled forwards to test its stability. The hook can also be used to sweep flaps from under the meniscus, to palpate the articular cartilage (Fig. 13.12), to assess the integrity of the anterior cruciate ligament, and to determine the extent of articular cartilage defects (Fig. 4.37).

DOUBLE PUNCTURE TECHNIQUE

Whenever operating instruments are used inside the knee, four basic rules must always be observed:

1. Identify the pathology precisely before inserting operating instruments.
2. Plan the approach carefully with a probing hook.
3. Keep the tip of the instruments in view at all times and never cut blindly.
4. Always rehearse the operation with a probing hook, before inserting a cutting instrument.

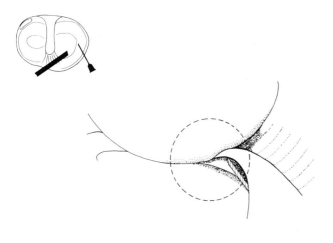

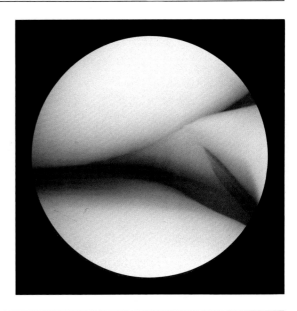

Fig. 4.36 Lifting the medial meniscus with a percutaneous joint-line needle to expose its under-surface and the inferior coronary ligament

Insertion of the instruments

The instruments are inserted through a short incision, just as the arthroscope is inserted, and the points of insertion are essentially the same as those for the arthroscope. Attempts to insert the instruments elsewhere are inadvisable and are likely to damage the articular cartilage of the femur. In particular, the instruments should never be inserted more than 2 cm from the edge of the patellar tendon when using the antero-medial or antero-lateral approach, because there is not enough space beyond these points either to insert the instrument easily or to manipulate it in the knee without damage to the articular cartilage.

Care must be taken to avoid striking the arthroscope with the instruments as they are inserted (Fig. 4.38) by keeping the knee flexed and the arthroscope lying so that its tip points downwards and backwards in the intercondylar notch. The patient's foot can then be rested on the surgeon's knee, and the

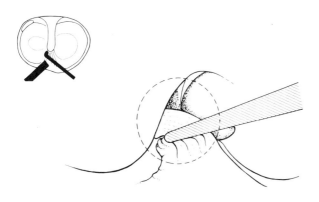

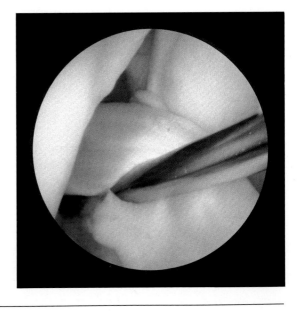

Fig. 4.37 Although this anterior cruciate ligament was apparently intact, the anterior drawer sign was positive and the hook demonstrated abnormal laxity

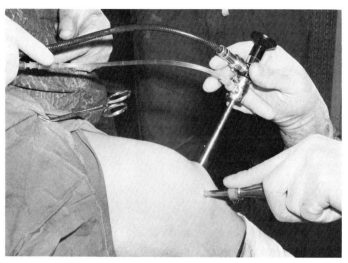

Fig. 4.38 Inserting the cannula for the operating instruments from the antero-medial approach

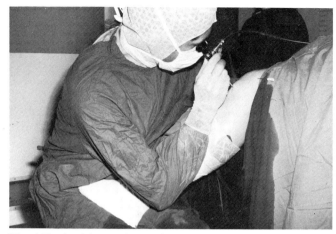

Fig. 4.39 Applying a valgus and external stress without an assistant

instrument aimed upwards, backwards and laterally towards the lateral femoral condyle so that it passes well above the arthroscope. When the instruments are to be inserted from the lateral suprapatellar approach, the knee should be straight and the instrument aimed well away from the arthroscope.

Manipulating the leg

The importance of holding and manipulating the leg correctly cannot be emphasised too strongly. An assistant can steady the arthroscope or manipulate the leg, but it is better if the surgeon is in full control of both. The most practical answer is for the surgeon to steady the patient's foot between his own knees and apply whatever stresses he wishes by pressure with his hand or knee, or by varying the height of the operating table. Although the various manoeuvres seem clumsy at first, with practice they will come naturally and without conscious thought.

Sitting on a wheeled stool and with the patient's foot resting on the surgeon's lap, the knee can be flexed or extended by moving the stool towards or away from the patient, or by raising or lowering the operating table. When the right knee is being examined, a valgus stress can be applied if the surgeon sits with his right leg crossed over his left to steady the patient's foot against the inner edge of his right thigh, and then applies the inner aspect of his left forearm to the outer side of the patient's calf (Fig. 4.39). The knee can be rotated internally or externally by movement of the patient's foot.

To open up the lateral compartment, a gentle varus stress is applied by pressure with the hand and wrist against the medial side of the knee, and a firmer pressure by using the edge of the operating table as a fulcrum and leaning gently against the outer side of the patient's ankle (Fig. 4.40). Although it is easy to describe these manipulations, only practice will bring confidence.

Manipulating the instruments and 'triangulation'

Manipulation of an operating instrument and an arthroscope inserted separately has become known as

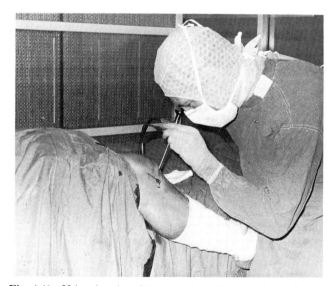

Fig. 4.40 Using the edge of the operating table as a fulcrum for a valgus strain to open up the lateral compartment

'triangulation', and forms the basis of the double puncture technique. Directing an instrument with one hand, while holding an arthroscope in the other and manipulating the patient's leg with the knees and body is a skill not acquired instantly. Assistants, however able, are little help unless they are both experienced and can see the operation on a television monitor, and the surgeon must therefore be able to manage without assistance.

At first, it is difficult enough to find the tip of the irrigating needle in the suprapatellar pouch, without trying to keep it in sight while it is moved from one side of the suprapatellar pouch to the other. It is of no consolation at this stage to know that triangulation in the suprapatellar pouch is much easier than in the intercondylar notch or in the medial or lateral compartment.

The beginner may rest assured that triangulation does become easier with practice, but until the cerebellum has acquired the necessary pathways to find the operating instruments without conscious effort, other methods of location may be used. The simplest is to look away from the eyepiece and place the tip of the instrument in front of the telescope by pointing the shafts of the instruments towards each other (Figs. 4.41, 4.42). An alternative is to slide the instrument along the sheath to the tip of the arthroscope. A third method is to use some easily

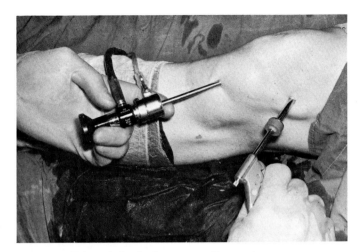

Fig. 4.42   Triangulation in the suprapatellar pouch

identifiable point in the knee, such as the intercondylar notch or the apex of the suprapatellar pouch, as a 'reporting base' where instruments can be placed for easy identification. As with routine diagnostic arthroscopy, orientation of the instrument within the knee is easier with the straightahead 0° telescope than with the 30°.

Triangulation with the arthroscope and one set of instruments is difficult enough (Fig. 4.43), but the manipulation of an arthroscope from the central approach and one instrument through each of the antero-lateral and antero-medial approaches de-

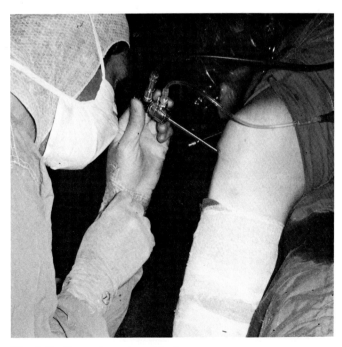

Fig. 4.41   External rotation of the leg

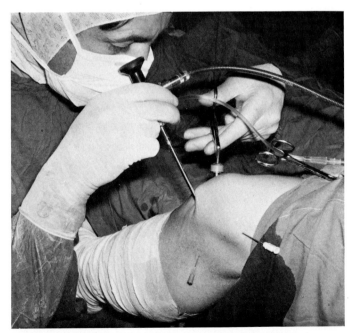

Fig. 4.43   Applying a varus strain while operating in the lateral compartment. The punch forceps are held correctly

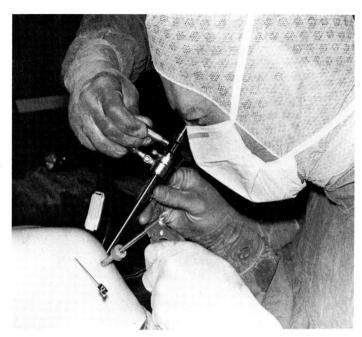

Fig. 4.44 Triple puncture technique with the arthroscope inserted from the central approach. Note the third hand

mands either a third arm or a skilled assistant (Fig. 4.44). Although the use of three approaches simultaneously complicates the procedure, the manipulation of two instruments as well as the arthroscope is sometimes unavoidable and is a skill that must be learned.

ARTHROSCOPY IN ACUTE TRAUMA

An acute haemarthrosis indicates a serious injury to the knee, and approximately 70% have a ruptured anterior cruciate ligament (Jackson et al 1980, Noyes et al 1980). In the past, the management of an acute haemarthrosis often consisted of two weeks' rest in a firm supportive bandage, followed by physiotherapy, an approach which was completely safe, but delayed rehabilitation and postponed definitive operations such as ligament reconstruction until the ideal time had passed. Arthroscopy of the acutely injured knee is almost exactly the opposite. Blood and debris can be removed from the joint so that rehabilitation is faster, and the precise diagnosis and treatment policy can be decided without delay, but the procedure can be dangerous. Partial ruptures of the anterior cruciate or medial ligament may be made complete by forceful manipulation, undisplaced fractures can become displaced, and in children the lower femoral

epiphysis can be loosened. Careful handling of the injured leg by an experienced arthroscopist is therefore essential, preferably without a leg holder.

Blood obscures vision in haemarthrosis, but, if a tourniquet is used and the joint is irrigated thoroughly (O'Connor 1974), the view should be entirely satisfactory (Fig. 12.16), unless the capsule of the knee is torn, when irrigating fluid may run through the defect into the soft tissues of the calf. Because the leg is covered with drapes the calf swelling may go unnoticed, while litre upon litre of saline is poured into the patient's calf, which can jeopardise the blood supply to the lower limb and make a wide fasciotomy necessary to restore a pulse to the foot.

These problems can be avoided if capsular rupture is suspected whenever the joint is slow to empty after it has been filled with saline. If, for example, 200 ml of saline is run into the knee and only 50 ml comes out, the other 150 ml must have gone somewhere else. Although the disparity between inflow and outflow may not be obvious the first time it occurs, if it happens a second or third time the capsule should be considered ruptured until proved otherwise.

To add to these technical problems, there is the administrative difficulty that acute knee injuries occur most commonly at nights and at weekends, when they are likely to be seen and treated by surgeons in training, who may be tempted to undertake an emergency arthroscopy without appreciating the hazards. Because of the dangers of arthroscopy in the acutely injured knee, these guidelines may be appropriate.

1. Arthroscopy of the acutely injured knee should only be performed by competent and experienced arthroscopists.
2. Arthroscopy should not be performed if the shaft of the femur or tibia is fractured, or if there is any suspicion of vascular damage.
3. If arthroscopy is performed on the acutely injured knee, the knee should be examined gently without forceful manipulation and the leg holder should not be used.
4. The aim of arthroscopy in the acutely injured knee is to evacuate blood, establish a diagnosis, and help to decide management. There is no sense in arthroscoping an acutely injured knee if the surgeon is not prepared to proceed with a definitive operation, if arthroscopy shows that it is necessary.

5. If a saline pump is used, it should be used with great caution.

ARTHROSCOPY IN CHILDREN

Arthroscopy in children presents surprisingly few technical problems. The child's knee is large in comparison with the rest of the body, and the ligamentous laxity of childhood means that tight knees do not occur. A standard 5 mm telescope can therefore be used in the normal way. The space between the cruciates and condyles is larger than in an adult, and entry to the postero-medial and postero-lateral compartments is actually easier in children.

The arthroscopic appearances are similar to those of the adult, but the articularis genu muscle is more easily seen, the articular cartilage is softer, and the articular margins are rounder and more vascular. The indications for arthroscopy in children are comparatively few (Suman et al 1984). Discoid menisci can be treated by excision of the central portion (p. 155), taking care not to damage the tibial plateau, osteochondritic lesions can be drilled, and synovial biopsy may be required for persistent effusions, if investigation and conservative management are unhelpful. In the adolescent, anterior knee pain is the main indication for arthroscopy and is described in Chapter 13.

AFTERCARE

Wound closure

A single stitch of monofilament nylon extending through skin and subcutaneous tissues is a convenient and effective wound closure. Adhesive tape can also be used, but a stitch closes the deeper layers of the wound more soundly. An absorbable subcutaneous stitch and adhesive tape is an alternative. Another approach is to inject the sites of proposed incision with Marcain (bupivacaine) 0.5% with added adrenaline and leave the wound unsutured; the Marcain will control pain, the adrenaline may diminish bleeding, and the absence of a stitch will encourage some patients with their rehabilitation.

When the wound has been closed, a gauze dressing should be applied, the knee supported with a few turns of light orthopaedic wool and a crepe bandage

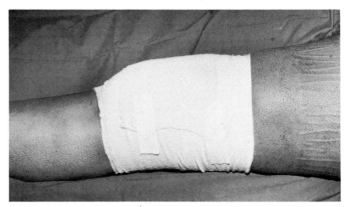

Fig. 4.45 The bandage should extend above the upper limit of the suprapatellar pouch and should not include the calf

applied around the knee – but not the calf. There is a tendency to extend the bandage halfway down the calf, which results in oedema of the ankle and foot, while not taking the bandage to the upper limit of the suprapatellar pouch. The bandage should extend at least 20 cm above the joint-line, and no more than 4 cm below it (Fig. 4.45). The bandage may be removed on the day after operation if necessary, but should be retained for one week if the joint is inflamed.

If the arthroscopy is followed by an open operation, the leg should, ideally, be re-prepared and re-draped. If, however, it is known that arthrotomy will definitely be necessary, it may be permissible to perform the arthroscopy through an additional large drape with a small opening for the arthroscope. The additional drape can be removed when the arthroscope is withdrawn and a Steridrape or similar product applied. This procedure is useful if the arthroscopy is done as a preliminary to ligament reconstruction or osteotomy.

Post-operative care

Patients can expect to lift the leg straight, to flex the knee to 90° on recovering from the anaesthetic, and to leave hospital either on the day of operation or the day after, provided they have received proper pre-operative instruction in quadriceps exercises.

Post-operative physiotherapy is helpful, but not mandatory. Ultrasound treatment to the wounds may help to speed the natural resolution of the swelling around them, and is helpful in athletes anxious to cut every imaginable corner on the road to recovery. Flexion to 90° and a good straight leg raise should always be possible within 24 hours of operation, except perhaps after the release of an ankylosis. Excessive exercise should be avoided by all patients for the first week in order to minimise synovial effusion.

Rehabilitation

The greatest single advantage of arthroscopic surgery is the dramatic reduction in the time required for return to work and normal everyday activities (Hamberg et al 1984). Using arthroscopic meniscectomy as an example, one-quarter of the first 60 patients needed physiotherapy after discharge and these 15 patients attended for an average of 5.1 treatments, making a total of 1.3 out-patient physiotherapy treatments after discharge for each patient in the whole group (Dandy 1979). Out-patient physiotherapy was usually required in knees locked for several weeks before operation, but gentle encouragement in full straight leg raising was also needed in some patients with comparatively small tears.

The time taken for patients to return to work is also reduced, but varies according to the intra-articular pathology and the patient's occupation. Patients engaged in light work are usually fit to return to work after 7 days, and those in heavy work after 14 days, but recovery is slower if there is osteoarthrosis or a major ligament injury (Dandy 1978, Oretorp & Gillquist 1979, Glinz 1980, Lysholm & Gillquist 1981, Tregonning 1983). The rate of recovery after open meniscectomy can be hastened by the administration of non-steroidal anti-inflammatory drugs (Muckle 1984), and the same is presumably true after arthroscopic surgery.

One unforeseen difficulty in achieving an early return to work in a welfare state is the understandable tendency of family practitioners unfamiliar with the technique to issue Certificates of Incapacity for six weeks, on hearing that the patient has undergone a meniscectomy. The patient may be content with this, if there is little or no incentive for an early return to work, and may even consider it his right and privilege. This difficulty can be resolved by an out-patient appointment one week after discharge from hospital so that a certificate of fitness can be issued.

Arthroscopic meniscectomy has sometimes attracted publicity because it enables athletes to return to sporting activities more quickly than journalists expect. The return to full sporting fitness varies according to the individual and the sport concerned, but some patients have been able to return to competitive football within 7 days. It is, however, possible to return to full activity too soon, and the risk of a low-grade chronic synovitis with persistent effusion following early mobilisation is real.

ARTHROSCOPY IN PRACTICE

Diagnostic versus operative arthroscopy

The transition between diagnostic and operative arthroscopy is not clear cut, and a diagnostic arthroscopy will often give enough information to make a small incision instead of a full arthrotomy. If, for example, the arthroscope shows only a locked bucket-handle fragment and no other abnormality, the fragment can be removed through a 2 cm incision and the rehabilitation will be almost as fast as after arthroscopic surgery (Hamberg et al 1984).

The border is blurred still more by the variation in the role of arthroscopy from one practice to another. Some surgeons will be content to restrict themselves to diagnostic arthroscopy and make a small arthrotomy when necessary, whereas others may stop short of the more complicated procedures, but feel happy with synovial biopsy and the removal of small flaps of meniscus. In the fullness of time it is likely that every knee surgeon will be able to do most arthroscopic procedures, but until then there is room for several levels of expertise and no surgeon should feel threatened or compelled to learn the more taxing arthroscopic techniques in order to practice diagnostic arthroscopy.

Duration of operation

The length of the operation is its greatest disadvantage in the early stages. If a meniscus can be removed neatly and without fuss through a small arthrotomy in 15 minutes, there has to be a good reason for turning to an operation that may take two hours to perform and is frustrating both for the surgeon and the operating theatre staff. Because the operation takes longer to perform, less patients can be treated, waiting lists lengthen, and morale falls.

Not surprisingly, tales of the length of operation are exaggerated but the following figures should destroy the myth of the four-hour meniscectomy. Of the first 30 meniscectomies (Dandy 1978), eight took more than one hour from the insertion of the irrigation needle to cutting the last stitch. The mean operating time was 43 minutes, with a range of 10–90 minutes. During this period, three attempts were abandoned and open meniscectomy was performed instead. Five of the second group of 30 took over an hour, with a mean operating time of 37 minutes and a range of 10–105 minutes, and no attempts at closed meniscectomy were abandoned. In the third group of 30 patients, three procedures took over one hour, the mean operating time was 34.5 minutes, with a range of 12–75 minutes, and there were no abandoned procedures. It is now most unusual for a meniscectomy to take more than 50 minutes, and the mean operating time has become steady at a little less than 20 minutes. Excision of a synovial shelf or a lateral release takes a very predictable 10–15 minutes from start to finish; other procedures, such as the removal of loose bodies, are variable, but rarely occupy more than 45 minutes. The operating time is prolonged by taking photographs, demonstrating to students and visitors, displaying the operation on television, or using powered instruments, pumps and miscellaneous gadgetry.

When planning an operating list, it is helpful to know that six arthroscopic procedures can easily be accommodated in a three and a half hour operating session, or seven if the list includes nothing more complicated than synovial biopsy, excision of a synovial shelf, or a lateral release.

Length of stay in hospital

Diagnostic arthroscopy and arthroscopic surgery can be performed safely and reliably as an out-patient 'day-case' procedure (Rosenberg & Wong 1982), but only if the surgeon is experienced. When learning arthroscopic surgery, it is sensible to warn the patient that however much effort is made to avoid opening the knee, this may be necessary, if the operation cannot be performed arthroscopically. It is also advisable to admit patients on the day before operation and warn them that although they will probably be able to return home on the day after operation, it may be necessary to delay their discharge for several days, although in practice delay in discharge is exceptional. Of the first 30 arthroscopic meniscectomies, 22 patients were able to return home on the day of operation or the day after

(Dandy 1978), seven on the second day, and one patient, who had a cystic lateral meniscus, on the fourth day. Of the second 30 patients, one stayed in hospital until the fourth day after operation, because of a severe attack of migraine, and one stayed until the second day, because of difficulties in arranging transport home. Since then, all patients have been able to return home within 24 hours of operation, and meniscectomy is done as an out-patient procedure when appropriate.

The rapid turnover of patients affects many departments in the hospital and the changes can cause unexpected difficulties. For the nurses on the ward and the physiotherapists, early discharge results in an uneven distribution of work, with peaks around the operating days and troughs at other times, including weekends, when the wards may be virtually empty.

The advantages of short-stay surgery depend on many factors, among them the pressure on hospital beds, the facilities for out-patient surgery, and the way in which health care is financed. Arthroscopic surgery reduces the overall bed occupancy so that fewer beds are needed to achieve the same patient throughput, but it is worth noting that the bed-occupancy figures which loom so large in the minds of some hospital administrators are usually based on the number of beds occupied at midnight, and do not include patients admitted and discharged on the same day. The result is that a large number of out-patient procedures can have a disastrous effect on the hospital statistics, if they depend on the bed occupancy rather than the number of patients treated.

References

Dandy D J 1978 Early results of closed partial meniscectomy. British Medical Journal 1: 1099–1100

Dandy D J 1979 Closed partial meniscectomy. Journal of Bone and Joint Surgery 61B: 128

Gillies H, Seligson D 1979 Precision in the diagnosis of meniscal lesions: a comparison of clinical evaluation, arthrography and arthroscopy. Journal of Bone and Joint Surgery 61A: 343–346

Gillquist J, Hagberg G 1976 A new modification of the technique of arthroscopy of the knee joint. Acta Chirurgica Scandinavica 142(2): 123–30

Gillquist J, Hagberg G, Oretorp N 1979 Arthroscopic visualisation of the posterior compartments of the knee joint. Orthopedic Clinics of North America 10: 545–547

Glinz W 1980 Arthroscopic partial meniscectomy. Helvetica Chirurgica Acta 47: 115–119

Halperin N, Axer A, Hirschberg E, Agas M 1978 Arthroscopy of the knee under local anaesthesia and controlled pressure. Clinical Orthopaedics and Related Research 134: 176–179

Hamberg P, Gillquist J, Lysholm J 1984 A comparison between arthroscopic meniscectomy and open meniscectomy. Journal of Bone and Joint Surgery 66B: 189–192

Iino S 1939 Normal arthroscopic findings in the knee joint in adult cadavers. Journal of the Japanese Orthopaedic Association 14: 467–523

Jackson R W, Abe I 1972 The role of arthroscopy in the management of disorders of the knee. Journal of Bone and Joint Surgery 54B: 310–322

Jackson R W, Dandy D J 1976 Arthroscopy of the knee. Grune & Stratton, New York

Jackson R W, Marshall D J, Fujisawa Y 1982 The pathological medial shelf. Orthopedic Clinics of North America 13: 307–312

Jackson R W, Peters R I, Marczyk R L 1980 Late results of untreated anterior cruciate rupture. Journal of Bone and Joint Surgery 62B: 127

Johnson L L 1977 The comprehensive examination of the knee. C V Mosby, St Louis, Mo

Joyce M J, Mankin H J 1983 Caveat arthroscopos: extra-articular lesions of bone simulating intra-articular pathology of the knee. Journal of Bone and Joint Surgery 65A: 289–292

Klein W, Schulitz K P 1979 Out-patient arthroscopy under local anaesthesia. Archives of Orthopaedic and Traumatic Surgery 96: 131–134

Lysholm J, Gillquist J 1981 Endoscopic meniscectomy. International Orthopaedics 5: 265–270

McGinty J B, Matza R A 1978 Arthroscopy of the knee. Evaluation of an out-patient procedure under local anaesthesia. Journal of Bone and Joint Surgery 60A: 787–789

McLean I D 1983 Arthroscopic surgery: triumph of technology over reason. Journal of Bone and Joint Surgery 65B: 672

Mayeda T 1918 Uber das Strangartige Gebilde inder Kniegelenkhole (chorda cavi articularis genu). Mitteilungen aus der Medizinschen Fakultat der Kaiserlichen Universitat zu Tokio 21: 507–553

Muckle D S 1984 Open meniscectomy: enhanced recovery after synovial prostaglandin inhibition. Journal of Bone and Joint Surgery 66B: 193–195

Noyes F R, Bassett R W, Grood E S, Butler D L 1980 Arthroscopy in acute traumatic haemarthrosis of the knee. Journal of Bone and Joint Surgery 62A: 687–695

O'Connor R L 1974 Arthroscopy in the diagnosis and treatment of cruciate ligament injuries. Journal of Bone and Joint Surgery 56A: 333–337

Oretorp N, Gillquist J 1979 Transcutaneous meniscectomy under arthroscopic control. International Orthopaedics 3: 19–25

Patel D 1978 Arthroscopy of the plicae-synovial folds and their significance. American Journal of Sports Medicine 6: 217–225

Patel D 1982 Superior lateral-medial approach to arthroscopic meniscectomy. Orthopedic Clinics of North America 13: 299–305

Pevey J K 1978 Arthroscopy of the knee under local anaesthesia. American Journal of Sports Medicine 6: 122–126

Rosenberg T D, Wong H C 1982 Arthroscopic surgery in a free-standing outpatient surgery centre. Orthopedic Clinics of North America 13: 277–282

Sakakibara J 1976 Arthroscopic study on Iino's band – plica synovialis mediopatellaris. Journal of the Japanese Orthopaedic Association 50: 513–522

Suman R K, Stother I G, Illingworth G 1984 Diagnostic arthroscopy of the knee in children. Journal of Bone and Joint Surgery 66B: 535–537

Tregonning R J A 1983 Closed partial meniscectomy: early results for simple tears with mechanical symptoms. Journal of Bone and Joint Surgery 65B: 378–382

Whipple T L, Bassett F H 1978 Arthroscopic examination of the knee. polypuncture technique with percutaneous intra-articular manipulation. Journal of Bone and Joint Surgery 60A: 444–453

5

Complications and technical problems

COMPLICATIONS

Remarkably few complications have been described (Dick et al 1978, Rosenberg & Wong 1982, Dandy 1983), but arthroscopic surgery is young and it is inevitable that new complications will be reported. Self-criticism is therefore essential and a careful record of patients and their progress should be kept. In 1982, Mulhollan compiled a list of the complications encountered by ten surgeons in a total of 9178 operations; this list is summarised in Table 5.1. Although such an estimate is little more than anecdotal, there is at present no better indication of the incidence of complications or their nature.

Broken instruments

The fracture of instruments within the knee was perhaps the greatest early anxiety. In the first 1000

Table 5.1 Percentage incidence of complications in 9178 operations performed by ten surgeons (after Mulhollan 1982)

Complication	Incidence (%)
Instrument breakage	0.3
Instrument breakage requiring arthrotomy	0.01
Infection	0.07
Non-pyogenic inflammation	0.3
Haemarthrosis *	9
Haemarthrosis requiring aspiration	5
Draining sinus	0.01
Draining sinus requiring re-operation	0
Wound granuloma	0.03
Tender scar	14
Neuroma pain at portal of entry	0.02
Persistent effusion	9
Hypoaesthesia below portal of entry	0.4
Thrombophlebitis	0.3
Pulmonary embolus	0.0

*Excluding lateral retinacular release.

procedures, five such incidents occurred (Dandy & O'Carroll 1982). In one, the tip of a small tenotomy blade introduced at the medial joint-line fractured as a meniscal fragment was divided. The fragment was so small and so firmly embedded in the medial ligament that the decision was made to leave it rather than proceed to an extensive dissection that would have done more harm than good. The practice of inserting a tenotomy knife at the joint-line was tried in the early stages of developing the technique, but it did not prove helpful and is not recommended.

In a second patient, the tip of a percutaneous hypodermic needle used to manipulate a flap of lateral meniscus was severed with the punch forceps used to remove the meniscal fragment. The patient, an athlete, was particularly anxious to avoid an arthrotomy and returned to competitive sport four days after operation; subsequent radiographs showed the fragment in the soft tissues of the intercondylar notch.

In another patient, a pair of scissors fractured when a synovial shelf was being divided. The distal end of the scissors separated and fell into the postero-lateral compartment, with the tips of the blades penetrating the posterior joint capsule and the other end wedged firmly in the intercondylar notch. A small lateral arthrotomy was necessary to remove the fragment. In a fourth patient, a fragment of steel measuring 2 mm × 2 mm × 0.5 mm separated from the tip of a guillotine and was successfully retrieved without opening the joint.

Fracture of the instruments is a real problem during the early stages, and great care must be exercised to prevent this complication by avoiding excessive loading or twisting of the instruments. In

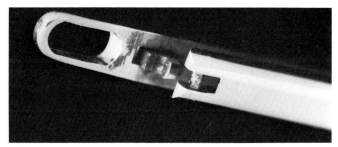

Fig. 5.1 A broken punch forceps with missing jaw

the fifth patient, the jaw of a pair of punch forceps fractured (Fig. 5.1) and became lodged in the synovial sheath surrounding the posterior cruciate ligament (Fig. 5.2). Figure 5.3 shows the jaw of an arthroscopic rongeur which fractured and shows the fracture line in the hinge mechanism. The fragment was retrieved arthroscopically.

The fracture of instruments can be avoided, to some extent, by improvements in design, and the consequences of fracture can be minimised by ensuring that the weakest point of the instrument lies

outside the knee in such a way that the fragments are not liberated into the joint cavity (Fig. 5.4).

Synovial fistula

One early patient (the ninth arthroscopic meniscectomy) developed a clear watery discharge from the antero-medial wound on the ninth post-operative day and was considered to have a synovial fistula. The wound became dry after immobilisation in a plaster cylinder for seven days and the patient's recovery was uneventful thereafter. Although the presence of a synovial fistula was not proved conclusively, the diagnosis seems likely. A fistula between the knee and a prepatellar bursa has also been described after a lateral retinacular release (Hadied 1984), but not after arthroscopy alone.

Medial collateral ligament rupture

The medial ligament can be ruptured, particularly through clumsy use of a thigh holder, but this

(a)

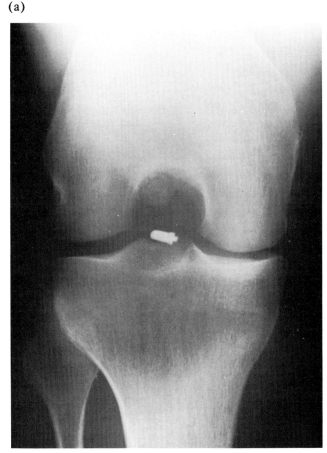

(b)

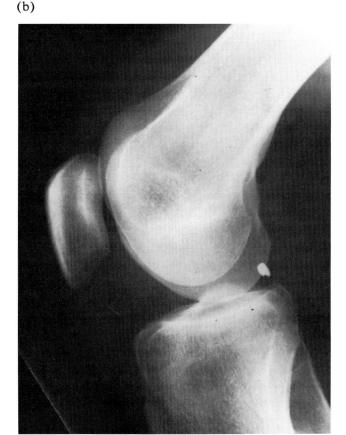

Fig. 5.2 Antero-posterior (A) and lateral (B) radiographs to show the position of the jaw missing from the instrument in Figure 5.1

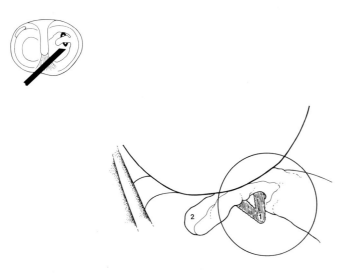

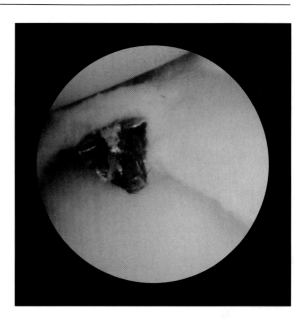

Fig. 5.3 The broken jaw of a pair of rongeurs (1) lying beneath a meniscal flap (2)

complication may become less common with experience (Rosenberg & Wong 1982, Jackson 1983).

Deep vein thrombosis

To determine the exact incidence of deep vein thrombosis is difficult, but it is probably in the region of one to three per thousand (Rosenberg & Wong 1982, Dandy & O'Carroll 1982). Although such evidence is insubstantial, deep vein thrombosis is not an important practical problem, but does occur occasionally.

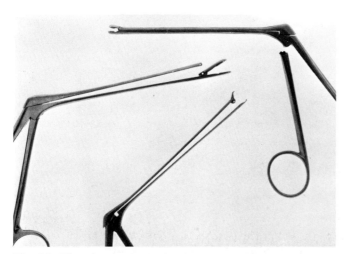

Fig. 5.4 These instruments broke during use, but were withdrawn without leaving a fragment of metal in the knee

Arterial damage

There are sporadic reports of arterial damage leading to amputation (Jackson 1983), and the author is aware of an incident in which the popliteal artery and vein needed surgical repair after a lateral meniscectomy.

Distension of soft tissues with gas

Henderson & Hopson (1982) report pneumoscrotum, following the use of a defective pump which drew air into the irrigation fluid through a split in the irrigation tube. Although an unusual and distressing complication, the patient made a good recovery.

Infection

The questionable sterility of arthroscopic surgery has already been mentioned and it is therefore reassuring to know that wound infection is almost unknown following arthroscopic procedures (Rosenberg & Wong 1982). Haematomata following lateral release can become infected and joint infections are seen very occasionally (Johnson et al 1982), but one patient is known to have died from acute gram-negative septicaemia (Jackson 1983). Although the infection rate is so low, this is no excuse for carelessness or for touching the tips of instruments entering the joint.

Effusion and haemarthrosis

The incidence of post-operative haemarthrosis depends, at least in part, on the criteria for its diagnosis. If a haemarthrosis is taken to be a tense effusion of blood in the knee which prevents straight leg raising, the incidence of haemarthrosis in the first 1000 operations (Dandy & O'Carroll 1982) was 1%. If a haemarthrosis is present and the patient cannot lift the heel off the bed, the joint should be aspirated because, if this is not done, rehabilitation will be just as slow and painful as after a wide arthrotomy.

Effusion is not a major problem, but the reported incidence varies; some surgeons have encountered an incidence in the region of 15%, whereas others report none at all (Mulhollan 1982), probably because the criteria for diagnosis are imprecise. Patients who exercise too vigorously during the first week after operation may develop a moderate effusion that can last for several weeks. If a persistent effusion does develop, the patient should be advised to stop all sport, wear a crepe bandage to minimise the risk of accidental injury, and take an anti-inflammatory drug.

Wound tenderness

A little thickening and tenderness is common around the wounds, particularly lateral suprapatellar incisions. The thickening, which is due to a small haematoma and feels like a dried pea under the skin, is seldom troublesome and settles within a few weeks of operation.

Articular cartilage damage

Scuffing of the articular cartilage becomes less common with experience, but is difficult to avoid completely (Fig. 5.5). Any irregularity of the articular surface, however slight, is magnified by the arthroscope and it is comforting to know that the defects may prove impossible to find at arthrotomy. No ill-effect has been observed from minor intra-articular cartilage damage and repeat arthroscopic examination later suggests that it can become smooth (Fig. 5.6), but the injury can do no good and care must be taken to avoid trauma to the articular cartilage during operation.

Intra-articular granuloma

A troublesome granuloma can form at the site of insertion of the instruments or arthroscope and may cause a block to extension, even when the meniscus has been removed. At re-arthroscopy, a small knot of proliferative synovium is seen, with all the appearances of pigmented villonodular synovitis. Lindenbaum (1981) suggested that the lesion may be a reaction to talc. Recovery is usual after excision of the pathological area. Lindenbaum also reported herniation of the fat-pad through the capsular incision as a cause of persistent wound pain following arthroscopy.

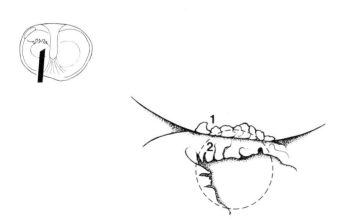

Fig. 5.5 Damage to the under-surface of the lateral femoral condyle (1) caused by attempts to trim the lateral meniscus (2) with cutting instruments passed directly across the joint space between the tibial plateau and femoral condyle

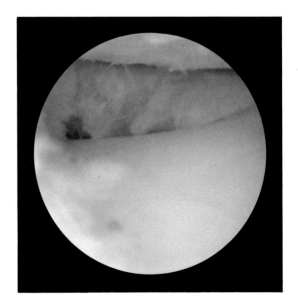

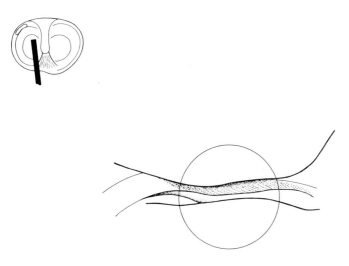

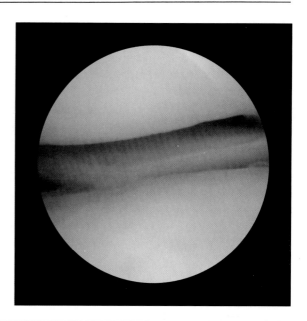

Fig. 5.6 The same knee as that in Figure 5.5 examined two years later. The meniscus has rounded and the articular cartilage defects are smooth

Medico-legal complications

It is a matter of professional responsibility for a surgeon only to attempt procedures within his ability and the surgeon who ignores this precept and attempts arthroscopic surgery before he is properly competent is a source of special anxiety. To embark on arthroscopic surgery immediately after purchasing a set of powered instruments and a video system is a recipe for disaster that can only bring the individual surgeon, and arthroscopic surgery in general, into disrepute.

Great expectations

Many patients have unreasonably high expectations of arthroscopic surgery and are disappointed with anything short of a total cure. The problem is most commonly seen in patients with knees hopelessly destroyed by osteoarthritis, ligamentous instability, multiple meniscectomy or patellectomy. Such patients have often received many good opinions, all of them pessimistic, and look to the innovation of arthroscopy as an answer to their insoluble problem. Although arthroscopy may be helpful in confirming the awful prognosis, and the removal of articular cartilage fragments or osteophytes can produce transient improvement, lasting relief is improbable. The patients are likely to transfer their dissatisfaction from the pathology to the surgeon, unless it is made crystal clear to them that their prognosis is poor and that arthroscopy cannot produce the lasting benefit they are seeking. Even if the surgeon is at his most gloomy in describing the prognosis, the patient may still fail to comprehend what is said and depart in a mood of misplaced optimism that can only lead to disappointment and possible recrimination. Unjustified euphoria on the part of the patient at the first post-operative consultation often means that the patient has failed to absorb, either at the conscious or subconscious level, the clinical information that has been given.

A similar problem is encountered in younger patients, often athletes, who have a serious injury with a poor prognosis. A young footballer with a torn lateral meniscus and articular cartilage damage in the lateral compartment has a poor prognosis, but because the incisions and the immediate post-operative course are identical to those of a straight-forward arthroscopic meniscectomy, patients can be forgiven for believing that the prognoses are also identical. Unless the prognosis is explained clearly to the patient and in writing both to the family practitioner and the club doctor, if appropriate, it is very likely that when the inevitable problems arise in the future they will be attributed to the surgeon. In the management of the professional athlete, the manager or 'owner' frequently needs more explanation and reassurance than the patient, and in this respect there is more than a little similarity with veterinary medicine.

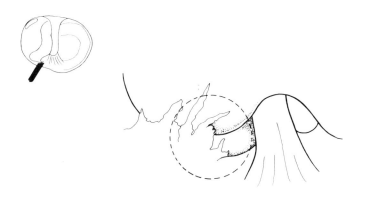

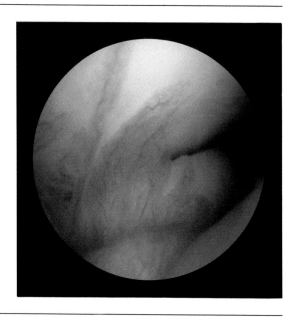

Fig. 5.7 Intense synovitis obscuring a locked bucket-handle fragment of the lateral meniscus

TECHNICAL PROBLEMS

Many technical problems are encountered in arthroscopy, but the following summary may be helpful.

'It has gone dark'

The light cable may have become disconnected, or the light source may have failed. If the light source has two cable sockets, the cable may be plugged into the wrong socket.

'The telescope won't stay locked in the sheath'

Some arthroscopes have an inadequate locking mechanism and become unlocked as the sheath is rotated. If the locking mechanism depends on a rubber 'O' ring, the ring probably needs replacing. Accidental unlocking can be prevented by holding the light post of the telescope and the sheath with thumb and forefinger, or by holding the two together with a small elastic band.

'I don't know where I am'

Orientation is a problem for everyone at first, but improves with practice. Orientation can be established by moving the eye away from the eyepiece of the arthroscope to find the area of transilluminated skin. In most fore-oblique arthroscopes, the line of vision is directed away from the light post, so that the field of view can be imagined as a flat 'slab' trailing behind the tip of the arthroscope, rather than a cone attached to its tip. This concept is particularly helpful when using the 70° telescope. The identification of a landmark such as the anterior cruciate ligament or the tip of the irrigation needle is also helpful, but if orientation with the 30° telescope is particularly difficult, the 0° telescope should be used until more experience has been gained.

'The fat-pad is in the way'

The fat-pad has probably been distended with saline, perhaps because the arthroscopic sheath has saline ports proximal to the end of the sheath. The problem can best be avoided by not using such a sheath in the first place, but turning off the saline as soon as the arthroscope slips out of the synovial cavity, or reversing the flow so that the fluid runs out of the knee through the arthroscope sheath is effective. If all visibility is lost, the medial or lateral mid-patellar approach can be used. Retractors for the fat-pad have been designed, but the best answer to the problem of the enlarging fat-pad is swift and gentle surgery.

An intense inflammatory response can cause a similar problem (Fig. 5.7). If a patient exercises vigorously with a knee that has been locked with a displaced bucket-handle fragment of meniscus for several weeks, a mass of inflamed synovium in the notch can be expected. It is wise to advise such a patient to take life easily and perhaps to take an anti-inflammatory drug for a few days before operation so that the engorged tissues will have time to subside.

'The field is cloudy'

There is more blood or debris in the knee than the irrigation can remove. Check that the irrigation fluid is flowing, and that the outflow needle is not blocked. If necessary, withdraw the telescope from the sheath and irrigate the joint until the effluent is clear, as if examining a patient with a haemarthrosis. If bleeding is a problem, check that the tourniquet is inflated to the correct pressure.

'The knee has deflated'

Check that the saline reservoir is full and that it is at least 1 m above the knee. If deflation of the joint is a persistent problem, use a smaller outflow needle and a larger inflow channel (see irrigation, pp. 38–9). If the patient has an acute haemarthrosis, the dire consequences of a capsular rupture must be remembered (p. 59).

'I can't get into the lateral compartment'

Crossing from the medial to the lateral side can be difficult if the infra-patellar fold is large, but the arthroscope can usually be passed over the top of the fold, if the edge of the intercondylar notch is followed closely to its apex. Alternatively, the arthroscope can be passed down the lateral gutter; if this also fails, an antero-medial insertion will solve the problem (p. 51).

'I can't see the posterior horn of the medial meniscus'

The posterior horn is best seen in 30° of flexion with a firm valgus strain and the foot externally rotated. If this does not bring the posterior horn of the medial meniscus into view, the knee is unusually tight and visibility will be difficult.

'I can't get into the posterior compartment'

Entry into the posterior compartment is sometimes impossible in tight knees or if there is an osteophyte or prominent tibial spine, but entry is usually possible from the antero-medial, antero-lateral, or central approaches, provided that the knee is held correctly (p. 51). If entry is not possible from one approach, try another.

'I can't see the anterior horns of the menisci'

If the anterior horn cannot be seen with a 30° telescope, try the 70° arthroscope from the antero-medial or antero-lateral approach, or use the mid-patellar approach.

'I can't find the instruments'

Triangulation, like orientation, is difficult at first, but improves with practice. Try the 0° telescope instead of the 30°.

'The instrument won't reach the lesion'

Either the instrument has been inserted in the wrong place, or the knee is being held incorrectly. Selecting the correct points of insertion and the technique of manipulation are essential and are described above (p. 57).

'The instruments are too big'

Quite large operating instruments can be made to reach the back of the medial and lateral gutters or the postero-medial and postero-lateral compartments, provided they follow the 'highways' of the knee, but they will not pass across narrow spaces. The problem can be anticipated by rehearsing the operation with a probing hook before inserting the instruments.

'I can't find the loose body/meniscal fragment'

Meniscal fragments and loose bodies are elusive, but techniques for finding these are described below (p. 86).

'The subcutaneous tissues are swollen'

Irrigation fluid escapes into the subcutaneous tissues if the synovium is breached by taking a large biopsy specimen, excising a wide synovial shelf, or perform-

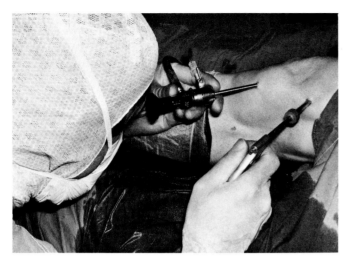

Fig. 5.8 Operating in the suprapatellar pouch. Saline has escaped into the subsynovial tissues to cause an unsightly distension of the subcutaneous tissue

ing a lateral release. Procedures in which the synovium is breached should therefore be planned carefully and completed as quickly as possible. The amount of fluid escaping depends on the pressure of saline within the knee and can be minimised by lowering the irrigation reservoir to reduce the hydrostatic pressure.

The subcutaneous saline is harmless and dis-appears within 12 hours of operation, but it is a minor insult to the tissues and worth avoiding for this reason alone, quite apart from the unpleasing appearance of a swollen and shapeless knee at the end of the procedure (Fig. 5.8)

References

Dandy D J 1983 Arthroscopy of the knee: some problems. Journal of the Royal Society of Medicine 76: 448–450

Dandy D J, O'Carroll P F 1982 Arthroscopic surgery of the knee. British Medical Journal 285: 1256–1258

Dick W, Glinz W, Hnche H R, Ruckstuhl J, Wruhs O, Zollinger H 1978 Complications of arthroscopy. A review of 3714 cases. Archives of Orthopaedic and Traumatic Surgery 92: 69–73

Hadied A M 1984 An unusual complication of arthroscopy: a fistula between the knee and the pre-patellar burse. Journal of Bone and Joint Surgery 66A: 624

Henderson C E, Hopson C N 1982 Pneumoscrotum as a complication of arthroscopy. Journal of Bone and Joint Surgery 64A: 1238–1239

Jackson R W 1983 Current concepts review. Arthroscopic surgery. Journal of Bone and Joint Surgery 65A: 416–419

Johnson L L, Shneider D A, Austin M D, Goodman F G, Bullock J M, De Bruin J A 1982 2% Glutaraldehyde: a disinfectant in arthroscopy and arthroscopic surgery. Journal of Bone and Joint Surgery 64A: 237–239

Lindenbaum B L 1981 Complications of knee joint arthroscopy. Clinical Orthopaedics and Related Research 160: 158

Mulhollan J S 1982 Complications and disasters. Read at Fourth International Seminar on Operative Arthroscopy, UCLA, Maui, October 1982

Rosenberg T D, Wong H C 1982 Arthroscopic surgery in a free-standing outpatient surgery centre. Orthopedic Clinics of North America 13: 277–282

6

Operations on synovium and joint capsule

Pathological synovium cannot be assessed accurately if the leg has been exsanguinated because the synovium will be unnaturally pale, but inflating the tourniquet after elevation of the leg does not have the same effect. Operations on synovium are therefore best done with the tourniquet inflated, but without exsanguination.

SYNOVIAL BIOPSY

Because synovial biopsy is the simplest arthroscopic operation, it is a good starting point for arthroscopic surgery, and can be done in several ways.

'Blind' synovial biopsy

Good specimens of synovium can be obtained with a small pair of cup or basket forceps passed along the sheath of the arthroscope (Fig. 6.1). When a representative area of synovium has been identified, the tip of the telescope is held against it, the telescope removed, biopsy forceps passed along the sheath and the specimen removed.

This technique does not allow the specimen to be taken under direct arthroscopic control, but a fair volume of high-quality tissue can be obtained. The technique is safe and uncomplicated, but only one, or at the most two, specimens should be taken from the same site, because repeated biopsy of the same area will penetrate synovium, capsule and eventually muscle and subcutaneous fat. Apart from unnecessary trauma to the soft tissues, histological reports on tissues other than synovium are embarrassing and unhelpful.

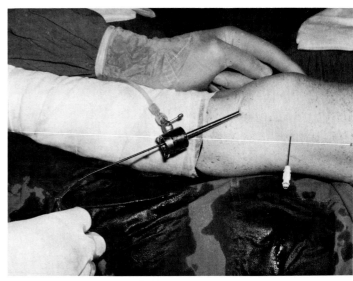

Fig. 6.1 Taking a specimen of synovium for histological study using fine forceps passed along the sheath of the arthroscope. The index of the left hand is used to apply counter pressure to introduce synovium into the jaws of the forceps

Biopsy by double puncture

Synovial specimens can also be taken with biopsy forceps or rongeurs inserted from the lateral suprapatellar approach (Fig. 5.8). The best point of insertion of the instruments is found with the irrigation needle; if the needle can reach the target easily, so will biopsy forceps inserted at the same point. The instrument should be inserted as described in Chapter 4, taking care not to damage either the patella or the arthroscope. With the knee straight, the forceps are identified through the arthroscope and the specimen taken under direct arthroscopic control (Fig. 6.2). This technique yields

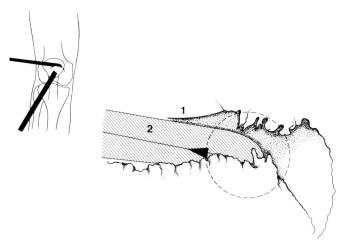

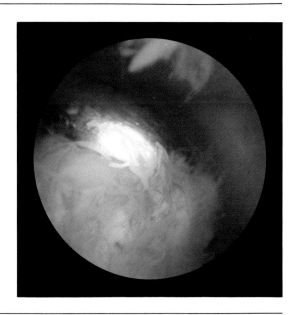

Fig. 6.2 Synovial biopsy by the double puncture technique using pituitary rongeurs (2) inserted from the lateral suprapatellar approach; under-surface of the patella (1)

the best specimens and a representative sample of tissue can be identified, but two incisions and a little expertise are required.

Biopsy using the operating arthroscope

Although an operating arthroscope makes it easy to take synovial specimens under direct vision through one incision, vision and orientation with the narrower telescope are more difficult, and the biopsy specimens, which are only 1–2 mm in diameter, may show only the histological appearances of surgical trauma. However much care is taken in the cleaning and maintenance of the biopsy forceps, specks of oil and debris can still contaminate the specimen and confuse the pathologist.

A complicated operating arthroscope is unnecessary. Biopsy forceps in place of the bridge in one of the older diagnostic arthroscopes is satisfactory for synovial biopsy under local anaesthesia (Fig. 2.9), and this may be the technique of choice for rheumatologists, who require nothing more than a good view of inflamed synovium and a decent specimen from the suprapatellar pouch.

SYNOVECTOMY

Plaques of pathological synovium can be widely excised without arthrotomy, but suitable lesions are rare. Localised areas of synovial chondromatosis or

pigmented synovitis, for example, can be removed with punch forceps or sharp dissection with scissors along the margin of the lesion, and patches of localised synovitis in the intercondylar notch can be plucked out with rongeurs. The procedure is more extensive than a biopsy, and might be described as a partial synovectomy.

Advances in the medical management of acute rheumatoid arthritis have narrowed the indications for surgical synovectomy. Patients over 40 years of age can be treated by an yttrium synovectomy, and chemical synovectomy is often successful in younger patients; if these techniques fail, synovectomy can be performed using a standard powered shaver (Fig. 6.3). These indications are more often met in younger patients with juvenile rheumatoid arthritis, Still's disease, haemophilia or pigmented synovitis than the older patient with active rheumatoid arthritis.

If a shaver is used, it should be introduced from the lateral suprapatellar route and used to remove as much exuberant synovium as possible (Highenboten 1982). As in other operations with powered instruments, a high flow rate is required, but in synovectomy this is particularly important because the outflow channel may become blocked by masses of soft synovium. In most powered instruments, the blade can be rotated in either direction and frequent changes of direction may be needed to keep the outflow channel open. If the synovium is unusually soft and friable, the whole of its thickness can be

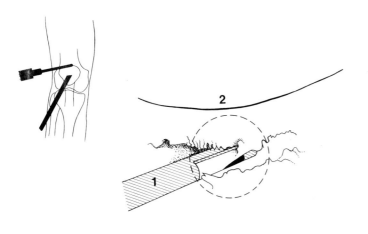

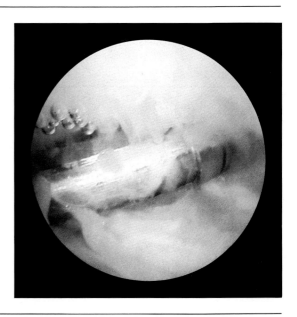

Fig. 6.3 Performing a synovectomy using the Stryker powered shaver (1); patella (2)

drawn into the sucker, leaving the fibres of the capsule exposed. This is seen particularly in conditions where the immune response is especially marked (Dandy 1984).

Although the synovium in the suprapatellar pouch is most easily reached, tissue can also be removed from the depths of the gutters, notch and posterior compartments with either powered instruments or rongeurs. Synovectomy using an electric resectoscope has also been described (Aritomi & Yamamoto 1979), but there is no evidence to suggest that it has any major advantages over other instruments.

For practical purposes, the suprapatellar pouch is the most important area for synovectomy and common sense should limit attempts to achieve a complete synovial clearance, if this would increase the surgical trauma. When a defect 1 or 2 cm in diameter is created in the synovium, the irrigating saline quickly distends the subcutaneous tissues (Fig. 5.8) whichever technique is used, and the procedure should be completed swiftly once the synovium has been breached.

Although a synovectomy performed arthroscopically may not be as complete as a synovectomy performed through a wide arthrotomy, the recovery period is so much shorter and less uncomfortable that it is greatly preferred by patients. As with other arthroscopic operations, patients can leave hospital within twenty-four hours of operation and resume normal activity in 1–2 weeks; the disability of one open synovectomy is therefore roughly the same as

five or six arthoscopic synovectomies. Rehabilitation after arthroscopic synovectomy is similar to that after any other arthroscopic surgery, but should take account of the patient's general condition and frailty.

ADHESIONS AND FIBROUS ANKYLOSIS

Arthroscopy of a knee that has undergone arthrotomy is often made difficult by fibrous adhesions between adjacent layers of synovium and articular cartilage, but the relationship of the adhesions to symptoms is not clear. Open meniscectomy, for example, is sometimes followed by adhesions between the synovium and femoral condyle, but these seldom give rise to serious problems unless they restrict flexion, even if they pucker the synovium on flexion. Adhesions are also seen between the tibial plateau and the residual rim that follows meniscectomy, and such adhesions can be broken down with a blunt hook. Although the results of dividing these isolated adhesions is unpredictable and often disappointing, the procedure is simple and is sometimes followed by remarkable relief of pain in patients with persistent pain.

Division of thicker adhesions can be rewarding in joints with limited flexion, particularly if the suprapatellar pouch has been obliterated by trauma, infection or arthrotomy (Sprague et al 1982), but arthroscopic release of adhesions does not replace physiotherapy as the mainstay of treatment for post-

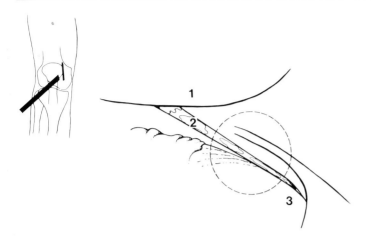

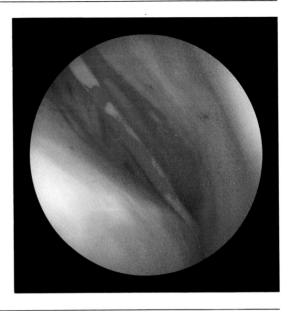

Fig. 6.4 Adhesion (2) between the medial femoral condyle (3) and the synovium of the suprapatellar pouch made tense by flexion of the knee; patella (1)

traumatic knee stiffness. Vigorous mobilisation of the knee after femoral fractures is still needed, and operation should not be considered until the fracture is soundly united and all improvement has ceased. If these requirements are met, arthroscopic division of the adhesions is indicated and stiffness of the knee becomes an indication for arthroscopy rather than a contra-indication.

Division of adhesions

Flimsy adhesions may rupture as the joint is distended with saline to produce a 'popping' sensation under the surgeon's fingers, and more may be ruptured by squeezing the irrigation reservoir. Some indication of the extent of the adhesions can be gauged by the volume of saline that the knee will hold; the normal knee will hold 60–80 ml of saline, but an ankylosed knee may take only 5–10 ml. After distension of the knee, the arthroscope should be inserted and the joint examined in the usual way, taking care not to bend the arthroscope by using it as a crow-bar. Taut isolated bands (Fig. 6.4) can be cut with scissors or avulsed with rongeurs until the arthroscope can be moved freely throughout the knee.

Release of fibrous ankylosis

If the adhesions are so dense that flexion is severely restricted and the synovial cavity is completely obliterated, insertion of the arthroscope from the antero-lateral route is often impossible. The trocar and cannula should then be inserted first from the lateral suprapatellar approach, without inflating the joint with saline, and the trocar used to rupture some of the adhesions. Although the trocar alone will not make enough space to restore flexion, it will usually create enough room to admit the arthroscope for a preliminary examination. The pouch can then be developed fully with a knife, ensuring that its tip remains in the suprapatellar pouch (Fig. 6.5). The lateral gutter is then freed, the trocar and cannula are inserted antero-laterally, and any adhesions lying in front of the femur are divided. If this does not restore movement, the medial gutter should be developed through a medial suprapatellar approach. Adhesions in the postero-medial compartment can also be broken down or divided with a knife from the postero-medial approach. Surprisingly, release of these posterior adhesions seldom results in any noticeable improvement in the range of movement, even if the symptoms are relieved.

When all accessible adhesions have been cut, the joint is irrigated thoroughly and re-examined, the tourniquet is released, and the joint is irrigated again. The improvement in the range of flexion is measured, a firm dressing is applied, and the knee is held in the position of maximum flexion with adhesive strapping, partly to prevent the contracture recurring and partly to convince the patient that the

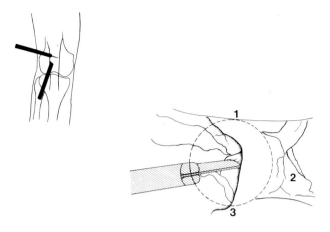

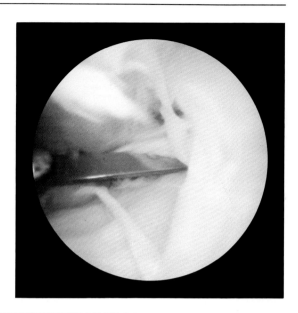

Fig. 6.5   Release of a dense fibrous ankylosis of the suprapatellar pouch using a knife inserted from the lateral suprapatellar route. Under-surface of the patella (1), dense fibrous adhesions in the suprapatellar pouch (2), anterior surface of the femur (3)

knee really will flex further than it did before operation.

An immediate improvement of about 40° is usual (Sprague et al 1982), but the improvement in symptoms is not proportional to the increase in the range of movement. It is not unknown for the patient to report a dramatic improvement in the symptoms after a disappointingly small increase in the range of flexion, but the reverse is also found. Physiotherapy should be continued as an out-patient, and may be followed by further improvement. If the contracture recurs, a second procedure is often more successful, and it is a tribute to the atraumatic nature of arthroscopic surgery that patients are willing to undergo this procedure for a second time.

SYNOVIAL SHELF EXCISION

The synovial folds of the knee are described in Chapter 13, together with the indications for shelf excision, but it is worth repeating that the medial synovial shelf lies in the coronal plane, arises in the fat-pad below the lower pole of the patella, and runs proximally for a variable distance. The medial suprapatellar plica is a quite different structure and crosses the shelf at a right angle (Fig. 2.16).

The aim of operation should be excision of a full-width segment of shelf at least 1 cm in length rather than simple division (Fig. 6.6). Division alone can

result in the development of a band of dense fibrous tissue in the place of the shelf and a recurrence of the symptoms (Fig. 6.7).

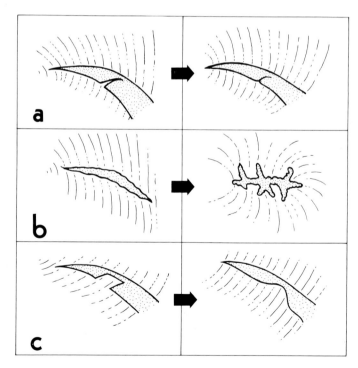

Fig. 6.6   Possible methods of excising the synovial shelf: (A) a simple cut down to the synovium can heal with a linear scar; (B) excision of a large area with the surrounding synovium can result in contracture; (C) excision of a 1 cm band does not heal or result in contracture

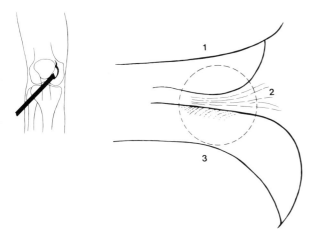

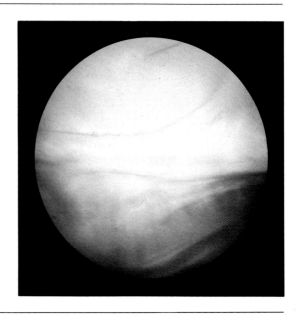

Fig. 6.7 A band of dense fibrous tissue (2) which had formed at the site of an earlier excision of the medial synovial shelf; patella (1), medial femoral condyle (3)

Excision of the shelf by the double puncture technique

The medial shelf can be excised with basket forceps from the lateral suprapatellar approach, but in some patients the shelf cannot be reached from this route, particularly if the patient has the excessive lateral pressure syndrome or just a tight patella. This difficulty can be anticipated by touching the shelf with the tip of an irrigation needle inserted from the lateral suprapatellar approach; if this can be done easily, the needle can be withdrawn and the operating instruments inserted at the same point with full confidence that the shelf can be reached. If the shelf cannot be touched with the irrigation needle, forceps will not reach it either; the operating arthroscope should be used or the arthroscope moved to the lateral suprapatellar approach and the instruments to the antero-lateral.

Excision of the shelf with the operating arthroscope

The shelf can also be excised with the operating arthroscope from the antero-lateral route (Figs. 6.8, 6.9). Two incisions are made with the scissors, at least 1 cm apart and extending into normal synovium. The irrigating saline will dissect a plane of cleavage beneath the shelf, which can then be excised neatly with scissors and basket forceps.

Alternatively, the shelf can be excised widely by applying gentle traction to its lateral edge with grasping forceps inserted from the lateral suprapatellar route, while the base is divided with the scissors of an operating arthroscope inserted from the antero-lateral route (Fig. 6.10). This technique allows the whole shelf to be excised (Fig. 6.11), but requires some expertise with the operating arthroscope.

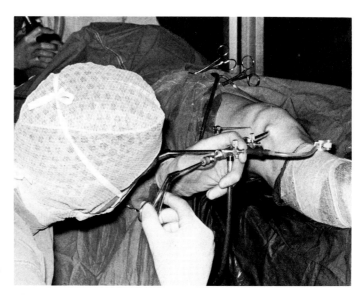

Fig. 6.8 Using the Wolf operating arthroscope to excise the medial synovial shelf

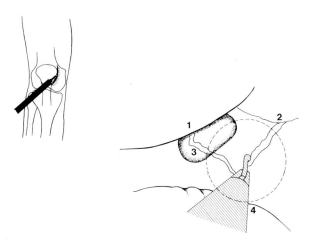

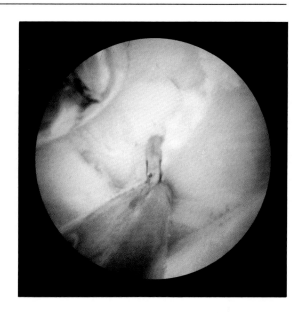

Fig. 6.9 Excision of the synovial shelf using a Wolf operating arthroscope. Patella (1), cut edge of synovium (2), air bubble (3), anterior surface of femur (4)

Aftercare

The wounds should be closed in the usual way and a firm dressing applied. As with other arthroscopic procedures, straight leg raising and flexion to 90° is usual within 24 hours of operation.

LATERAL RETINACULAR RELEASE

Of all the arthroscopic operations at present practised, arthroscopic lateral release (Fig. 4.14) prob-ably has the greatest morbidity. The aim of opera-tion is to release the vastus lateralis tendon and the lateral edge of the patella by making an incision in the capsule extending to a point 4 cm above the upper pole of the patella, including the whole of the patellar insertion of vastus lateralis (Fig. 6.12). Some believe that the synovium should be divided as well as the capsule, but there is no evidence to suggest that division of the synovium influences the quality of the clinical result. The indications for arthros-copic lateral release are described below (p. 186).

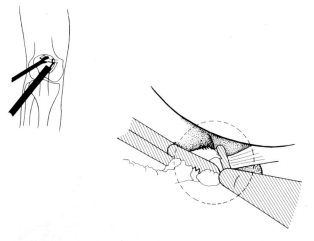

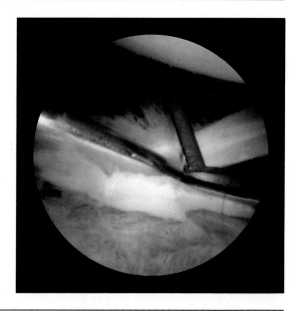

Fig. 6.10 Excising the medial synovial shelf using the scissors of the operating arthroscope, while applying traction to the shelf with tendon tunnelling forceps

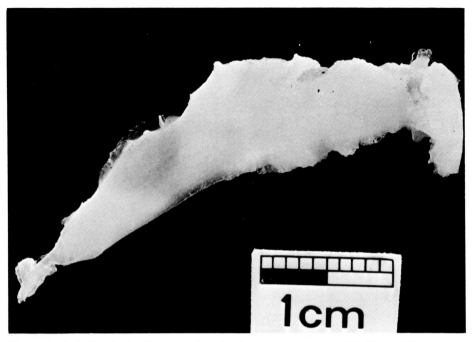

Fig. 6.11 A shelf excised arthroscopically using the technique illustrated in Figure 6.10

Technique

There are several ways to perform an arthroscopic lateral release, but whichever is used, it is advisable to infiltrate the line of capsular incision with bupivacaine 0.5% containing adrenaline to reduce

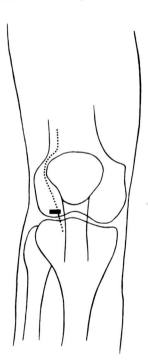

Fig. 6.12 The line of capsular incision for lateral release of the extensor mechanism

post-operative pain and minimise bleeding from the superior branch of the lateral geniculate artery.

The simplest technique is to use a Smillie meniscectomy knife or a similar blade from the antero-lateral approach (Fig. 6.13). The 'V' of the blade should be placed carefully over the cut edge of the capsule, which can then be divided as far as necessary both proximally and distally (Fig. 6.14). Special care should be taken to keep the blade as close to the edge of the patella as possible in order to minimise bleeding, and to curve the incision over the supero-lateral corner of the patella. The soft tissue is released until the patella can be tilted upwards and its under-surface felt with the thumb (Fig. 6.15). The criticism is sometimes made, quite correctly, that lateral release performed in this way is a 'blind' rather than an arthroscopic procedure. If the surgeon particularly wants to make the incision under direct vision (which is not necessary), this is possible from the antero-medial approach.

A combination of blind and arthroscopic technique has been developed by Dr R. Metcalf (1982). A pair of Metzenbaum scissors is introduced from the antero-lateral approach to develop a subcutaneous tissue plane as far as the lateral edge of the patella. A second skin incision is made over the tips of the scissors, and the subcutaneous tissue plane is extended medially in front of the patellar tendon.

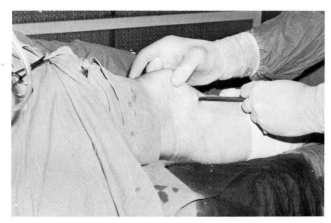

Fig. 6.13 Dividing the lateral attachments of the patella with a Smillie's knife, while stretching the tissues by tilting the patella

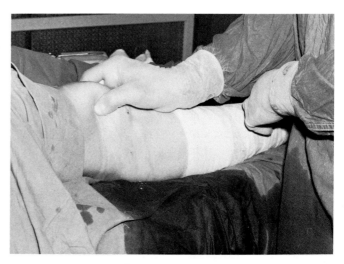

Fig. 6.15 At the conclusion of the procedure, the patella can be turned vertically, demonstrating that the tissues have been divided

The distal part of the capsule is then divided with the Metzenbaum scissors, and the proximal part with the scissors of the operating arthroscope. Saline tracks through the incision and produces a boggy swelling in the subcutaneous tissues, which is absorbed within 12 hours with either technique.

Electrocautery can be used to perform a lateral release (Miller et al 1982) (p. 24). Bleeding vessels can be coagulated under direct vision and this is said to reduce pain in the post-operative period.

Haematoma

The line of capsular incision involves more soft tissue damage than other operations and creates a wide communication between the synovial cavity and the subcutaneous tissues. If there is bleeding from either the superior lateral geniculate artery or from the vastus lateralis muscle, a large subcutaneous haematoma can form. The incidence of haematoma formation is variable, but the criteria for determining the presence of a haemarthrosis or haematoma are vague, and comparison of one series with another is difficult. Metcalf (1982) has reported only 10%, but other surgeons have found the incidence to be much higher and some have returned to open lateral release.

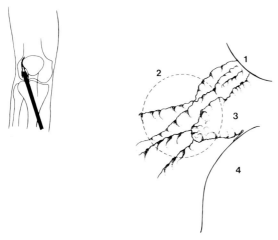

Fig. 6.14 Arthroscopic view of the line of lateral release of the synovium and capsule: patella (1), synovium (2), cut edge of capsule (3), lateral femoral condyle (4)

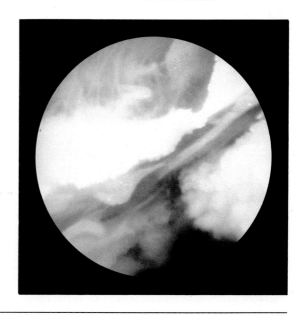

Haematoma formation can be kept to the minimum by the following measures:

1. The line of capsular incision is infiltrated with 0.5% bupivacaine (Marcain) containing added adrenaline (epinephrine), taking special care to infiltrate the region of the superior lateral geniculate artery thoroughly.
2. The capsular incision is kept as close to the patella as possible by using a curved blade closely applied to the lateral margin of the patella so that the vessels are avoided.
3. A suction drain is placed in the line of the capsular incision. If the drain is passed distally from the upper limit of the capsular incision, the holes in the drain can be tucked neatly into the capsular defect opposite the lateral superior geniculate artery.
4. A pressure dressing is applied to the line of capsular incision and the area marked with a skin pencil so that the pressure dressing can be correctly re-applied, if it should slip (Fig. 6.16).
5. In other procedures the tourniquet is released before the wounds are closed, but after a lateral release the tourniquet should not be released until the drapes have been removed, the pressure dressing has been applied, and the suction drain connected and seen working. The drain should remain in position until the following day, or longer if drainage continues, which may mean a hospital stay of two nights following operation.

Despite the precautions outlined above, problems do occur. In the author's practice, the indications for aspiration of the knee or evacuation of the haematoma are severe pain and inability to achieve a straight leg raise; patients with mild discomfort along the line of incision who are able to raise the leg fully are managed conservatively.

Aftercare

Good quadriceps function is essential after a lateral release. If the quadriceps is weak, the knee will feel insecure and unsteady when running or descending stairs, and physiotherapy is essential to maintain both good quadriceps power and the patient's confidence in the knee. The risk of haematoma, infection, persistent pain and quadriceps weakness make lateral release a less predictable operation than other arthroscopic operations, and careful supervision is vital. In particular, the patient should not be allowed to let the quadriceps wither in the immediate post-operative period by walking with crutches, rather than bearing his entire body weight on the leg.

Apart from these problems, some discomfort at the site of the capsular division is usual and tenderness at the upper limit of the capsular incision may persist for several months, but it always settles eventually.

EXCISION OF FAT-PAD

The fat-pad can be removed with rongeurs from the antero-medial route, but the jaws of the instrument lie so close to an arthroscope inserted from the antero-lateral or central approach that control is difficult. The procedure is easier if the arthroscope is transferred to the lateral suprapatellar approach, and the fat-pad removed piecemeal with a combination of straight and curved rongeurs inserted from the antero-lateral or antero-medial approach (Fig. 6.17). The powered shaver can also be used.

A powered shaver is used by some to remove the fat-pad when it obscures the arthroscopic view, but the removal of healthy tissue simply because it makes life difficult for the surgeon is not in keeping with the atraumatic spirit of arthroscopic surgery. If the surgeon cannot see everything he wishes down the arthroscope, he should concentrate on improving his technique rather than disguise his deficiencies by taking a powered tool to normal tissue.

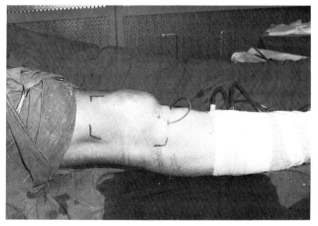

Fig. 6.16 A suction drain is placed in the line of capsular incision and the area for the pressure dressing marked in case the dressing should slip

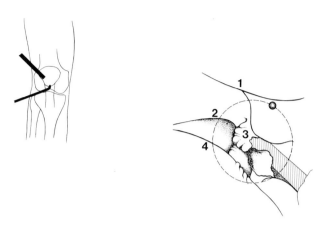

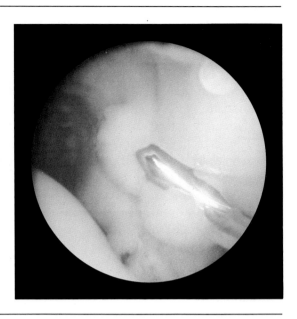

Fig. 6.17 Removing a hypertrophic fat-pad (3) with instruments inserted from the antero-lateral route and seen from the lateral suprapatellar approach; patella (1), medial synovial shelf (2), femur (4)

LIPOMATA AND SYNOVIOMATA

The arthroscopic appearances of pedunculated lipomata causing symptoms very similar to those of a torn meniscus or a loose body were first described by Burman & Mayer in 1936. These tumours can be removed neatly by avulsing them with a pair of pituitary rongeurs applied to their base (Fig. 6.18) leaving a small defect in the synovium (Fig. 6.19).

If the pedicle cannot be identified precisely, which is a problem if the tumour is particularly large, a short incision can be made over the tumour so that it can be lifted out of the knee and divided at its base under direct vision. Histological study of these lesions usually shows them to be either a lipoma or a benign synovioma.

GANGLIA

Ganglia in the intercondylar notch are easy to remove. Pedunculated ganglia can be avulsed and

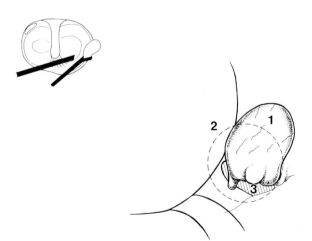

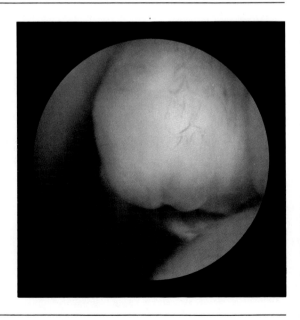

Fig. 6.18 A pedunculated benign synovioma (1) in the medial gutter grasped at its base with curved rongeurs (3); medial femoral condyle (2)

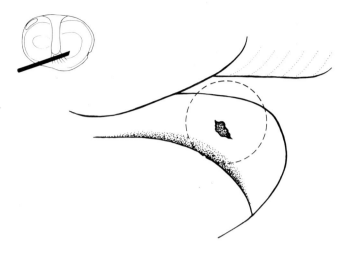
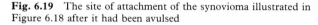

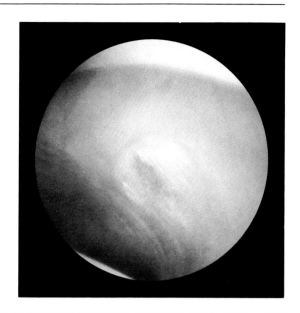

Fig. 6.19 The site of attachment of the synovioma illustrated in Figure 6.18 after it had been avulsed

sessile ganglia removed by incising the synovium around the edge of the lesion with a sharp knife and excising the ganglion with the overlying synovium, taking care to preserve the anterior cruciate ligament. Ganglia are also seen around the posterior horns of the menisci and in the stubs of ruptured ligaments (Fig. 6.20) (Dandy 1984), and can be avulsed.

CRYSTAL SYNOVITIS

Although irrigation of the joint can scarcely be considered an arthroscopic operation, the pain and effusion of crystal-induced synovitis (Fig. 6.21) is almost always relieved dramatically by simple joint irrigation and such relief can last for more than a year (O'Connor 1973). Not all calcification in the

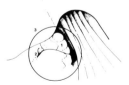

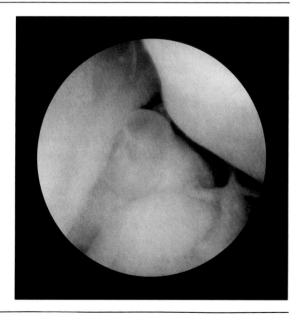

Fig. 6.20 A cluster of ganglia (1) at the posterior attachment of the lateral meniscus (2) beneath the lateral condyle (3)

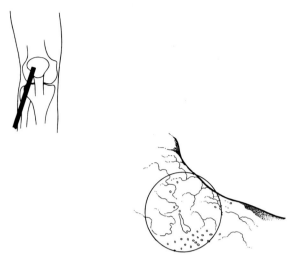
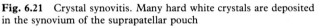
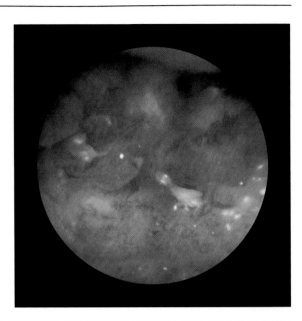

Fig. 6.21 Crystal synovitis. Many hard white crystals are deposited in the synovium of the suprapatellar pouch

knee can be regarded as crystal synovitis (Altman 1976), but the symptoms of other types of synovitis, including that of osteoarthritis, may nevertheless be relieved by irrigation (Burman et al 1934). It is not known whether this relief of pain is due to the removal of abnormal synovial fluid and joint debris, lavage of the synovium, temporary hypothermia of the synovium from irrigation with cold saline, or to some metabolic alteration induced by contact with irrigation fluid. The fact that we cannot explain the mechanism of this pain relief is taken by some as proof that it does not exist and by others as proof of our ignorance.

SEPTIC ARTHRITIS

Septic arthritis is commonly managed by thorough irrigation and joint lavage. The irrigation can be accompanied by arthroscopy, but apart from assessing the state of the articular surfaces and the synovium, diagnostic arthroscopy alone has little to offer in the management of septic arthritis. If septic arthritis is to be managed arthroscopically, it must not be done half-heartedly. The joint should be irrigated thoroughly until the effluent fluid is clear, which may take two or three litres of saline, and adhesions should be broken down to open up loculi and pockets of infection (Jarrett et al 1981). At the conclusion of the procedure, the joint should be filled with an antibiotic solution, and an intermittent drainage system set up. Alternatively, a continuous suction/drainage system can be set up (Mason 1984), but it is probably better to keep the joint distended rather than allow it to deflate by applying suction.

HAEMOPHILIA

Arthroscopy is helpful in the management of haemophilia at two stages. First, the blood can be aspirated more thoroughly than with an aspirating needle, which minimises synovial irritation (Guttmann & Handal 1982). Second, if synovectomy is required, it can be done arthroscopically. Haemophiliac synovium is dark in colour, and the subsynovial layers are fibrotic (Dandy 1984).

References

Altman D 1976 Arthroscopic findings of the knee in patients with pseudogout. Arthritis and Rheumatism 19: 286–292
Aritomi H, Yamamoto M 1979 A method of arthroscopic surgery. Clinical evaluation of synovectomy with the electric resectoscope and removal of loose bodies in the knee joint. Orthopedic Clinics of North America 10: 565–584
Burman M S, Mayer L 1936 Arthroscopic examination of the knee joint. Archives of Surgery 32: 846–874
Burman M S, Finkelstein H, Mayer L 1934 Arthroscopy of the knee joint. Journal of Bone and Joint Surgery 16: 255–268
Dandy D J 1984 Arthroscopy of the knee: a diagnostic atlas. Gower–Butterworth, London
Guttmann G G, Handal J 1982 Arthroscopy in the management of haemophiliac haemarthrosis. Orthopaedic Review 11: 105–107
Highenboten C L 1982 Arthroscopic synovectomy. Orthopedic Clinics of North America 13: 399–405

Jarrett M P, Grossman L, Sadler A H, Grayzel A I 1981 The role of arthroscopy in the treatment of septic arthritis. Arthritis and Rheumatism 24: 737–739

Mason L 1984 Arthroscopic management of the infected knee. In: Grana W A (ed) Update in arthroscopic techniques, pp. 66–67. Edward Arnold, London

Metcalf R W 1982 An arthroscopic method for lateral release of the subluxating and dislocating patella. Clinical Orthopaedics and Related Research 167: 11–18

Miller G K, Dickason J M, Fox J M et al 1982 The use of electrosurgery for arthroscopic subcutaneous lateral release. Orthopaedics 5: 309–314

O'Connor R L 1973 The arthroscope in the management of crystal-induced synovitis of the knee. Journal of Bone and Joint Surgery 55A: 1443–1449

Sprague N F, O'Connor R L, Fox J M 1982 Arthroscopic treatment of post-operative knee fibrarthrosis. Orthopedic Clinics of North America 13: 399–405

7

Loose bodies

Loose bodies are the 'banana-skins' of arthroscopic surgery. Even quite large loose bodies can be difficult to find and the difficulty of removing them should never be underestimated. Furthermore, it is not uncommon to remove one loose body only to find that the post-operative radiograph shows that another remains, usually because the first loose body was transradiant. Transradiant loose bodies are not unusual; in one study (Dandy & O'Carroll 1982), 24% of loose bodies more than 1 cm in diameter were transradiant.

Most loose bodies are recognised from the clinical history, examination and radiographs, but arthroscopy is useful in determining the true size of partly calcified loose bodies, finding uncalcified loose bodies and identifying the site from which they arose. The patella and femoral condyles often have a defect that corresponds with the loose body, and experience of arthroscopy leads to the conclusion that osteochondral fractures are more common than is generally believed, whereas idiopathic loose bodies and 'osteochondritis dissecans' are less common. Arthroscopy is also helpful in assessing those isolated areas of calcification along the joint margins and in the intercondylar notch, often reported by radiologists as 'loose' bodies, which are in fact osteophytes.

The arthroscopic removal of loose bodies has three stages:

1. finding the loose body
2. catching the loose body
3. removing the loose body

FINDING THE LOOSE BODY

Because the entire joint can be examined arthroscopically and the loose body chased from one compartment to another, loose bodies are more easily found at arthroscopy than arthrotomy. A plain radiograph before operation is helpful, but does not exclude the possibility of the loose body moving when the limb is draped.

The suprapatellar pouch is the first place to look, and usually the most rewarding. Table 7.1 shows the

Table 7.1 Site of loose bodies (after Dandy & O'Carroll 1982)

Site	Number of cases	Percentage
Suprapatellar pouch	32	36
Intercondylar notch	22	25
Postero-medial compartment	9	10
Medial gutter	9	10
Medial compartment	4	5
Lateral gutter	4	5
Lateral compartment	3	3
Postero-lateral compartment	2	2
Under lateral meniscus	2	2

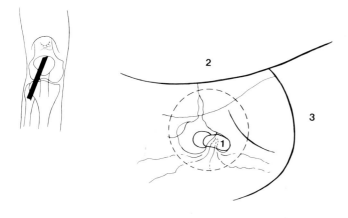

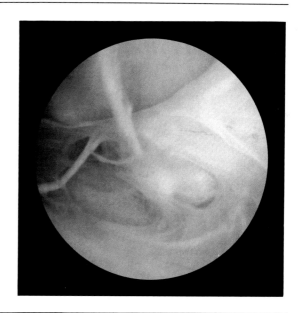

Fig. 7.1 Three loose bodies (1) concealed behind a fold of synovium at the apex of the suprapatellar pouch, above the medial suprapatellar plica (3); under-surface of the patella (2)

site in which loose bodies were found in one series (Dandy & O'Carroll 1982). A large medial suprapatellar plica can conceal the loose body and the space beyond it should be examined carefully (Fig. 7.1). While examining the suprapatellar pouch, the under-surface of the patella should be examined for defects.

Because loose bodies sink in saline, any in the suprapatellar pouch will fall into the medial or lateral gutter when the knee is flexed and can then slip into one of the posterior compartments, from which retrieval is difficult. The possibility of a loose body lying in one of the gutters should therefore be excluded before the knee is flexed. The recess

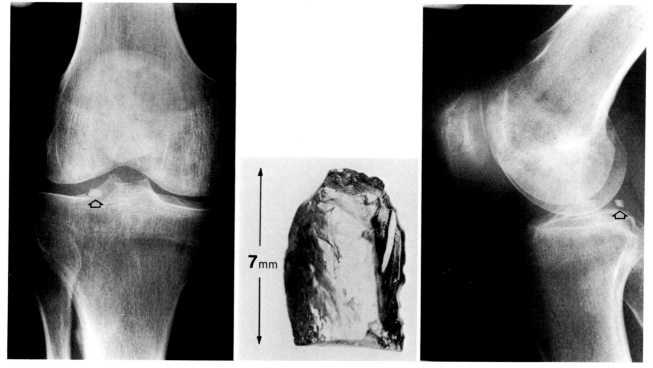

Fig. 7.2 A fragment of glass which had entered the knee anteriorly and come to rest beneath the posterior horn of the lateral meniscus. The fragment, shown in the centre, is clearly seen on both the anterior and lateral radiographs

proximal to the fold of synovium in the lateral gutter can also hide quite large loose bodies and should be examined carefully before the knee is flexed, as should the entrance to the tunnel for the popliteus tendon, a favourite refuge for smaller loose bodies. If both gutters are clear, the knee can be flexed and the rest of the joint examined; if, however, a loose body is present in either gutter, palpation through the skin from below upwards will push it back up into the pouch.

Special problems are found in the intercondylar notch. Large loose bodies may become jammed and obstruct the arthroscope, while small flat ones can skate away to the lateral compartment or, worse, the postero-medial compartment. Care must therefore be taken not to nudge a loose body into the posterior compartments with the tip of the telescope. There is little room to hide in the lateral compartment but loose bodies, and sometimes foreign bodies, can slip beneath the posterior third of the meniscus (Figs. 7.2, 7.3).

The postero-medial and postero-lateral compartments should be examined next with 30° or 70° telescopes, as described in Chapter 4, but if the postero-medial compartment cannot be entered through the notch and the loose body has still not been found, a postero-medial insertion is advisable. If the loose body is not in the postero-medial compartment, the lateral suprapatellar insertion can be used again to examine the pouch and popliteus

tunnel more closely and the routine examination repeated.

If this routine has been followed correctly without finding a loose body, the lateral suprapatellar incision can be enlarged and one sterile finger cautiously inserted into the suprapatellar pouch to search for any recesses that might have escaped notice. However carefully the suprapatellar pouch is examined, there is always the possibility of an anomalous pouch of synovium large enough to conceal a loose body. If palpation with a sterile finger is unsuccessful, there is no alternative but to seek the help of the radiologist.

CATCHING THE LOOSE BODY

When the loose body has been found, it must be held still, grasped and removed. This is simple in theory, but more difficult in practice, because of the ease with which loose bodies can escape.

As soon as a loose body is sighted, the 'loose body procedure' should be put into operation. The first step is to switch off the irrigation and hold the leg completely still so that the loose body sinks to the bottom of the compartment in which it lies. Loose bodies in the suprapatellar pouch can be held there by blocking the medial and lateral gutters with thumb and forefinger (Fig. 7.4), and those in the notch remain stationary unless disturbed by the jet

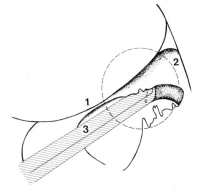
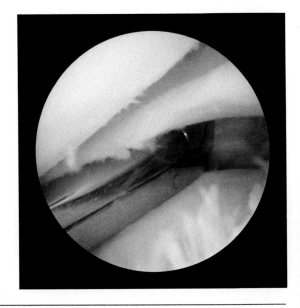

Fig. 7.3 Small angled rongeurs (3) passed beneath the posterior horn of the lateral meniscus (2) and seen from the antero-medial approach; lateral femoral condyle (1)

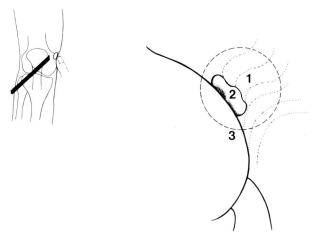

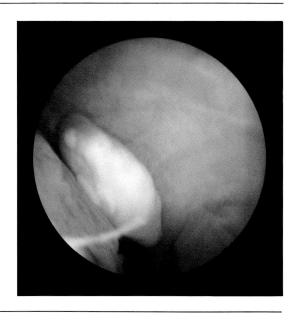

Fig. 7.4 A loose body (2) is prevented from slipping from the suprapatellar pouch into the medial gutter by external finger pressure applied to the medial wall of the knee (1); medial femoral condyle (3)

of irrigation fluid, the tip of the arthroscope or another instrument. If the loose body lies in a gutter, it can be pushed back up into the pouch or transfixed with a percutaneous needle, but the needle must be put into soft tissue rather than bone. The leg should be held still while plans are made for removing the loose body, even when it seems to be securely transfixed (Fig. 7.5).

REMOVING THE LOOSE BODY

The technique for removing loose bodies depends on their site, size and number. As a general rule, the smallest should be removed first to defer the largest incision until last and thus minimise the loss of saline from the knee, but large loose bodies obscure vision and this policy is hard to follow (Fig. 7.6).

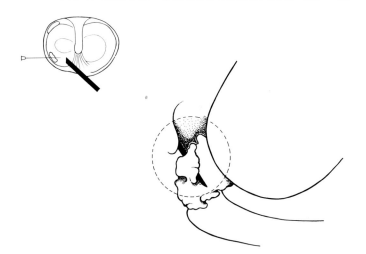

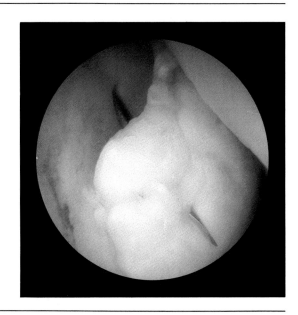

Fig. 7.5 An osteochondral fragment lying in the lateral gutter and transfixed with a percutaneous needle

Small loose bodies can be washed up the instrument cannula by placing the tip of the arthroscope against them and withdrawing the telescope so that they are swept along the cannula with the escaping fluid. For a larger loose body, the surest method is to catch it in the suprapatellar pouch, lock a pair of grasping forceps fairly and squarely across its middle (Fig. 7.7), and pull it out through a short skin incision. If no special arthroscopic grasping forceps are available, small Kocher's forceps can be used, but the hinge must be placed at the level of the incision or the jaws will not open. As the loose body is withdrawn, it will tent the capsule and skin, which can be cut carefully with a small No. 15 blade in the manner of an episiotomy. The loose body should be held firmly between the jaws of the forceps so that it does not slip away or break into several smaller fragments, but if this does happen, the resulting crumbs of bone must be removed one by one.

Straight grasping forceps will only grasp bodies lying in the middle of the pouch, and those lying in the gutters can be tantalisingly out of reach. Bouncing the loose bodies out of the gutter into the pouch by external pressure will usually bring them within range of the forceps, but there are times when only curved instruments will be successful. Curved rongeurs or artery forceps are suitable.

If the loose body is in the notch, it can either be nudged into the pouch or removed from the notch itself. Moving the loose body from the notch to the pouch runs the risk of allowing it to escape into the postero-medial compartment, and the decision to play the ball as it lies or move it to a better spot depends very much on the surgeon's familiarity with the postero-medial approach. If the decision is made to remove the loose body from the notch, the usual problems of operating in the notch can be expected. Structures lie so close to the lens that they are difficult to assess, the fat-pad is everywhere, and the operating instruments lie uncomfortably close to the tip of the instrument. To make matters worse, the capsular and subcutaneous tissues are thicker in this area than in the lateral suprapatellar region, making it easy to lose the loose body in the subcutaneous fat. If this occurs, the loose body will never be found with the arthroscope, because it lies outside the knee. When the surgical team has re-scrubbed, re-gowned and the leg has been re-prepared and re-draped, the loose body will be found lying in the subcutaneous tissues to the delight of the nurses and the embarrassment of the surgeon.

Loose bodies are more difficult to remove from the postero-medial compartment than elsewhere and the average loose body will be able to elude the

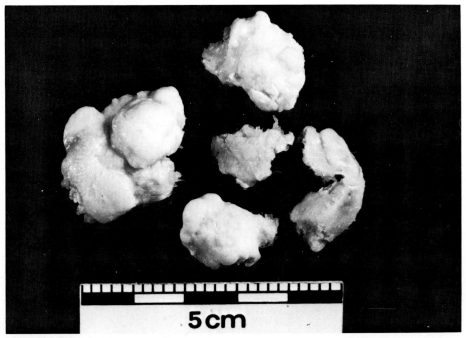

Fig. 7.6   Multiple loose bodies of differing sizes

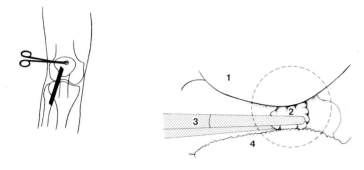

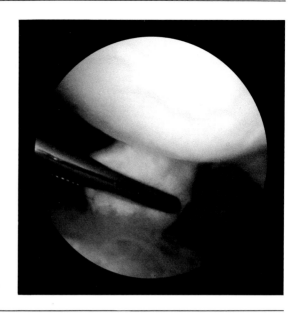

Fig. 7.7 A loose body (2) is grasped in Kocher's forceps (3) inserted from the lateral suprapatellar route; patella (1), anterior surface of the femur (4)

inexperienced surgeon and escape there without difficulty, making an arthrotomy unavoidable, unless the postero-medial approach is used. At operation, the postero-medial compartment is the most dependent part of the knee, making it very difficult for a loose body to move elsewhere. The compartment is small, with a well-defined inferior recess where loose bodies settle predictably; this can actually make it easier to remove the loose body from the postero-medial compartment than anywhere else, provided

always that the surgeon is familiar with the postero-medial insertion (Fig. 7.8).

If the arthroscope cannot be passed through the intercondylar notch and the loose body is found only after a postero-medial insertion, it can either be removed 'blind' by passing grasping forceps through a short incision or by making a second postero-medial incision for the grasping forceps just beside the arthroscope.

If the outer edge of the foot is rested on the table

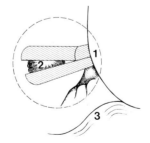

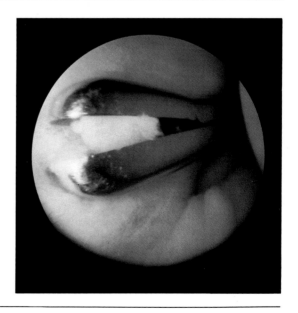

Fig. 7.8 A loose body grasped with pituitary rongeurs inserted from the postero-medial approach and seen from the antero-lateral approach: medial femoral condyle (1), loose body (2), medial meniscus (3)

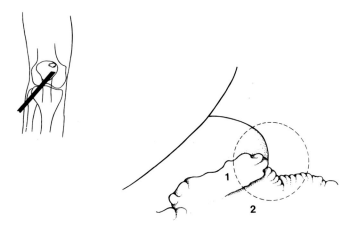

Fig. 7.9 A 'loose body' (1) which proved to be firmly adherent to the synovium (2) overlying the anterior surface of the medial femoral condyle (see Fig. 7.10)

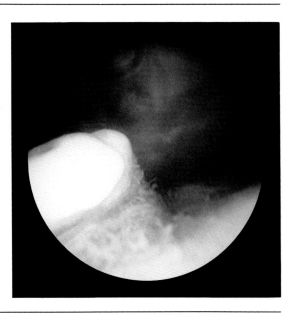

during examination of the lateral compartment (Fig. 4.23), the postero-lateral compartment becomes the most dependent part of the knee and loose bodies will gravitate there instead of the postero-medial compartment. Loose bodies often drop into the postero-lateral compartment when this technique is used, but can sometimes be moved to an easier area of the joint by manipulation with a hook or a jet of saline. If this is not possible, a postero-lateral insertion will be needed. Loose bodies that lie beneath the lateral meniscus can be removed with

small angled rongeurs inserted from the antero-lateral route, and those in the popliteus tunnel can be removed with rongeurs from the lateral suprapatellar approach.

RE-EXAMINATION AND WOUND CLOSURE

When the loose body has been withdrawn, the joint should be searched again to be sure that no more loose bodies are left behind and all articular surfaces, including the classical birthplace of osteochondritic fragments on the medial condyle, should be examined for defects that might indicate the site of origin. The tourniquet can then be released, the joint irrigated and the wounds closed in the usual way.

PEDUNCULATED LOOSE BODIES

'Loose bodies' are sometimes attached to the synovium either by fibrous adhesions (Fig. 7.9) or, in the case of osteochondral fractures, by a strip of soft tissue at the margin of the fracture. Because the pedicle must be divided first, tethered loose bodies are often more difficult to remove than those which are completely loose. Attempts to avulse the loose body usually fail, because the bone is so soft that it will break into fragments rather than tear its soft tissue attachment (Fig. 7.10), but if it does break

Fig. 7.10 The loose body shown in Figure 7.9, which was broken in an attempt to avulse it before it had been completely mobilised

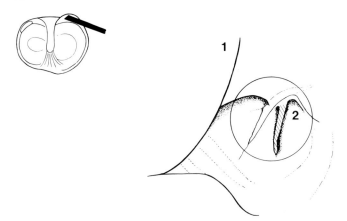

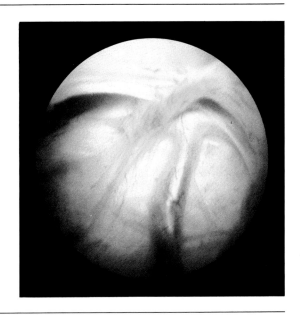

Fig. 7.11 The tip of a needle, which came to rest beneath the synovium of the posterior capsule (2), is seen from the postero-medial approach; medial femoral condyle (1)

away, any bone still adherent to the synovium must be picked off with pituitary rongeurs.

The stalk of a pedunculated fragment can be cut with scissors or a knife, but 'loose' bodies bound to synovium by fibrous adhesions must be mobilised with scissors or knife and removed in the usual way. Fortunately, most of these attached loose bodies lie in the suprapatellar pouch and do not need removing, but some interfere with joint movement or cause pain.

FOREIGN BODIES

Most foreign bodies provoke a soft tissue reaction that tethers them to the joint wall (Fig. 7.11) with fibrous tissue which must be divided before the foreign body can be removed. If the foreign body is of a firm and smooth material such as steel or glass, the fibrous covering needs to be cut at only one edge and the foreign body slipped out of its pocket; pieces

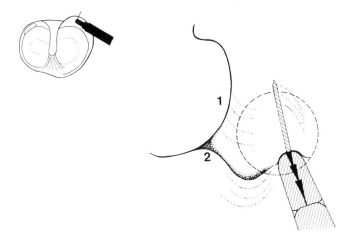

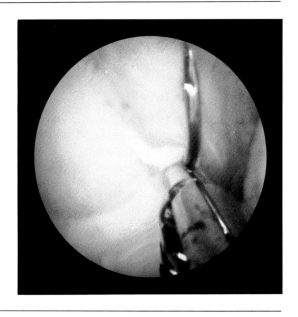

Fig. 7.12 The fragment of needle shown in Figure 7.11 is grasped in the forceps of the Wolf operating arthroscope inserted from the postero-medial approach; medial femoral condyle (1), posterior edge of medial meniscus (2)

of wood and fibrous material, however, are more tedious and usually need to be avulsed.

Arthroscopic instruments are designed to grasp soft tissue rather than metal or glass (Fig. 7.12), and the foreign body can easily slip out of the jaws as it is being pulled through the subcutaneous tissues. Apart from making a large enough hole in the subcutaneous tissue and synovium to accommodate the foreign body, and taking a firm grip, there is no easy solution to this problem.

Broken instruments (McGinty 1982) and internal fixation devices present a slightly different problem. Fragments of instruments are often large, and have not had time to become adherent to the joint lining. The basic rule should be to freeze, switch off the irrigation fluid, and think before doing anything. The greatest error that can be made is to poke hopefully at the fragment with a hook; this can only drive the fragment into a corner, from which it may be irretrievable. Magnetic retrievers (p. 22) (Fig. 2.42) are available, but will only attract ferrous metals. Even this is no guarantee of success, because some instruments are made of non-magnetic steel.

Internal fixation devices can also be removed arthroscopically. Screws are easier to remove than pins, and staples are even simpler. Staples can be withdrawn from the bone with a bone spike from almost any angle, but screws need to be approached perpendicularly with a screwdriver. The ideal point of insertion of the screwdriver can be found with a needle, and it must be exact. Self-retaining screwdrivers are attractive, but bulky, and it is often better to convert the screw to a loose body and remove it as such, if possible with a magnet.

References

Dandy D J, O'Carroll P F 1982 The removal of loose bodies from the knee under arthroscopic control. Journal of Bone and Joint Surgery 64B: 473–476

McGinty J B 1982 Arthroscopic removal of loose bodies. Orthopedic Clinics of North America 13: 313–328

8

Operations on bone and articular cartilage

OSTEOCHONDRITIS DISSECANS

The cause, pathology and progress of osteochondritis dissecans is controversial. Many localised disorders of bone, including subchondral bone necrosis and osteochondral fractures, are often erroneously included under the heading of osteochondritis dissecans, perhaps because the radiological appearances are similar (Aichroth 1971). For the arthroscopist, this is confusing because the arthroscopic appearances are so distinct that arthroscopy makes it easy to separate one condition from another.

As the name implies, osteochondritis dissecans is a chronic dissecting process quite different from an acute osteochondral fracture. Nobody has expressed this more clearly than Paget (1870):

> But how can such pieces of articular cartilage be detached from bone? The question has been asked in many similar cases. They cannot be chipped off; no force can do this; and they are not like the fragments of condyle which are sometimes, in violent fractures, broken off the femur or left pendulous in the joint.

The gradual dissection and separation of a fragment of bone from the medial wall of the intercondylar notch is quite different from an acute osteochondral fracture, which is usually caused by a single injury, is often accompanied by a haemarthrosis, and seldom involves the intercondylar notch. As the 'dissection' of osteochondritis dissecans proceeds (Figs. 8.1, 8.2), a block of bone gradually separates and causes pain and discomfort, which is most marked when the knee

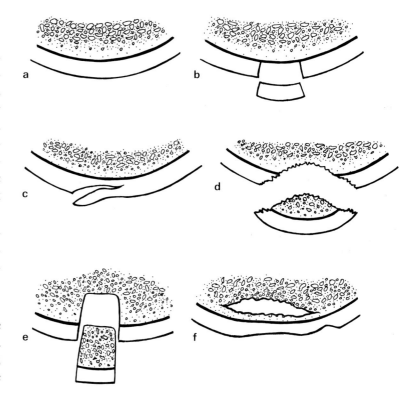

Fig. 8.1 Different lesions of articular surface: (A) normal; (B) chondral separation; (C) chondral flap; (D) osteochondral fracture; (E) osteochondritis dissecans; (F) spontaneous osteonecrosis

is extended and the tibia rotated internally so that the patient walks with the foot externally rotated – Wilson's sign (Wilson 1967). Later, the block becomes a loose body and the surfaces of both the fragment and its crater quickly acquire a cartilaginous covering that makes it impossible to replace the fragment precisely.

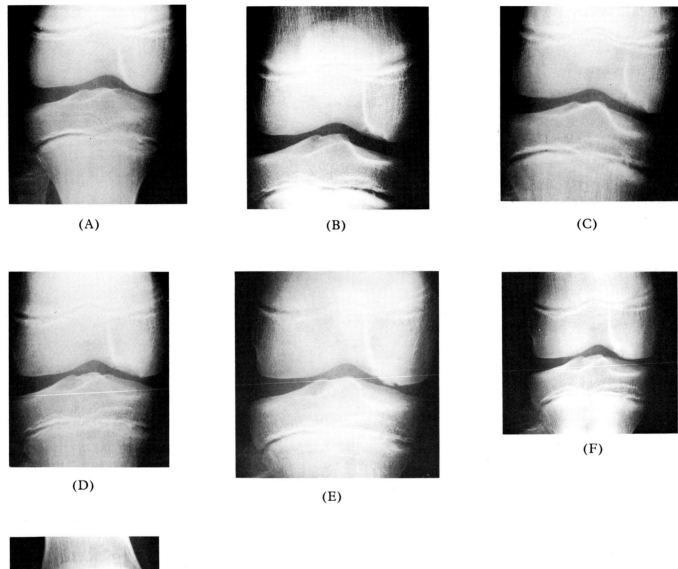

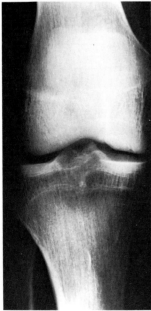

Fig. 8.2 Osteochondritis dissecans. (A) Radiograph of a 12-year-old boy with pain in the knee. There is a very slight irregularity of the medial femoral condyle. (B) The pain persisted and six months later the appearances were typical of early osteochondritis dissecans. (C) Aged 13, one year after the initial presentation, the pain persisted and the lesion had progressed. The decision was made to drill the lesion. (D) Two months later, the drill holes can be seen in the condyle. (E) Six months after drilling, the fragment is united and there are signs of healing. (F) Two years after drilling, the plane of separation between the fragment and condyle is no longer visible. (G) A different patient, showing an un-united osteochondritic fragment in a mature skeleton

Osteochondritis dissecans can present in three ways:

1. intact articular cartilage
2. broken articular cartilage
3. complete separation.

Intact articular cartilage

Perhaps the commonest presentation is the child aged between 10 and 13 years, with pain and a classical lesion on the lateral side of the medial femoral condyle. Although the radiograph may suggest that the fragment is loose, at arthroscopy the articular surface overlying the fragment is usually intact. Gentle probing or stroking with a hook will find the lesion, which is felt as a hard area surrounded by a moat of softened cartilage. As the hook is drawn over the surface of the condyle, a distinct depression is felt as its tip passes over the bony defect and the hook may leave a small dent in the articular surface, a little like a finger-mark on pitting oedema. Dimming the light source by turning down the voltage with the control knob, or more simply by loosening the attachments of the light cable to the arthroscope, is also helpful and will often show up irregularities in the joint surface that were not previously apparent.

The natural history of these lesions is unknown, although Aichroth (1971) found that 25% of them developed into loose bodies, if left untreated. If we knew that all such lesions healed spontaneously, there would be no need to treat them. On the other hand, if we knew that each lesion progressed to a loose body, it would be better to prevent detachment of the fragment by screwing or pinning in every patient. Simple drilling of the lesion carries little morbidity, and is probably advisable in the hope that bone bridges will form along the pin tracks and secure the fragment to the femur.

The technique of drilling is simple. Once identified with the probing hook, the correct point of insertion is selected with a needle and five or six holes are drilled through intact articular cartilage with a 1.5 mm Kirschner wire. As the drill crosses the space between the fragment and the bone, a distinct 'jump' is felt. The post-operative care does not differ from that required for an open drilling of bone, except that the patient can leave hospital within 24 hours of operation. Early mobilisation is important, but the role of early weight-bearing is unclear.

Broken articular surface

Patients also present when the articular surface is broken and the bone block has begun to separate. The fragment can then be reattached, provided that it has not separated completely as a loose body, using a threaded wire passed through the fragment and femoral condyle to leave the femur on its medial side (Guhl 1979, 1982). The pin is screwed into the condyle so that it lies just below the articular cartilage and is not visible on the articular surface. Alternatively, ordinary Kirschner wires can be used.

Once in position, the pin protruding from the medial side of the femur is cut to length. If the pin is left long, it will be easier to remove at a later date but will cause pain and tenderness when the knee is flexed. If the pin is cut flush with bone, removal will be difficult. It is usual practice to immobilise knees for 6–8 weeks after pinning, but the effects of immobilisation on the nutrition of joint cartilage may outweigh the advantages of fixation, and no harm seems to arise from early mobilisation and weight bearing of joints following this procedure.

Arthroscopic screwing is also possible. With a percutaneous needle, the point at which the drill or pin can be inserted at right angles to the bone surface is selected carefully, and an initial hole is made with a 1.5 mm Kirschner wire. The hole is then enlarged to take either a small ASIF cancellous screw or a Herbert double-pitched screw.

Complete separation

Sadly, patients with fragments suitable for reattachment are less common than those who present in early adult life with a loose body. Once separated from its bed, the loose body grows by accretion, the crater begins to fill, and accurate reposition quickly becomes impossible. Although it is perfectly possible to screw such fragments back into their bed and even insert bone grafts under arthroscopic control (Guhl 1982), these procedures must be followed by a period of plaster immobilisation of several weeks. The great advantage of arthroscopic surgery is early mobilisation, and there is no point in performing a procedure arthroscopically unless it either enables the knee to be mobilised more quickly or makes it possible for the procedure to be completed more precisely and effectively than by other means. Neither of these conditions applies to the screwing and grafting of old osteochondritis dissecans lesions, and simple removal of the loose body is probably the treatment of choice.

OSTEOCHONDRAL FRACTURES

Osteochondral fragments in which subchondral bone has broken away with the overlying cartilage (Fig. 8.1) in a single traumatic episode are easily recognisable on a plain radiograph, yet often pass unnoticed until they present as loose bodies (Matthewson & Dandy 1978) (Fig. 8.3). The fragment can be reattached if the lesion is recognised within two weeks of injury, but after this the cancellous bed will have begun to fill and the fragment to remodel so

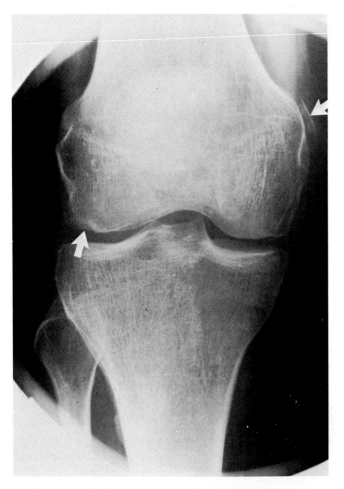

Fig. 8.3 An undiagnosed osteochondral fracture (marked). The fragment arose from the point marked on the lateral femoral condyle

that exact reposition is impossible. If the decision is made to reattach the fragment of articular cartilage, it is sensible to remove it arthroscopically in order to check that the procedure is technically possible before opening the joint. Some fragments have only a thin flake of bone and such a large flap of unsupported articular cartilage that accurate reposition may be impossible; in this instance early mobilisation of the joint would be the treatment of choice.

Arthroscopic reattachment of the fragment is technically possible, but unless the procedure allows either more accurate reposition or more rapid rehabilitation, it is not indicated. To struggle for several hours to achieve imperfect reposition of the fragment, when it can be replaced precisely in a fraction of the time through a short arthrotomy is silly, particularly if the knee is to be immobilised in a cast after either technique. At some stage, equipment may become available to reattach these fragments precisely and quickly without arthrotomy, but none is yet available.

The screws and pins used for fixation of osteochondral fragments can be removed arthroscopically (p. 94).

CHONDRAL SEPARATIONS

Full-thickness lesions with complete separation of articular cartilage (Figs. 8.1, 8.4) from the underlying bone cause similar symptoms to those of a torn meniscus (Johnson-Nurse & Dandy 1985). The lesions usually result from a sharp twisting injury under load, and the patient will often be aware of a tearing sensation in the knee, followed by an effusion. The chondral fragment will either remain intact as a loose body or become ground into small cartilage fragments within the joint, in which case the effusion will persist until all the fragments have been absorbed. In practical terms, the patient will present with an apparently classical meniscal tear, but after three or four weeks the effusion and other symptoms may well have disappeared and the diagnosis can then only be confirmed by arthroscopy.

At arthroscopy, the bed of subchondral bone will be visible, perhaps covered by a thin layer of fibrous tissue. If the lesion is fresh, healing can be encouraged by drilling (Fig. 8.5) or abrasion of the

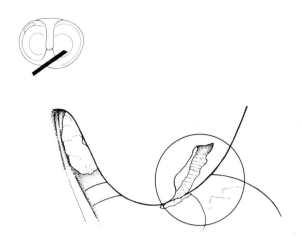

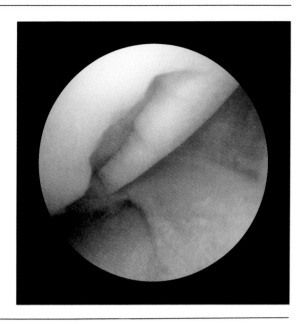

Fig. 8.4 A chondral separation of the medial femoral condyle. The lesion has steep sides and there is exposed subchondral bone at its base

underlying bone, but no firm evidence is yet available to establish the indications for either of these procedures. At present, it would seem sensible to drill articular cartilage lesions up to 1 cm in width (using the technique described on p. 104), provided that the surrounding articular cartilage is normal.

CHONDRAL FLAPS

Partial-thickness flaps of articular cartilage (Figs. 8.1, 8.6–8.8) can cause symptoms similar to those of a torn meniscus (Johnson-Nurse & Dandy 1985) and may be seen on either condyle, the patella or the intercondylar groove where it articulates with the patella. The characteristic features of a chondral flap are catching on flexion and extension of the knee without true locking, but the lesions are so rare that it is unwise to make the diagnosis on clinical grounds alone. The area of articular cartilage separation is seldom more than 1 or 2 mm in depth, and light debridement of these lesions will relieve symptoms. The lesions are seen on the patella, when they can cause 'locking' in extension, or the femoral condyles,

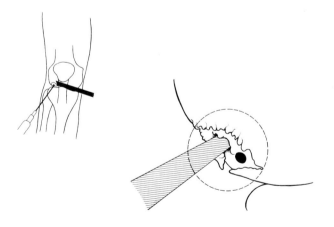

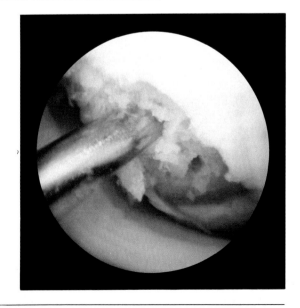

Fig. 8.5 Drilling the subchondral bed of a full-thickness chondral fracture of the lateral femoral condyle with a thick Kirschner wire

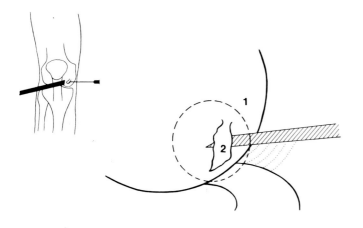
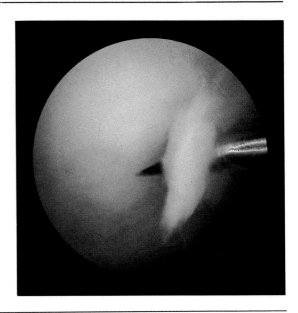

Fig. 8.6 A flap of articular cartilage (2) raised from the medial femoral condyle (1) is manipulated with a percutaneous needle inserted from the antero-medial approach

when they can mimic a torn meniscus. Flaps are also seen, although much more rarely, on the tibial plateau.

Small flaps of articular cartilage are often seen adjacent to the intercondylar notch on the medial femoral condyle of older patients with no other sign of joint degeneration and can be regarded as a normal finding in the elderly.

OSTEONECROSIS AND STEROID NECROSIS

Spontaneous subchondral osteonecrosis (Fig. 8.1) is not uncommon in the medial femoral condyle of patients over 60 (Ahlback et al 1968, Bauer 1978), and is well described by Insall et al (1984). The cause is unknown, but the condition can be recognised

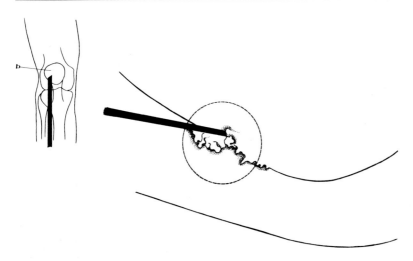
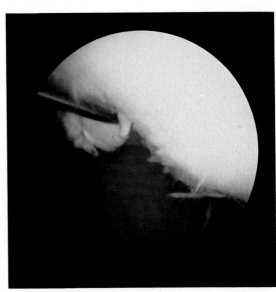

Fig. 8.7 Probing a chondral fracture of the lateral margin of the patella using the irrigation needle

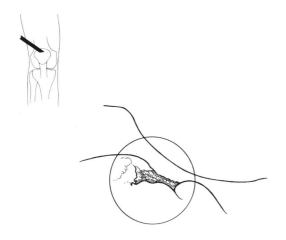

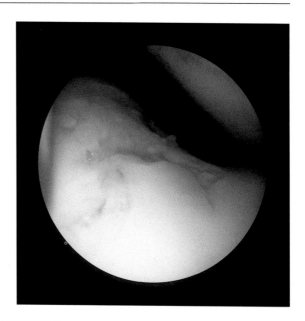

Fig. 8.8 A chondral separation surrounded by chondral flaps on the intercondylar groove of the femur, seen from the lateral suprapatellar approach. The joint is distended with gas

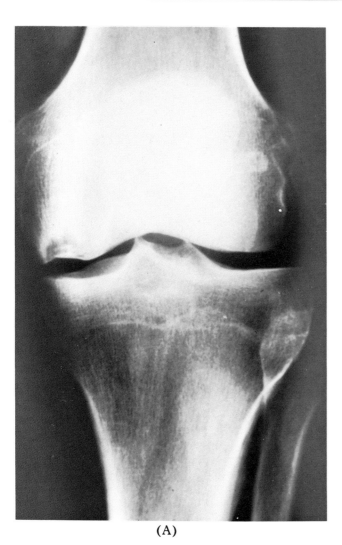

(A)

radiologically either by plain radiographs (Fig. 8.9) or tomograms, and the diagnosis confirmed by radionuclide scintigraphy. The arthroscopic changes, however, are said to be visible before any abnormality can be detected on the plain radiolograph (Koshino et al 1979).

The symptoms of osteonecrosis may be due at least in part to the mechanical instability of the unsupported articular cartilage flap overlying the bony defect, and these symptoms can be relieved by removing the articular cartilage flap and debriding its base with a power-driven or hand burr (Fig. 8.10). If a large segment of the articular surface is involved, a weight transference osteotomy may be required, but simple debridement and drilling of the underlying bone is often helpful if the defect is less than 1 or 2 cm in diameter.

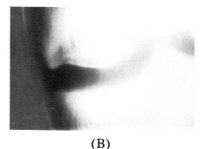

(B)

Fig. 8.9 Spontaneous osteonecrosis of the medial femoral condyle. The lesion is clearly seen on the antero-posterior film (A), and the tomogram (B) shows an intact plate of cortical bone collapsed into a defect in the bone

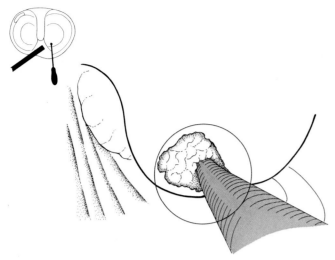

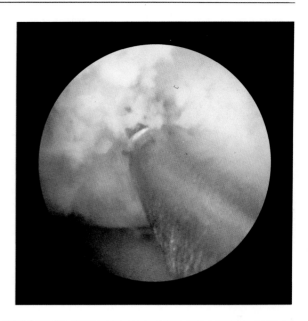

Fig. 8.10 An osteonecrotic lesion of the medial femoral condyle being debrided arthroscopically with a hand burr. The bed of the lesion is soft necrotic bone

A very similar condition occurs in patients with organ transplants and others who have received large doses of steroids (Bauer 1978, Fisher & Bickel 1971, Cruess 1977, Elmstedt 1981). In these patients, the plane of separation is more extensive and a large segment of femoral condyle can become detached (Fig. 8.11). Removing the bony fragment and drilling its base is a simple and elegant arthroscopic procedure, but there is no published evidence that it does any good and the lesions are perhaps best left alone.

CHONDROMALACIA

'Chondromalacia patellae' will be described later (p. 187). Similar changes are seen on the femoral condyles and probably represent an early stage of articular cartilage breakdown leading to eventual osteoarthritis.

OSTEOARTHRITIS

The point at which chondromalacia becomes osteoarthritis is hard to determine precisely, but for practical purposes it can be said that if both joint surfaces are involved, the patient has osteoarthritis. Degenerative changes in the joint can be graded in

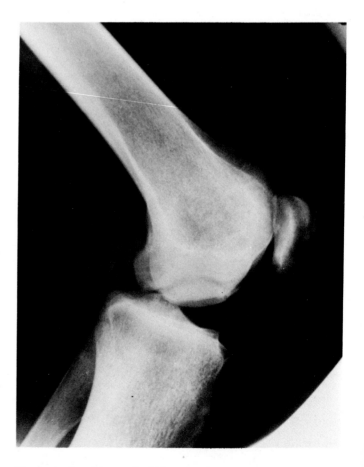

Fig. 8.11 Steroid necrosis. This patient had received large doses of steroids following renal transplantation and there is a large separated fragment of bone

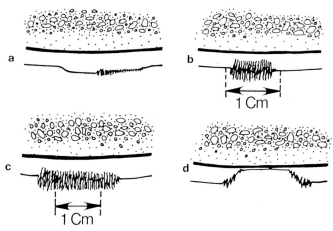

Fig. 8.12 Grading of chondral lesions: (A) grade I with fine fibrillation; (B) grade II – coarse fibrillation in an area less than 1 cm in diameter; (C) grade III – coarse fibrillation more than 1 cm in diameter; (D) grade IV – exposed bone

several ways, but the variation in the appearances from one area to another makes classification difficult. The following grading, based on that of Outerbridge (1961) for chondromalacia, is simple and easily reproducible.

Grade I. Fine fibrillation over an area less than 1 cm in diameter (Fig. 8.12A).

Grade II. Coarse fibrillation with vertical fissuring over an area less than 1 cm in diameter or fine fibrillation over an area of more than 2 cm in diameter, on one surface of the joint only (Fig. 8.12B).

Grade III. Coarse or fine fibrillation over an area more than 1 cm in diameter. Areas of exposed bone less than 2 mm in diameter can also be included as grade III change (Fig. 8.12C).

Grade IV. Exposed subchondral bone more than 2 mm in diameter on either surface (Fig. 8.12D).

LINEAR FISSURES

Fissures are sometimes seen on otherwise normal condyles, perhaps the result of direct impact or a fragment of bone becoming caught between the condyle and patella and acting as a rasp. These lesions should be carefully probed and any obviously loose flaps of articular cartilage removed without damaging the surrounding healthy tissue. A hole drilled into the centre of the lesion either with a small (2 mm) drill or a bone awl may be helpful in preventing further spread of the lesion.

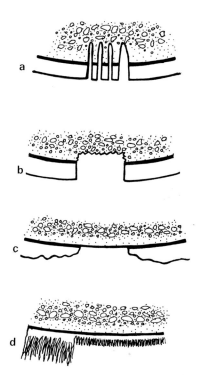

Fig. 8.13 Procedures that can be performed on articular surfaces: (A) drilling through articular cartilage with large- or small-diameter holes; (B) spongiolisation; (C) abrasion; (D) shaving

THE 'IMPINGEMENT' LESION

The articular cartilage lesion at the point of impingement of the medial femoral condyle and the anterior horn of the meniscus has already been mentioned (Figs. 4.20, 4.21). The lesion can be trimmed with basket forceps or rongeurs, but a ragged base is left and it is very probable that the lesion will re-form. The full significance of this lesion is not known.

OPERATIONS ON ARTICULAR CARTILAGE

Anything that can be done to articular cartilage at arthrotomy can be done just as well arthroscopically (Fig. 8.13). Surface irregularities can be levelled with rongeurs, basket forceps or powered instruments, and exposed subchondral bone can be drilled. Because the procedures are performed without the additional trauma of arthrotomy, the results can be expected to throw much-needed light on the management of chondral lesions.

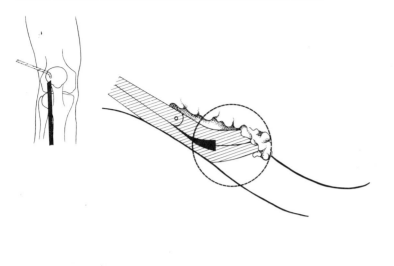
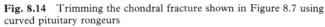
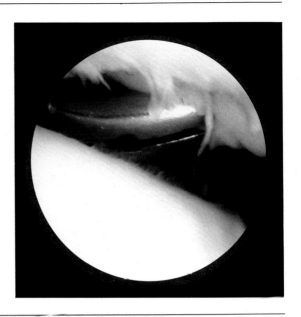

Fig. 8.14 Trimming the chondral fracture shown in Figure 8.7 using curved pituitary rongeurs

Patellar shaving

The indications for shaving are described in Chapter 13. In general, 'crab meat' lesions with a localised area of flaking articular cartilage do better after shaving than the finer fibrillation or generalised irregularity of degenerative joint disease (Fig. 8.13). Lesions suitable for shaving are comparatively rare, and many patellae are being shaved quite unnecessarily only because the surgeon is the proud owner of a powered shaver.

Shaving with rongeurs and basket forceps

Pituitary rongeurs (Fig. 8.14) can be used to level irregular areas, and side-biting forceps (Fig. 8.15) will remove all softened articular cartilage until subchondral bone is exposed and the edges of the lesion are vertical, which is not possible with the powered shaver. If desired, holes can be drilled down to the underlying cancellous bone through the subchondral bed. A knife can also be used to shave the lesion, but damage to healthy articular cartilage at the margin of the lesion is unavoidable.

Powered shavers

Powered shavers and their use are described in Chapter 2, but a few points are worth noting here.

Although the side-cutting window of the shaver will only admit tissue that stands proud of its surroundings, clumsy handling will harm healthy articular cartilage. The damage is usually caused by gouging with the edge of the cutting window and can be avoided by selecting the point of insertion with care. This can be difficult if the patello-femoral joint is tight, but the correct point can be found by touching the area to be shaved with the side of the irrigation needle; if the needle will not lie flat against the joint surface, the shaver will not do so either and another point of insertion must be found. Once inserted, the shaver should be pressed evenly against the lesion and moved gently across it from side to side until a smooth lawn-like surface remains (Fig. 8.16), but this is not always possible (Fig. 8.17), particularly when a chondral flap is levelled. It is essential with this instrument, as with all others, to keep the cutting tip in view at all times. To use the shaver 'blind' is likely to cause grievous damage not only to structures better preserved intact, but also to the arthroscope (Fig. 2.44).

If it is necessary to collect the fragments for inspection, this can be done by placing a gauze swab over the end of the outflow tube where it enters the suction bottle (Fig. 8.18).

Drilling

Articular cartilage lesions of the patella and femur can be treated by drilling into cancellous bone (Fig.

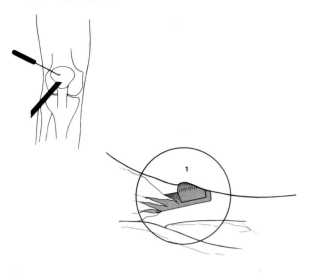

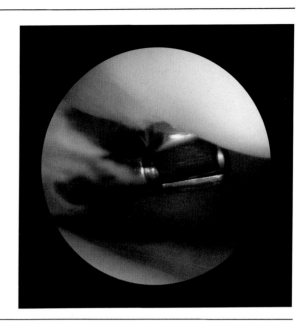

Fig. 8.15 Shaving a chondral lesion on the back of the patella (1) with side-biting rotary basket forceps

8.13) either directly through the damaged area itself (Fig. 8.19) or into the subchondral bone after removing the overlying cartilage (Fig. 8.5). A full Pridie procedure (Insall 1967) arthroscopically is also possible, although difficult, but the drilled areas do show signs of healing if examined later (Fig. 8.20).

Drilling under arthroscopic control is simple provided that the point of insertion has been chosen so that the drill is perpendicular to the joint surface. If the drill strikes the bone at an angle, its tip will 'wander' across the bone and cause needless damage. The correct point of insertion is found by passing a needle just above the meniscus and flexing the knee until it lies against the lesion. If the knee is flexed to 60° or more, which is often necessary, there may be little space at the front of the joint and visibility may be poor. Further problems arise if soft tissue

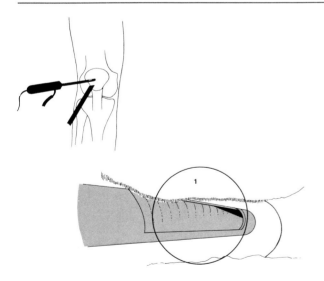

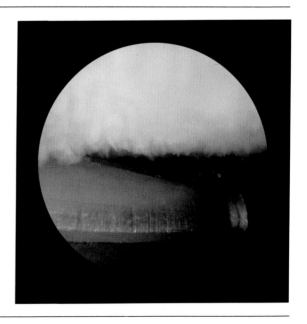

Fig. 8.16 Shaving the back of the patella (1) with a powered shaver

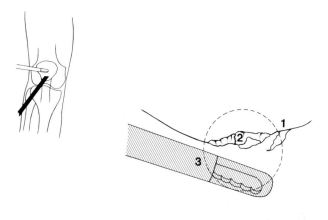

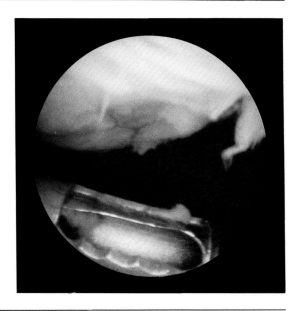

Fig. 8.17 The result of shaving an area of softened articular cartilage (2) on the under-surface of the patella (1) with a power tool (3); a smooth surface could not be obtained in this patient

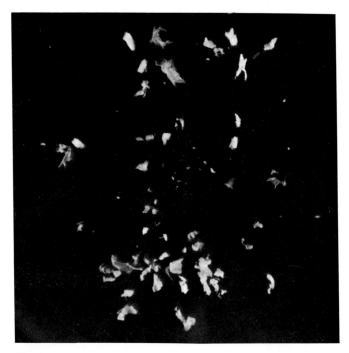

Fig. 8.18 Articular cartilage shavings obtained with the Dyonics shaver

becomes caught up on the drill, but this can be avoided by using a smooth-sided drill, Kirschner wire or a hand burr with a counter-helical groove (p. 22), rather than a twist bit.

Spongiolisation

Spongiolisation, the removal of cortex to expose cancellous bone (Fig. 8.13) (p. 191), can be done arthroscopically with a hand or power burr by drilling holes around the margin of the lesion, and completing the defect with rongeurs, osteotomes or gouges, just as would be done at arthrotomy. The procedure is difficult on the patella unless it is mobile and can be subluxed over the edge of the femoral condyle and approached from below.

ARTHROSCOPY AND THE DEGENERATE KNEE

Arthroscopy is helpful at several stages in the management of the degenerate knee.

Assessment

In patients with degenerative joint disease, particularly the younger patients, it is helpful to know the precise extent of the osteoarthritis. If, for example, a patient with exposed bone on the medial plateau has unsuspected grade III change on the tibial plateau, it might be anticipated that the benefits of osteotomy will be shortlived, as Coventry (1979) has stressed, but this is not universally agreed. Keene & Dyreby (1983) found that the extent of the degeneration had no bearing at all on the results after 2–3 years, and concluded that 'the arthroscopic findings prior to osteotomy appeared to have little, if any, predictive

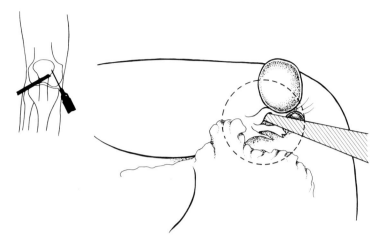

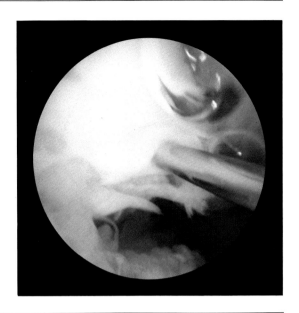

Fig. 8.19 Drilling into cancellous bone through a patch of softened and degenerate articular cartilage on the medial facet of the patella using a percutaneous Kirschner wire

value in evaluating patients for this procedure'. Whatever the outcome of this controversy, it can be said that if it is thought helpful to know the full extent of the damage to a joint surface, arthroscopy will supply that information.

Irrigation and debridement

Irrigation and debridement is a worthwhile procedure which can bring relief of symptoms for months or years. The symptoms of osteoarthritis are also helped by a simple diagnostic arthroscopy, as Burman first noted over fifty years ago:

> It was in the group of arthritic cases that we had the pleasant surprise of seeing a marked improvement in the joint following arthroscopy. This unlooked-for therapeutic effect was so marked in the case of one patient (A.B.) that after his one knee had been examined he begged us to do the same for his other knee (Burman et al 1934).

Many patients since 'A.B.' have benefited from this

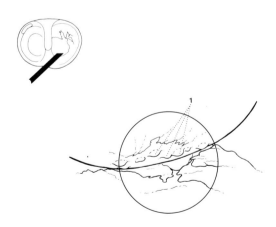

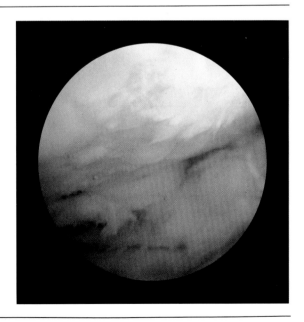

Fig. 8.20 The appearance six months after drilling an area of exposed bone in a patient with osteoarthritis. Small 'blisters' of fibrocartilage have appeared at the site of the drill hole

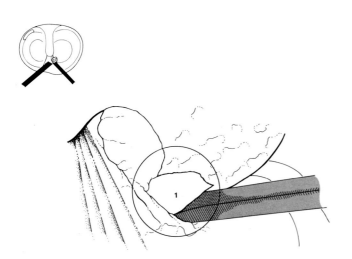

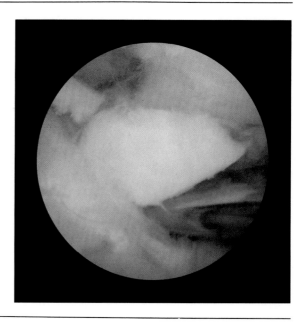

Fig. 8.21 Removing an osteophyte (1) from the intercondylar notch with a narrow osteotome

phenomenon, and arthroscopists are grateful for it, but it does create problems in the evaluation of other intra-articular procedures.

Debridement of irregular menisci and the removal of small meniscal flaps (Figs. 10.33, 10.34, 10.47) will also bring relief out of proportion to the extent of the procedure (Jackson & Rouse 1982). Care must be taken, however, not to remove healthy tissue, because this is likely to accelerate the degeneration (Jones et al 1978).

Osteophytes can be removed with a sturdy osteotome about 5 mm wide (Fig. 8.21). Osteophytes in the intercondylar notch are the easiest to remove, but those along the margins of the femur and patella are also possible. To remove an osteophyte from the intercondylar notch, the osteotome should be inserted from the antero-medial or antero-lateral approach, whichever gives better access, and the anterior cortex of the osteophyte divided. The osteotome can then be used to lever up the osteophyte, which is then avulsed with rongeurs. An alternative is to convert the osteophyte into a loose body, but this runs the risk of losing it in the joint and it is easier to avulse the posterior cortex than divide it.

Abrasion chondroplasty

Johnson has advocated abrasion of the superficial layer of osteoarthritic bone (Fig. 8.13) on the grounds that the superficial layer is dead and that the natural repair processes will resurface the lesion with either hyaline or good-quality fibro-cartilage. Regeneration of normal articular cartilage in osteoarthritis would seem on first principles to be unlikely, particularly as the pathology of osteoarthritis is one of abrasion. A final verdict on the long-term results of this procedure must await detailed studies. Johnson's post-operative regime also includes restricted weight-bearing with crutches for several weeks and this, together with the 'A.B.' effect and accompanying debridement of meniscal flaps (Jackson & Rouse 1982), which also contribute to the result, make accurately controlled studies difficult to achieve.

Despite these reservations, there is no evidence to show that abrasion chondroplasty does not work; if it proves to be more effective than debridement and irrigation alone, it will indeed be a great advance.

To perform an abrasion chondroplasty, a powered burr with a protective sheath to avoid damage to the opposite joint surface is applied lightly to the affected area until bleeding bone is reached. Only the superficial millimetre of bone is removed and not the full cortical thickness, the aim of the operation being to expose live bone and bring new blood supply to the joint surface. A high flow of irrigation fluid is required when this and other power tools are used (p. 39).

Knee prostheses

Arthroscopy has a small part to play in the management of patients with total knee prostheses,

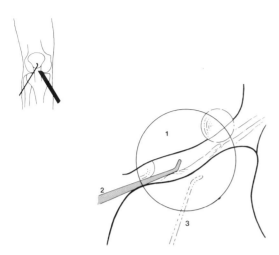

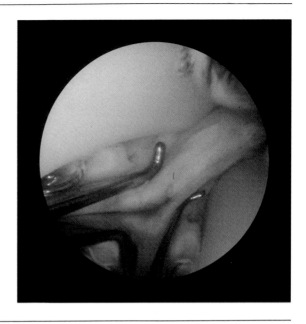

Fig. 8.22 An artificial knee joint. The patella (1) is above, and the hook (2) is reflected by the femoral component (3)

but this is likely to increase. Arthroscopic mobilisation is helpful in patients with a stiff knee following joint replacement. The technique is the same as that described above for the division of adhesions (p. 75), except that special care must be taken to maintain complete sterility and to avoid damage to the prosthetic surface. Fragments of cement can also be removed from the gutters if necessary, and inflamed synovial polyps removed.

A practical difficulty met when operating on a prosthetic knee is the reflection from the prosthesis, which can make orientation difficult (Fig. 8.22).

Replacement of uncemented prostheses is also possible, and in the author's experience (one case) is surprisingly straightforward. An uncemented MacIntosh prosthesis had slipped forwards to lie in front of the femoral condyle. At arthroscopy (Fig. 8.23), the prosthesis was manipulated into the

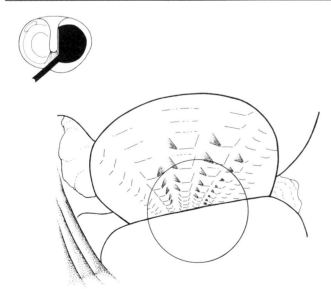

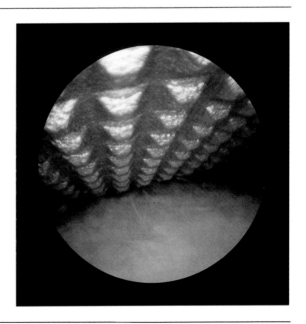

Fig. 8.23 The under-surface of a loose MacIntosh prosthesis

suprapatellar pouch, while the tibial surface was re-prepared with osteotomes and rongeurs, and a build-up of bone at the back of the tibia removed. The prosthesis was then re-seated on the tibia. If this procedure is possible, it must also be possible to prepare bone surfaces as a primary procedure, and even to insert cement.

Fractures

The arthroscope has also been used to confirm the diagnosis and determine the management of tibial plateau fractures. Depressed tibial plateaux can also be elevated and the arthroscope used to confirm that the reduction is correct (Reiner 1982). Fracture separations of the lower femoral epiphysis can be pinned under arthroscopic control and critical reports of the results of such treatment are eagerly awaited.

Loss of saline through the fracture line is inevitable, vision is obscured by blood, and the possibility of displacing the fracture further by the manipulation of arthroscopy must not be forgotten. The procedure is hazardous and difficult, but brings the advantage of anatomical reduction without arthrotomy.

References

Ahlback S, Bauer G C H, Bohne W H 1968 Spontaneous osteonecrosis of the knee. Arthritis and Rheumatism 11: 705–733
Aichroth P 1971 Osteochondritis dissecans of the knee. Journal of Bone and Joint Surgery 53B: 440–447
Bauer G C H 1978 Osteonecrosis of the knee. Clinical Orthopaedics and Related Research 130: 210–217
Burman M S, Finkelstein H, Mayer L 1934 Arthroscopy of the knee joint. Journal of Bone and Joint Surgery 16: 255–268
Coventry M B 1979 Upper tibial osteotomy for gonarthrosis. Evaluation of the operation in the last eighteen years and long term results. Orthopedic Clinics of North America 10: 191–210
Cruess R L 1977 Cortisone induced avascular necrosis of the femoral head. Journal of Bone and Joint Surgery 59B: 308–317
Elmstedt E 1981 Avascular bone necrosis in the renal transplant patient: a discriminant analysis of 144 cases. Clinical Orthopaedics and Related Research 158: 149–157
Fisher D E, Bickel W M 1971 Corticosteroid induced avascular necrosis. Journal of Bone and Joint Surgery 53A: 859–873
Guhl J F 1979 Arthroscopic treatment of osteochondritis dissecans: preliminary report. Orthopedic Clinics of North America 10: 671–683
Guhl J F 1982 Arthroscopic treatment of osteochondritis dissecans. Clinical Orthopaedics and Related Research 167: 65–74
Insall J N 1967 Intra-articular surgery for degenerative arthritis of the knee: a report on the work of the late K H Pridie. Journal of Bone and Joint Surgery 49B: 211–228
Insall J N, Aglietti P, Bullough P G, 1984 Osteonecrosis. In: Insall J N (ed) Surgery of the knee. Churchill Livingstone, New York
Jackson R W, Rouse D W 1982 The results of partial meniscectomy in patients over 40 years of age. Journal of Bone and Joint Surgery 64B: 481–485
Johnson-Nurse C, Dandy D J 1985 Fracture separation of articular cartilage in the adult knee. Journal of Bone and Joint Surgery 67B: 33–35
Jones R E, Smith E C, Reisch J S 1978 Effects of medial meniscectomy on patients older than forty years. Journal of Bone and Joint Surgery 60A: 783–786
Keene J S, Dyreby J R 1983 High tibial osteotomy in the treatment of osteoarthritis of the knee. The role of pre-operative arthroscopy. Journal of Bone and Joint Surgery 65A: 36–42
Koshino T, Okamoto R, Takamura K, Tsuchiya K 1979 Arthroscopy in spontaneous osteonecrosis of the knee. Orthopedic Clinics of North America 10: 609–618
Matthewson M H, Dandy D J 1978 Osteochondral fractures of the lateral femoral condyle: a result of indirect violence to the knee. Journal of Bone and Joint Surgery 60B: 199–202
Outerbridge R E 1961 The aetiology of chondromalacia patellae. Journal of Bone and Joint Surgery 43B: 752–757
Paget J 1870 On the production of some of the loose bodies in joints. St Bartholomew's Hospital Reports 6: 1–4
Reiner M J 1982 The arthroscope in tibial plateau fractures: its use in evaluation of soft tissue and bony injury. Journal of the American Orthopaedic Association 81: 704–707
Wilson J N 1967 A diagnostic sign in osteochondritis dissecans of the knee. Journal of Bone and Joint Surgery 49A: 477–480

9

Principles of meniscal surgery

THE IMPORTANCE OF THE MENISCUS

The meniscus is an essential part of the mechanical structure of the knee. Oretorp (1978) has shown that the peripheral fibres of the medial meniscus blend intimately with the medial ligament, and that total medial meniscectomy removes part of the medial collateral ligament complex. Seedhom et al (1974) reported that the medial meniscus transmits 50% and the lateral meniscus 70% of the load across the joint when the knee is straight. Hargreaves & Seedhom (1979) later used a four-spring knee model to show that when the knee was in full extension the proportion of the load across the joint taken by the meniscus fell from 85% to 35% after partial medial meniscectomy, and from 75% to 50% after partial lateral meniscectomy. Shrive (1974) reported similar results.

Histological study of the menisci (Fig. 9.1) shows that they are essentially complex ligaments (Bullough et al 1970), differing from other ligaments in their fine structure, ground substance, the smooth surface that is necessary because the meniscus articulates with the femur and tibia, and their crescentic shape. The attachment to bone at each end allows the circumferential fibres to act as a hoop, resisting the bursting force imposed by the downward thrust of the femoral condyle. By removing this protective shock-absorbing hoop, total meniscectomy increases the load taken by the articular cartilage and can only accelerate degenerative joint changes.

The risk of degenerative joint disease following meniscectomy is more than theoretical. Meniscectomy is not a benign procedure. Huckell (1965)

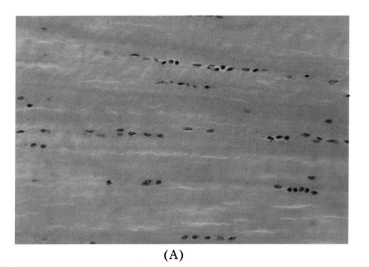

(A)

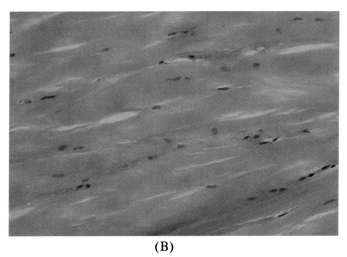

(B)

Fig. 9.1 The histological appearance of the anterior cruciate ligament (A) and meniscus (B). The similarity of appearance reflects the similar function of the two structures

found that 30% of patients have some clinical symptoms and signs of degenerative arthritis ten years after operation, and that more than half have radiological changes. Similar findings have been reported by Gear (1967) and J.P. Jackson (1968). It is difficult to distinguish between the long-term effects of the injury that damaged the meniscus, the effect of a loose meniscal fragment in the knee, the trauma of operation, and the absence of the meniscus itself, but Zaman & Leonard (1978) showed that the long-term effects of removing normal menisci from children are poor, with over 70% developing the clinical and radiological features of osteoarthritis in the second or third decades of life.

With this and other evidence available, there is no longer any reason to regard the meniscus as an unnecessary and troublesome appendage that can be excised with impunity. Indeed it might even be argued that excision of a normal meniscus is a surgical error comparable with the amputation of a normal finger.

ANATOMY OF MENISCUS IN RELATIONSHIP TO TEARS

The fine structure of the meniscus has a strong influence on the pattern of meniscal tears. The meniscus is composed of parallel circumferential fibres held together by ground substance and fibres that run both vertically and obliquely through the

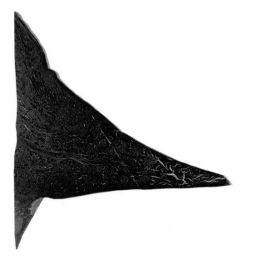

Fig. 9.2 A transverse section of meniscus stained to show fibrous tissue. There is a horizontal plate of fibrous tissue at the centre of the meniscus which is visible in the peripheral rim following meniscal lesions

meniscal body. In addition, there is a condensation of horizontal fibres at its periphery that probably acts as a 'spine' for the meniscus, and the meniscal surfaces are covered by a superficial layer of fibres separate from the main circumferential bundles (Fig. 9.2). A few radial fibres are also present. With this anatomy in mind, it is easy to understand how bucket-handle fragments arise from circumferential splits developing between the main bundles of circumferential fibres, how superior and inferior flap tears develop by the separation of the superficial layers, and how the deep horizontal condensation explains the deep fissure seen in the peripheral rim of a torn meniscus.

Popliteus tendon

The posterior third of each meniscus runs free behind the femoral condyle and is not attached to the capsule by a superior menisco-synovial junction like the anterior two thirds. The point at which the superior menisco-synovial junction ends is a stress raiser in both the medial and lateral compartments, and influences the pattern of tears. In the lateral compartment, the popliteus bridge lies at this point and acts as a localised peripheral separation that determines the pattern of complex oblique tears. Oblique, or parrot-beak, tears are centred upon the popliteus tunnel, and the exact positions of the anterior and posterior limits of the tear on the upper and lower surfaces of the meniscus determine the mobility, and therefore the stability, of the meniscal fragments. Although there is no comparable tunnel on the medial side, the junction of the posterior and middle thirds is nevertheless a point of weakness, and many tears start in this position.

It is possible that, as well as dictating their pattern, the popliteus tendon also initiates some tears of the lateral meniscus. In full extension, the space between the popliteus tendon and the femoral condyle is filled by the lateral meniscus, and in hyperextension the meniscus is driven up into the 'crutch' between the popliteus tendon and the femoral condyle so that it is fixed to the tibia as if by a staple (Fig. 9.3). A twisting strain applied to the femur with the meniscus jammed against the tibia in this way could cause a complex oblique tear based on the popliteus tendon.

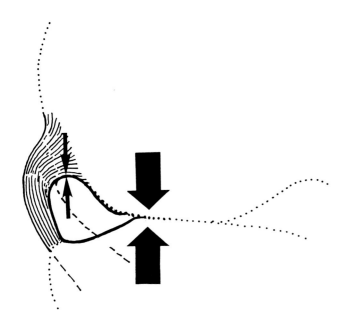

Fig. 9.3 When the lateral compartment is loaded in full extension, the popliteus tendon compresses the lateral meniscus and forces it onto the tibia. This may be responsible for initiating complex oblique tears

ASSESSMENT

History and clinical examination

The symptoms of a true meniscus lesion are usually caused by the loose fragment becoming caught between the joint surfaces when the knee is flexed and twisted, often during such gentle activities as putting on a pair of shoes or turning over in bed. These symptoms are quite different from sudden instability under stress, as when twisting sharply in a game of football; symptoms in the latter situation are usually due to ligament injuries. The predominantly mechanical nature of meniscal symptoms is hardly surprising, because the body of the meniscus has no sensory nerves and cannot 'hurt'. In this respect a loose meniscal fragment is like a loose body, except that it is tethered at the joint-line. Although a distorted meniscus can stretch synovium, irritate capsule, and cause pain and tenderness at the joint-line, these symptoms seldom overshadow the repeated locking or jamming that are the essential features of a true meniscal lesion.

Clinical examination will often demonstrate a mechanical click, a palpable mobile fragment, or a tender joint-line, but the findings of clinical examination are generally less helpful than the history. Although there are several studies to show that the accuracy of clinical diagnosis is between 60% and 70% (Dandy & Jackson 1975, Hirschowitz 1976, Korn et al 1979, Tregonning 1981), there have been many experienced surgeons in the recent past who have claimed near infallibility for their own clinical judgement. It is therefore reassuring to know that in 1909 Sir Robert Jones compared his clinical diagnosis with the findings at arthrotomy and found that, for meniscus lesions, his diagnostic accuracy was only 61.6%.

Arthrography

Double-contrast arthrography is an excellent technique, and in expert hands is almost as accurate as arthroscopy for the diagnosis of meniscus lesions, particularly those of the posterior third, but is less helpful than arthroscopy in assessing synovium, ligaments or articular cartilage. False positives are sometimes reported if a deep menisco-synovial sulcus is created by the firm valgus strain applied to the knee during arthrography; Figure 9.4 shows both a deep sulcus and a peripheral tear for comparison. Furthermore, although irregularities of articular cartilage are sometimes seen, the arthrogram can give no information about the mobility of chondral flaps, their depth, or the hardness of articular surface. Moreover, arthrography may be followed by a low-grade synovitis, which can last a few days or even weeks.

Daniel et al (1982) found a 98% accuracy for arthroscopic diagnosis of meniscus lesions when taken in conjunction with arthrography, compared

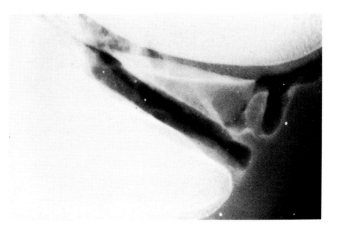

Fig. 9.4 An arthrogram demonstrating a peripheral tear of the meniscus as well as a deep sulcus at the menisco-synovial junction, itself often interpreted as a peripheral tear

with 89% for arthrography and 74% for clinical diagnosis alone (Carruthers & Kennedy 1980). Other studies have found a similar accuracy for arthroscopy, but when a probe is not used the diagnostic accuracy of arthroscopy is no better than arthrography (McGinty & Matza 1978, Ireland et al 1980).

For these reasons arthrography is, in general, less helpful than arthroscopy, but it does have the advantage that it is an out-patient procedure and adds to the workload of the radiology department rather than the orthopaedic department; its role will vary from place to place. In a centre where there is an experienced arthroscopist, but a busy radiology department and no radiologist with a specific interest in the knee, the technique probably has little part to play as a routine investigation, although it is still useful in assessing patients with popliteal cysts or persistent symptoms following either meniscectomy or arthroscopy. On the other hand, in a unit where there is a keen and experienced arthrographer, but no arthroscopist, arthrography is an essential part of the investigation of any internal derangement, and should always be performed before any arthrotomy for an internal derangement.

SELECTIVE SURGERY OF THE MENISCUS

Meniscal lesions can be treated by reattachment of the meniscal fragment, excision of the fragment alone, or complete meniscal excision. All these procedures have enjoyed periods of popularity in the past which have come and gone with the tides of surgical fashion, and the belief that any one operation is the correct solution for all meniscal lesions is a dangerous over-simplification. We are at present emerging from a period when total meniscectomy enjoyed widespread popularity (Watson-Jones 1940), and entering a period in which the arthroscope is used to select the operation appropriate for the individual lesion.

There are now several reports comparing the early and late results of partial and total meniscectomy (Bonnin 1956, Tapper & Hoover 1969, McGinty et al 1977, Northmore-Ball & Dandy 1982, Northmore-Ball et al 1983); all favour partial meniscectomy. Not only is partial meniscectomy a simpler operation than total meniscectomy, but the postoperative rehabilitation is shorter and the long-term results are better (Lysholm & Gillquist 1981).

These reports and that of Fahmy et al (1983), who found meniscal lesions in 57% of routine necropsies, are encouraging to arthroscopists, who have become increasingly sceptical of the clinical importance of some of the meniscal lesions for which total meniscectomy has been performed in the past. Some lesions, such as minor splits or fissures that cannot be related to the patient's symptoms, can probably be left alone altogether, particularly if there is doubt about the clinical relevance of the lesion (Noble & Erat 1980). Tiny fissures and irregularities in the meniscus are often seen in patients whose symptoms arise from obvious disorders elsewhere, and degenerative changes in the meniscus are almost universal in patients with early degenerative osteoarthritis, in whom the meniscus is often healthier than the articular cartilage (Noble & Hamblen 1975). It is difficult to understand how excision of such a meniscus can do anything but accelerate the degenerate process by increasing the load upon the already damaged articular surface, and such menisci should probably be left undisturbed (Jones et al 1978). Arthroscopic surgery of the meniscus, which restricts meniscectomy to the excision of unstable fragments only, is essentially conservative and this is probably the best approach in the present state of our knowledge (Goodfellow 1983).

Meniscal reattachment

Reattachment of the meniscal fragment with catgut was first reported in 1885 by Thomas Annandale, Regius Professor of Clinical Surgery in Edinburgh, but the case he described was very odd indeed. The patient was a 30-year-old miner with a ten-month history of recurrent locking of the knee, following a twisting injury in flexion, which caused a tense and painful effusion. Although he 'was able, by a little manipulation, to unlock the joint', the knee locked so frequently that he had not worked since the injury. At operation, on 16 November 1883, Annandale made a transverse incision above the medial meniscus, when:

It was seen that this semilunar cartilage was completely separated from its anterior attachments, and was displaced backwards about half an inch. The anterior edge of this cartilage was now seized by a pair of artery catch forceps, and it was drawn forwards into its natural position, and held there until three stitches of chromic catgut were passed through it and through the fascia and periosteum covering the margin of the tibia.

The knee was immobilised in plaster of Paris for seven weeks, and the patient discharged from hospital three weeks later. In April 1884, the patient was demonstrated to a group of distinguished visitors, 'who all expressed the opinion that the result was everything that could be desired'.

From the history, a classical bucket-handle tear might have been expected, but the lesion Annandale described sounds more like the antero-central separation described by Stone in 1979. Whatever the lesion, it would seem that one case with a five-month follow-up did not convince Annandale's visitors, because the operation of meniscal reattachment did not gain acceptance and was replaced by very conservative partial meniscectomy, as described by Sir Robert Jones: 'It is only necessary to remove the loose portion of cartilage, be it a fragment of the border, a circumferential tear or a detached anterior portion' (Jones 1909).

Reattachment of the meniscus is now being re-examined (Stone 1979, Heatley 1980, De Haven 1981, Hamberg et al 1984, Barber & Stone 1985) and is the treatment of choice for separations of the anterior horn and peripheral tears of the medial meniscus that involve the vascular tissue at the menisco-synovial junction (Arnoczky & Warren 1982). At present, meniscal reattachment is usually followed by plaster immobilisation; thus there is no great advantage in reattaching the meniscus arthroscopically, unless it can be done more neatly or more quickly.

Partial meniscectomy

Excision of localised 'bucket-handle' fragments of meniscus has never fallen entirely from favour, despite claims that the symptoms recur unless the intact rim is also excised. Although excision of the bucket handle is recognised as an acceptable procedure, there has been less enthusiasm for the open excision of isolated flaps or tags of meniscus, but it is hard to find a good reason for removing the whole meniscus if the symptoms are due only to a small flap. The aim of partial meniscectomy, performed by either open or arthroscopic techniques, is to leave an intact and stable rim of healthy tissue.

Multiple tears of the meniscus are common, and to remove one bucket handle, but leave another is to do an incomplete rather than a partial meniscectomy. Great care must always be taken to ensure both that the remaining meniscal tissue is intact and stable, and that only the minimum of tissue is removed.

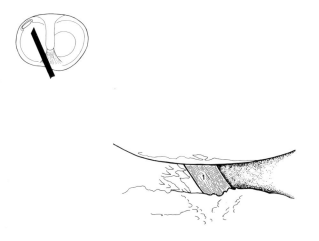

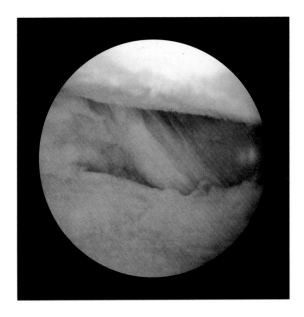

Fig. 9.5 The lateral compartment of a knee 20 years after lateral meniscectomy. There is extensive osteoarthritis, and the popliteus tendon is clearly seen (1). There is no sign of meniscal regeneration

Table 9.1 Indications for meniscal surgery

Meniscal reattachment	Full-thickness peripheral tears within 3 mm of the menisco-synovial junction
	Antero-central detachments
Total meniscectomy	Cystic degeneration
	Completely shattered menisci with no intact peripheral fibres
Leave alone	Horizontal fissures seen as incidental finding
	Some radial tears of the lateral meniscus
	Most asymptomatic tears
Partial meniscectomy	All other lesions with an unstable meniscal fragment

Total meniscectomy

Although total meniscectomy is deservedly in decline as the routine procedure for all meniscal tears, it is still the treatment of choice for cystic degeneration. Although isolated peripheral cysts of the lateral meniscus can be excised without disturbing the peripheral fibres of the meniscus, the whole meniscus must be removed when it is degenerate and swollen throughout its substance. Total or subtotal meniscectomy is also required if the meniscal rim is completely ruptured, or if the meniscus is so badly torn that no healthy meniscal tissue can be found.

The suggestion has sometimes been made (Smillie 1970) that total excision of the meniscal rim leads to regeneration of a new meniscus. In 1943, Smillie went so far as to say 'Total excision of a meniscus is invariably followed by replacement by a structure consisting of fibrous tissue which is almost a replica of the original'. On the other hand, Sir Robert Jones commented, 'In cases that have come to me with the history of removal of a cartilage, I have found no trace of any new structure even 10 years after operation' (King 1936).

Although a small whitish crescent will develop at the site of the former meniscus (Fig. 10.43), histological study of this structure shows that it consists of flimsy fibrous tissue with only a superficial macroscopic resemblance to the original, and even this is not always seen (Fig. 9.5). In contrast, Hargreaves & Seedhom (1979) have shown that the intact rim left after removing a bucket-handle fragment is capable of transmitting 35% of the load across the joint.

References

Annandale T 1885 An operation for displaced semilunar cartilage. British Medical Journal 1: 779

Arnoczky S P, Warren R F 1982 Microvasculature of the human meniscus. American Journal of Sports Medicine 10: 353–343

Barber F A, Stone R G 1985 Meniscal repair: an arthroscopic technique. Journal of Bone and Joint Surgery 67B: 39–41

Bonnin J G 1956 In: Platt H (ed) Modern trends in orthopaedics, 2nd series. Butterworth, London

Bullough P, Munuera L, Murphy J, Weinstein A 1970 The strength of the menisci as it relates to their fine structure. Journal of Bone and Joint Surgery 52B: 564–570

Carruthers L C, Kennedy M 1980 Knee arthroscopy: a follow-up study of patients initially recommended for further surgery. Clinical Orthopaedics and Related Research 147: 275–277

Dandy D J, Jackson R W 1975 The impact of arthroscopy on the management of disorders of the knee. Journal of Bone and Joint Surgery 57B: 349–352

Daniel D, Daniels E, Aronson D 1982 The diagnosis of meniscus pathology. Clinical Orthopaedics and Related Research 163: 218–224

De Haven K E 1981 Peripheral meniscal repair: an alternative to meniscectomy. Journal of Bone and Joint Surgery 63B: 463

Fahmy N R M, Williams E A, Noble J 1983 Meniscal pathology and osteoarthrosis of the knee. Journal of Bone and Joint Surgery 65B: 24–28

Gear M 1967 The late results of meniscectomy. British Journal of Surgery. 54: 270–272

Goodfellow J W 1983 Closed meniscectomy. Journal of Bone and Joint Surgery 65B: 373–374

Hamberg P, Gillquist J, Lysholm J 1984 A comparison between arthroscopic meniscectomy and open meniscectomy. Journal of Bone and Joint Surgery 66B: 189–192

Hargreaves D J, Seedhom B B 1979 On the 'bucket-handle' tear: partial or total meniscectomy? A quantitative study. Journal of Bone and Joint Surgery 61B: 381

Heatley F W 1980 The meniscus – can it be repaired? An experimental investigation in rabbits. Journal of Bone and Joint Surgery 62B: 397–402

Hirschowitz D 1976 Clinical assessment, arthrography, arthroscopy and arthrotomy in the diagnosis of internal derangement of the knee. Journal of Bone and Joint Surgery 58B: 367

Huckell J 1965 Is meniscectomy a benign procedure? A long-term follow-up study. Canadian Journal of Surgery 8: 254–260

Ireland J, Trickey E L, Stoker D J 1980 Arthroscopy and arthrography of the knee: a critical review. Journal of Bone and Joint Surgery 62B: 3–6

Jackson J P 1968 Degenerative changes in the knee after meniscectomy. British Medical Journal 2: 525–527

Jones R 1909 Notes on derangement of the knee: based upon personal experience of over five hundred operations. Annals of Surgery 50: 969–1001

Jones R E, Smith E C, Reisch J S 1978 Effects of medial meniscectomy on patients older than forty years. Journal of Bone and Joint Surgery 60A: 783–786

King D 1936 Regeneration of semilunar cartilages. Surgery, Gynecology and Obstetrics 62: 167

Korn M W, Spitzer R M, Robinson K E 1979 Correlation of arthrography with arthroscopy. Orthopedic Clinics of North America 10: 535–543

Lysholm J, Gillquist J 1981 Endoscopic meniscectomy. International Orthopaedics 5: 265–270

McGinty J B, Geuss L F, Marvin R A 1977 Partial or total meniscectomy. A comparative analysis. Journal of Bone and Joint Surgery 59A: 763–766

McGinty J B, Matza R A 1978 Arthroscopy of the knee. Evaluation of an out-patient procedure under local anaesthesia. Journal of Bone and Joint Surgery 60A: 787–789

Noble J, Erat K 1980 In defence of the meniscus. A prospective study of 200 patients. Journal of Bone and Joint Surgery 62B: 7–11

Noble J, Hamblen D L 1975 The pathology of the degenerate meniscus lesion. Journal of Bone and Joint Surgery 65B: 180–186

Northmore-Ball M D, Dandy D J 1982 Long-term results of arthroscopic partial meniscectomy. Clinical Orthopaedics and Related Research 167: 34–42

Northmore-Ball M D , Dandy D J, Jackson R W 1983 Arthroscopic, open partial, and total meisectomy. Journal of Bone and Joint Surgery 65B: 400–404

Oretorp N 1978 On the diagnosis and treatment of meniscus and ligament injuries in the knee. Linkoping University Medical Dissertation No. 63, I: 3–19

Seedhom B B, Dowson D, Wright V 1974 Functions of the menisci – a preliminary study. Journal of Bone and Joint Surgery 56B: 381

Shrive N 1974 The weight-bearing role of the menisci of the knee. Journal of Bone and Joint Surgery 56B: 381

Smillie I S 1943 Observations on the regeneration of the semilunar cartilage in man. British Journal of Surgery 31: 398

Smillie I S 1970 Injuries of the knee joint, 4th edn. Churchill Livingstone, Edinburgh

Stone R G 1979 Peripheral detachment of the menisci of the knee: a preliminary report. Orthopedic Clinics of North America 10: 643–657

Tapper E, Hoover N 1969 Late results after meniscectomy. Journal of Bone and Joint Surgery 51A: 517–526

Tregonning R J 1981 Diagnostical arthroscopy of the knee joint. Meniscal findings in a prospective study of 200 examinations. New Zealand Medical Journal 94: 81–83

Watson-Jones R 1940 Fractures and other bone and joint injuries. E & S Livingstone, Edinburgh

Zaman M, Leonard M A 1978 Meniscectomy in children: a study of fifty-nine knees. Journal of Bone and Joint Surgery 60B: 436

10

Operations on the medial meniscus

Arthroscopic management of either meniscus proceeds in three distinct stages:

1. identification of the exact anatomy of the lesion
2. reattachment or removal of the fragment
3. trimming the rim and checking its stability.

Of these three stages, identifying the exact anatomy is the most important and removing the fragment the easiest, but checking the rim requires the most experience. Accurate assessment of the anatomy and the establishment of a workable classification of meniscal lesions is a vital first step towards arthroscopic meniscectomy.

CLASSIFICATION OF THE LESIONS

Many systems have been devised for the classification of meniscus lesions, based on the site, pattern, shape, size of the fragment or the force responsible. These classifications are of overpowering academic interest, but the arthroscopic surgeon is more concerned with a classification which will make the operation easier. The classification which follows (Fig. 10.1) is based on the patterns of tears as they appear at arthroscopy, and the way in which the fragments can best be removed.

Lesions of the medial meniscus can be broadly divided into the following types:

1. circumferential tears which give rise to bucket-handle fragments
2. horizontal tears which give rise to flaps and tags
3. degenerative lesions in patients with osteoarthrosis

The presence of one lesion does not exclude the presence of others, and double, triple and even quadruple tears have to be considered, as must the possibility of a tear in the other meniscus.

CIRCUMFERENTIAL TEARS

Identifying the anatomy

Circumferential tears of the medial meniscus start in the posterior third and extend anteriorly for a variable distance to produce a bucket-handle fragment. For practical purposes, bucket-handle fragments of the medial meniscus always begin at the posterior insertion, however far anteriorly they may run, and can be divided into three types, according to the extent of the tear.

Complete (type I) circumferential tears

If the tear extends right up to the anterior insertion, the bucket-handle fragment (Figs. 10.1, 10.2) may cause remarkably few symptoms and the fragment can lie so comfortably in the intercondylar notch that full extension is still possible. Even when there is some loss of extension, the knee may gradually straighten over a period of years, as the surrounding tissues accommodate themselves to the fragment by stretching the anterior cruciate ligament or developing a groove in the articular cartilage of the femoral condyle.

This type of tear can be missed altogether at arthroscopy by slipping the arthroscope under the fragment. If an apparently intact meniscus seems to be unusually narrow and manipulation of the

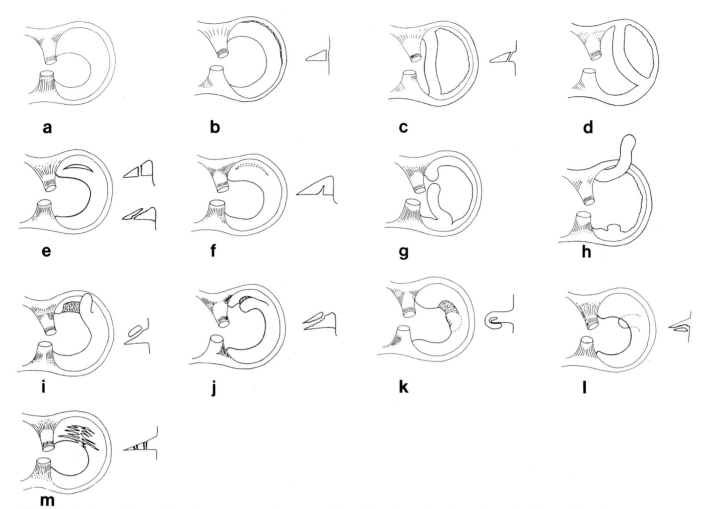

Fig. 10.1 Lesions of the medial meniscus: (A) normal meniscus; (B) peripheral separation of posterior half; (C) type I (complete) circumferential tear; (D) type II (incomplete) circumferential tear; (E) type III (concealed) circumferential tear, which may have either a very vertical or oblique split (inset); (F) partial-thickness tear of the posterior third, involving the inferior surface of the posterior third only; (G) detached bucket-handle fragment with long anterior segment; (H) detached bucket-handle fragment with long posterior portion; (I) horizontal superior flap tear of the posterior third dislocated into the gutter; (J) horizontal superior flap of posterior third in almost reduced position; (K) horizontal superior flap tear rolled under the meniscal body to produce an inverted flap; (L) inferior flap tear; (M) degenerate medial meniscus with many lacerations

arthroscope unexpectedly difficult, the possibility of a complete bucket-handle fragment lying on top of the arthroscope should be considered.

Incomplete (type II) circumferential tears

In the commonest pattern of bucket-handle fragment, the anterior extent of the tear falls short of the anterior insertion, but lies in front of the condyle and can be seen easily (Figs. 10.1, 10.3). Fragments of this type cause locking and loss of extension, the amount depending on the thickness of the fragment and the extent of the tear.

Concealed (type III) circumferential tears

If the anterior limit of the tear lies behind the medial femoral condyle, it will not be seen from the antero-

lateral approach (Figs. 10.1, 10.4) and there is a real risk that it will be missed, as Ireland et al (1980) and Daniel et al (1982) described. A concealed tear should be suspected if there is a history of definite locking of the knee in full flexion, particularly if the patient is apprehensive when the knee is bent during examination or is unwilling to squat with the knee fully flexed. The preliminary examination under anaesthetic may demonstrate either locking in full flexion, with a marked thud as the fragment is reduced on extension, or simply a block to flexion.

At arthroscopy, the meniscus may at first sight seem intact, but a valgus strain with the tibia externally rotated will produce a characteristic forward bulging of the meniscus. The presence of the tear can be confirmed by probing with a needle

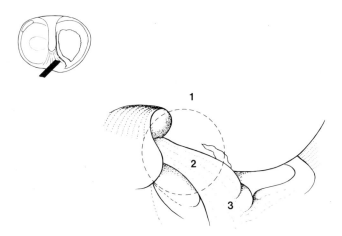

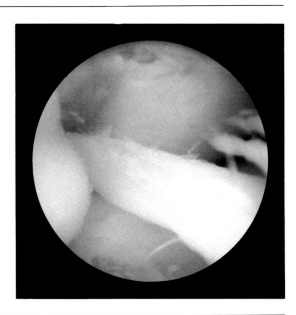

Fig. 10.2   A complete (type I) bucket-handle tear of the medial meniscus (2) lying locked in the intercondylar notch beneath the medial femoral condyle (1). The anterior attachment of the fragment (3) is at the anterior horn of the medial meniscus

(Figs. 10.5, 10.6), or by traction with a hook inserted from the antero-medial approach (Fig. 10.7).

Partial-thickness posterior horn tears

If the split in the meniscus does not extend completely through its full thickness, and the blunt hook demonstrates that the free edge is abnormally mobile, but not mobile enough to come in front of the femoral condyle within reach of the operating instruments, a partial-thickness tear may be present (Fig. 10.1). The probe may then demonstrate a cleft on the under-surface of the meniscus that has not extended through to its upper surface, and the line of cleavage can usually be identified on the upper surface as a slight depression that can be felt with the hook. These tears cause pain and discomfort from abnormal stretching of the capsule and synovium, rather than true locking, and probably progress to a complete tear if left untreated.

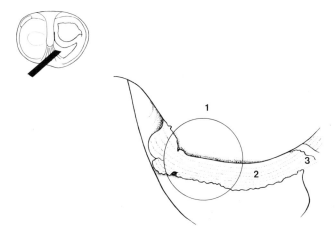

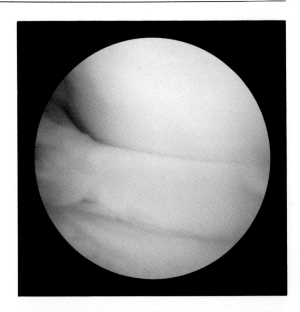

Fig. 10.3   An incomplete (type II) bucket-handle tear of the medial meniscus (2) with the anterior limit of the tear (3) falling short of the anterior attachment; medial femoral condyle (1)

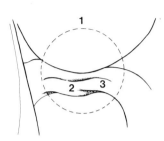

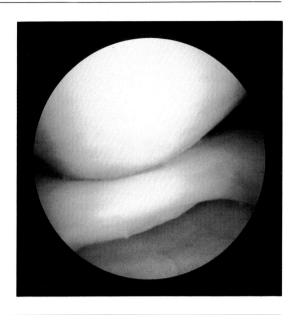

Fig. 10.4   A concealed (type III) circumferential tear of the medial meniscus (3) lying in the posterior part of the joint below the medial femoral condyle (1) produces a characteristic forward bulging (2) of the anterior margin of the meniscus

Posterior menisco-synovial detachments

Separation of the posterior third of the meniscus at the menisco-synovial junction is often found with anterior cruciate ligament injuries (Fig. 10.1), and can only be seen if the postero-medial compartment of the knee is entered and the meniscus probed, or if the joint is distended with saline under pressure. In some patients, the menisco-synovial junction may be inflamed, but intact (Fig. 10.8), and can be left untouched. Excision of the mobile segment is possible, but reattachment of the meniscus is probably the treatment of choice.

Detached bucket-handle fragments

Fragments resulting from circumferential tears can rupture to form a large tag (Fig. 10.1). In the medial compartment, bucket-handle fragments seldom become detached anteriorly, although this does occur

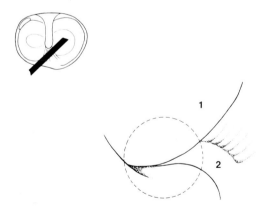

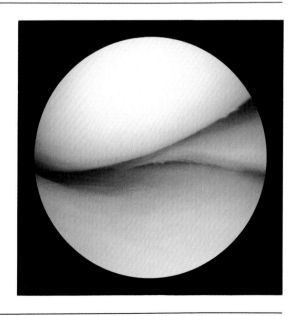

Fig. 10.5   An apparently normal medial meniscus (2) seen from the antero-lateral route; medial femoral condyle (1)

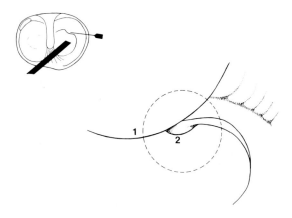

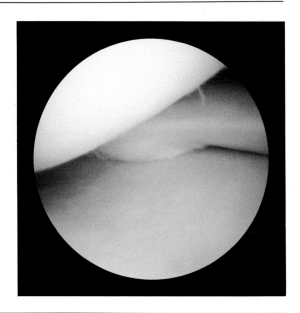

Fig. 10.6 The meniscus illustrated in Figure 10.5, using a percutaneous needle to demonstrate a tear of the inferior surface of the medial meniscus (2); medial femoral condyle (1)

in the lateral compartment. The fragment usually ruptures just less than 1 cm from its posterior attachment, leaving a finger of meniscal tissue that can be felt flicking backwards and forwards in the medial gutter like a 'loose body' tethered at one end. The length of the fragment varies according to the anatomy of the tear from which it arose, the fragments being longer the further forward the tear extends (Figs. 10.9–10.12). Double and triple fragments are sometimes seen (Fig. 10.13).

Detached bucket-handle fragments are easily seen at arthroscopy, but those in the posterior half of the joint may need to be lifted out of the gutter before the exact anatomy can be demonstrated. The end and the free edges of the fragments are usually smooth and rounded, and the fragments are thicker and longer than flaps arising from horizontal tears.

Although rupture of bucket-handle fragments in the medial compartment usually occurs near the posterior attachment, ruptures of the anterior limit

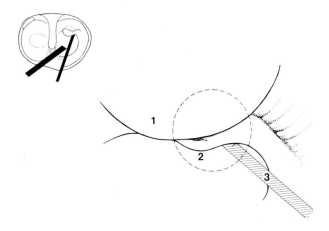

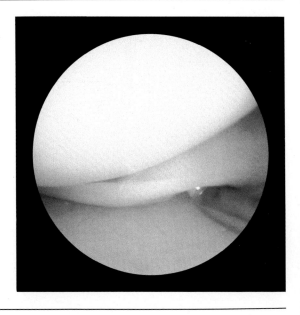

Fig. 10.7 A flap tear of the medial meniscus (2) is pulled from beneath the medial femoral condyle (1) using a blunt hook (3)

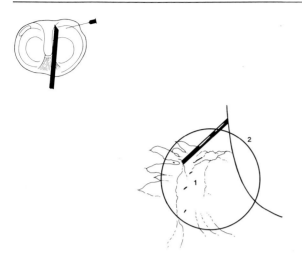

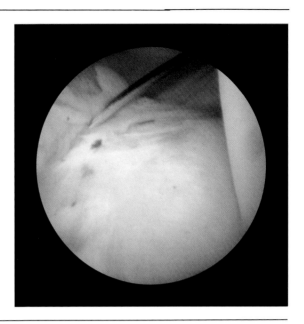

Fig. 10.8 The posterior horn of the medial meniscus (1) probed with a needle inserted behind the medial femoral condyle (2)

are also seen and produce a long tag that falls back into the posterior compartment and causes a block to flexion. These fragments can be removed either by pulling them forward into the front of the joint with a hook or forceps, or from the postero-medial approach. The approach for these lesions is the same as for bucket-handle fragments that have fallen into the postero-medial compartment after being detached anteriorly during arthroscopic meniscectomy.

Meniscal reattachment

The indications for reattaching the fragment are outlined in Chapter 9, but can be summarised as a sound intact fragment resulting from a tear at or near the menisco-synovial junction. Before describing arthroscopic meniscal reattachment in more detail, it must be said that there are some doubts about the way in which this operation is sometimes performed.

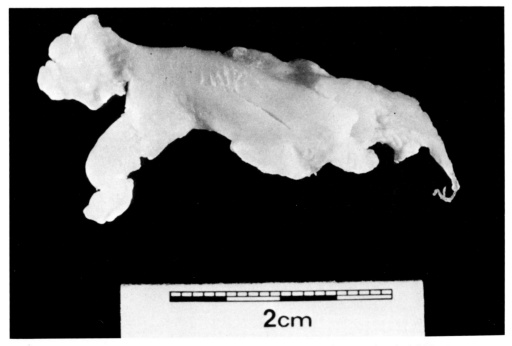

Fig. 10.9 Long detached bucket-handle fragment. The free end of the fragment (on the left) has become rounded

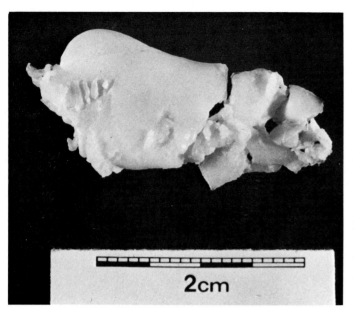

Fig. 10.10   Shorter detached bucket-handle fragment. The bulk of the fragment was removed intact and the base trimmed with rongeurs

First, the ideal lesions for meniscal reattachment are seen in patients with anterior cruciate sufficiency, in whom the operation can be combined with cruciate reconstruction. Tears of the middle third are much less common, and antero-central separations (Stone 1979) even rarer.

Intact menisci can tear in patients with cruciate insufficiency, and reattached menisci are likely to do the same unless the cruciate is reconstructed. If the

knee is to be opened for the ligament reconstruction, there is little point in reattaching the meniscus arthroscopically. For these reasons, arthroscopic reattachment in the cruciate-deficient knee seems unlikely to succeed in the long term, but only time will resolve this question.

Secondly, there is the problem that the posterior third of the meniscus, behind the femoral condyle, is much more difficult to reach than the middle third, and there is a grave temptation to reattach the middle third and leave the posterior third untouched, which is likely to be followed by a recurrence. On the other hand, suture of the posterior third is hazardous (Barber & Stone 1985), but few reports of the technique mention this. A substantial grain of doubt exists about the objectivity of some reports.

Posterior third detachments

Detachment of the posterior third at the posterior menisco-synovial separation is most often found in patients with anterior cruciate disruption. It can only be seen if the arthroscope is placed in the postero-medial compartment via the notch, or through a postero-medial insertion.

Access to the posterior third is difficult, but can be achieved by passing a long flexible needle through the meniscus from the front. Stone et al (1984) have described a technique in which the needle is pushed

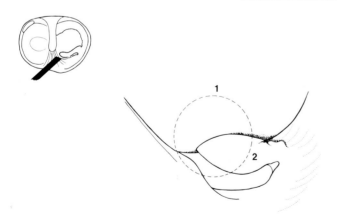

Fig. 10.11   A detached bucket-handle fragment of meniscus (2) has come to lie in front of the medial femoral condyle (1) and close to the lens in such a way that it appears larger than its true size

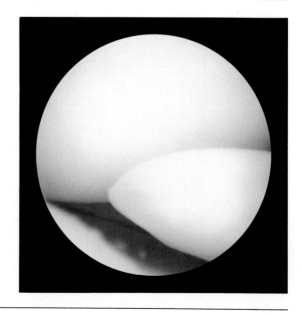

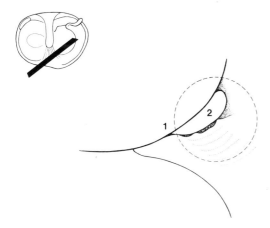

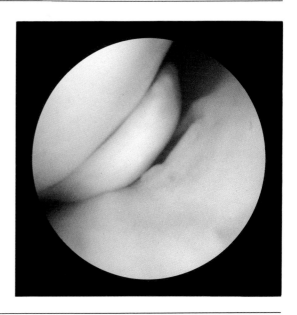

Fig. 10.12   A ruptured bucket-handle fragment (2) of medial meniscus which has turned back on itself to lie in the medial gutter beside the medial femoral condyle (1)

blindly through the soft tissues to leave the knee on the medial side. By repeating the process, a series of square stiches can be placed across the lesion. Once the sutures are in position, the threads are exposed through a short incision and tied firmly. This technique includes soft tissue in the knot, as well as the potential complications of pushing a needle blindly through the soft tissues at the back of the knee.

If an incision is to be made, it is better to open the postero-medial compartment and tie the knots under direct vision. Guides are available (Fig. 10.14) for passing the needles accurately, but the problem of tying the knot in the back of the knee remains.

Alternatively, a short curved 'fish-hook' needle can be passed through the postero-medial insertion on a small needle holder and the sutures placed under the control of a 70° arthroscope passed through the notch. This technique is difficult, and the needle tends to break at its eye.

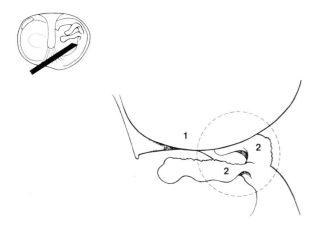

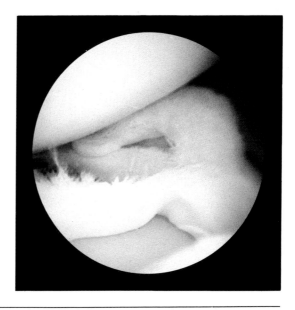

Fig. 10.13   Two detached bucket-handle fragments of medial meniscus (2) lying in the medial compartment beneath the medial femoral condyle (1)

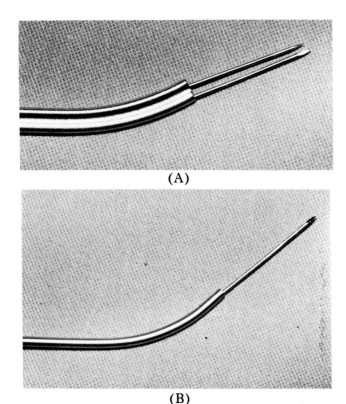

(A)

(B)

Fig. 10.14 Instruments for resuturing the meniscus: (A) curved insertor with two channels for inserting flexible needles; (B) single channel insertor

Tears of the middle third

Tears of the middle third are less difficult. Sutures can be placed accurately with a needle guide from within, or a standard intravenous needle can be used

as a guide by passing the needle through skin and meniscus and using it as a channel for a nylon suture. The nylon can then be used to pull the definitive suture of Vicryl or Dexon through the meniscus (Fig. 10.15). The knot is tied either over a roll of gauze, or subcutaneously through a short incision.

The suture material can be absorbable or unabsorbable. There is evidence to show that tight sutures (Heatley 1980) produce cell death in the rabbit's meniscus, and such lesions are probably compounded if an unabsorbable suture is used. Vicryl appears to be satisfactory.

The aftercare can include splintage or plaster immobilisation, but if the knots have been well tied, there does not seem to be any good reason why a sensible patient should have the knee immobilised. Immobilisation may, however, be advisable in the pathological athlete who will begin training unless physically restrained.

Because most of the lesions suitable for reattachment occur in cruciate deficient knees, reattachment can often be combined with cruciate reconstruction and the indications for arthroscopic meniscal reattachment alone may well become narrower with time.

Removing the fragment

When the anatomy has been properly defined, removing the fragment is comparatively easy. Several methods will be described.

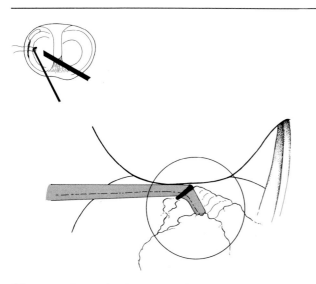

Fig. 10.15 Resuturing the peripheral rim of a lateral meniscus. A hook has been passed beneath the suture

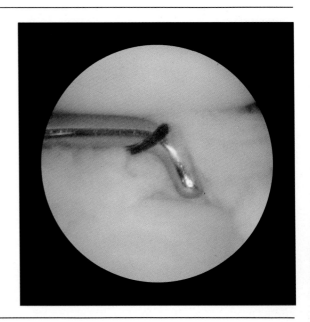

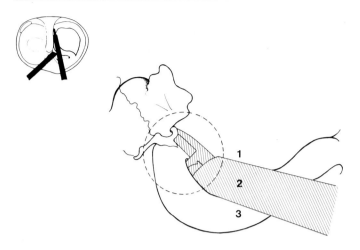

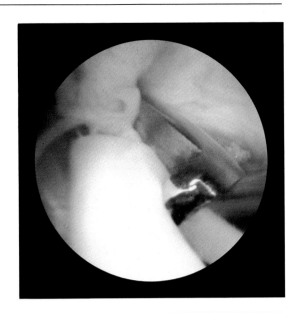

Fig. 10.16 A locked incomplete (type II) bucket-handle fragment of medial meniscus (3) being divided at its posterior attachment using the arthroscopic scissors (2); medial femoral condyle (1)

Double puncture technique

Type I tears These fragments can be removed with instruments inserted at the medial edge of the patellar tendon, about 1 cm above the meniscus (Fig. 4.7) (Dandy 1982). The fragment should be dislocated into the notch, if it is not already locked, and the posterior attachment divided first. Straight scissors will cut the posterior attachment easily if a blade is slipped into the 'axilla' of the tear between the femoral condyle and the fragment (Fig. 10.16).

The fragment can then be moved to the medial gutter and the cut posterior stub (Fig. 10.17) trimmed back with punch forceps or rongeurs. Excessive trimming will damage the meniscal rim and is potentially harmful.

With the fragment divided, excision can continue in one of two ways. The end of the fragment can be grasped and withdrawn through the skin (Fig. 10.18). Firm traction is then applied and the anterior attachment divided in the subcutaneous tissues with

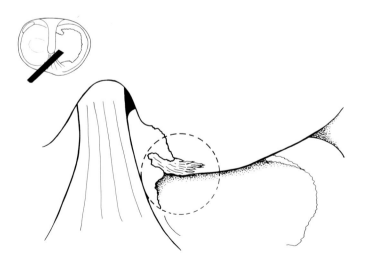

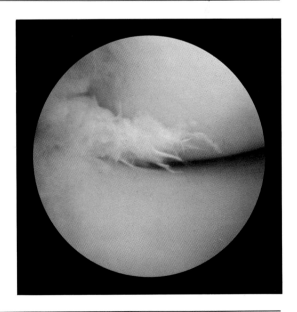

Fig. 10.17 The stump of medial meniscus left after division of its posterior attachment

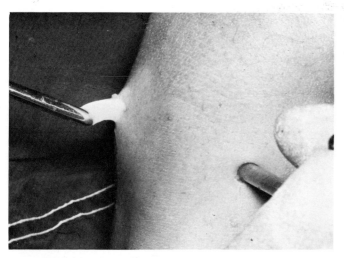

Fig. 10.18 A bucket-handle fragment of medial meniscus has been divided posteriorly with arthroscopic scissors and drawn through the skin with pituitary rongeurs

a No. 15 blade passed through the wound and under the fragment, which is then removed intact (Fig. 10.19). If the blade is passed above the fragment instead of below, a long anterior tag will remain. Alternatively, the fragment can be divided inside the joint as described below.

Type II tears Type II fragments require a different approach. After cutting the posterior attachment as described above, the anterior attachment is divided inside the knee from the antero-medial approach, transposing the instruments from medial to lateral side if necessary.

The simplest way to divide the fragment anteriorly is to avulse it with rongeurs applied to its base (Fig. 10.20). An alternative is to divide the anterior attachment with scissors, knife or guillotine (Fig. 10.21), but complete division of the fragment leaves it free as a particularly slippery loose body that can be elusive. Figure 10.22 shows this lesson being learned; as soon as the photograph had been taken, the fragment escaped to the postero-medial compartment. This problem can be avoided either by grasping the fragment with a second instrument, such as tendon forceps inserted through a third channel, or by leaving a few strands of meniscal tissue intact so that the fragment can be avulsed. To judge the amount of meniscal tissue that can be avulsed easily with forceps requires some experience, and attempts to grub out the meniscus by its roots should be avoided.

Alternatively, the anterior attachment can be cut before the posterior. Although the anterior attachment is the easier of the two to divide, cutting this first brings the very real danger that the meniscal fragment will drop back into the postero-medial compartment (Fig. 10.23). If the fragment should

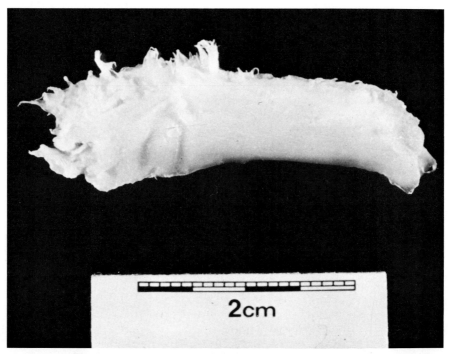

Fig. 10.19 A bucket-handle fragment of meniscus removed intact

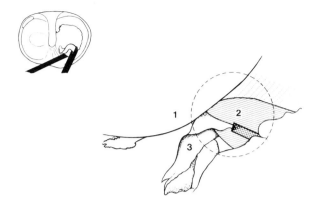

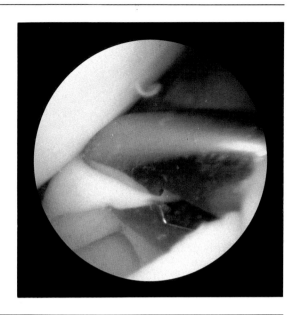

Fig. 10.20 Having divided a bucket-handle fragment of medial meniscus posteriorly, the fragment (3) is grasped with pituitary rongeurs (2) at its anterior attachment; medial femoral condyle (1)

escape in this way, it can either be fished out of the postero-medial compartment with a blunt hook from the antero-medial or central approach, or it can be removed neatly with curved rongeurs from the postero-medial approach under control of the arthroscope passed through the intercondylar notch.

Both these techniques may be impossible if the fragment is so tightly jammed in the front of the femoral condyle that the blade of the scissors cannot be insinuated between the fragment and the condyle. If this is a problem, the fragment can be divided at its centre with a knife and the two ends removed piecemeal (Fig. 10.24), or the fragment can be put back in the medial gutter and divided at each end.

Detached bucket-handle fragments These fragments, which can be regarded as bucket-handle fragments with one attachment already divided, can either be avulsed or divided at their base from the antero-medial route. If the guillotine or scissors are used rather than rongeurs, special care must be taken to prevent the fragment escaping as a loose body.

Type III tears There is no easy way of dealing with

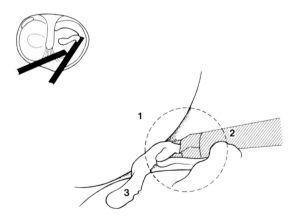

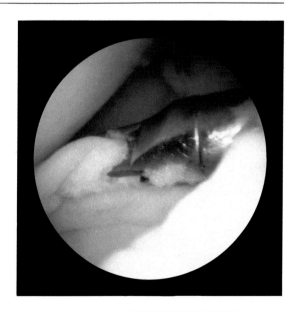

Fig. 10.21 A detached bucket-handle fragment of medial meniscus (3) is divided with the arthroscopic guillotine (2) as it lies beneath the medial femoral condyle (1)

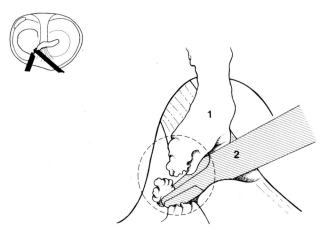

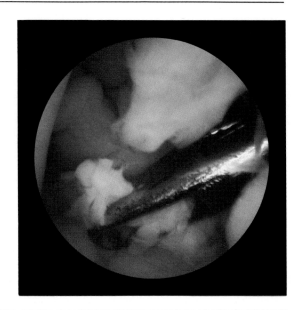

Fig. 10.22 A lateral meniscal fragment (1), having been detached posteriorly, is then detached anteriorly with the punch scissors (2) to create a loose body which floated off to the postero-medial compartment and proved difficult to remove

concealed (type III) fragments or posterior third menisco-synovial separations. The fragment cannot be reached directly across the joint between tibial and femoral condyles unless the joint is unusually lax, and attempts to remove fragments by a frontal assault are bound to damage articular cartilage. Neither end of the tear is visible, the fragment lies in the least accessible part of the knee, it cannot be dislocated into the joint, and the postero-medial approach is unhelpful except to confirm the diagnosis.

These problems can be reduced, but not eliminated, by accurate placement of the arthroscope and instruments, and correct manipulation of the knee. For a tear of the posterior third, the instruments should be inserted immediately above the anterior horn of the meniscus, about 1 cm medial to the edge of the patellar tendon so that they lie flat on the tibial plateau (Fig. 4.7). The blunt hook can then be slipped under the meniscus just in front of the femoral condyle, slid sideways behind the condyle, and turned so that its tip lies in the tear to pull the

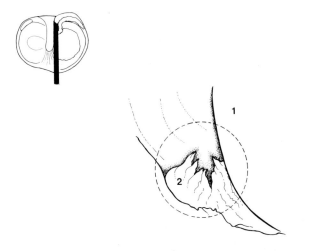

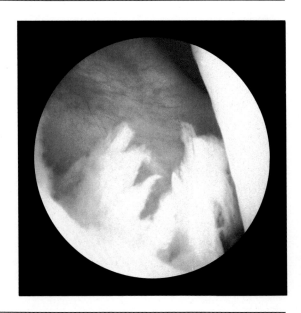

Fig. 10.23 A large fragment of medial meniscus (2) lying in the postero-medial compartment behind the medial femoral condyle (1)

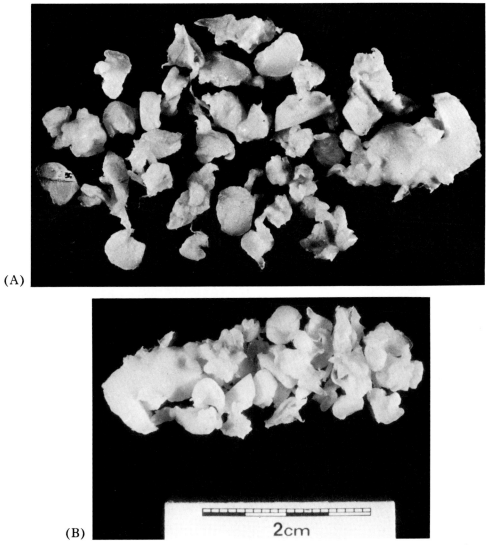

(A)

(B)

2cm

Fig. 10.24 (A) Fragments of meniscus removed piecemeal and (B) reassembled to demonstrate the volume of meniscus removed

fragment forward, while a strong valgus and external rotation force is applied to the tibia. The fragment usually stays dislocated and can either be divided at its posterior and anterior attachments or removed piecemeal. If it slips back under the femoral condyle, the attachments must be divided with the fragment reduced, using either a retractable knife or a guillotine.

Partial-thickness tears Excision of the mobile segment arising from a partial-thickness posterior third tear is even more difficult, because the fragment cannot be brought within range of the operating instruments.

If the tear has extended well through the meniscus so that the line of cleavage can be identified with a probing hook from the upper surface, the hook can be pushed through into the plane of cleavage and used to complete the tear by pulling the fragment forwards. The tear can then be removed like any other concealed (type III) tear of the meniscus.

If the split has not extended far enough to be completed with a hook, but the fragment is still mobile, the guillotine or a backward-cutting knife can be used to divide the fragment at its anterior limit. The fragment can then be grasped with forceps or rongeurs and pulled forwards so that it 'tears along the dotted line' and becomes a posteriorly based tag, which can be removed in the usual way. This method has the disadvantage that if the fragment does not tear as expected, either it must be removed with small nibblers passed between the tibia and femur, which is impossible in all but the loosest knees, or the plane of cleavage must be developed with a knife inserted from the postero-medial approach, so that the fragment can be removed as if a total meniscectomy were being performed (p. 133).

Using the operating arthroscope

To remove a bucket-handle fragment with the operating arthroscope, the diagnostic arthroscope is removed from the antero-lateral approach and the operating arthroscope inserted from the antero-medial. The fragment is then held with forceps inserted from the antero-lateral approach so that it cannot fall back into the postero-medial compartment; it is lifted with slight tension, and the posterior attachment is divided with the scissors of the operating arthroscope (see Fig. 10.28). Division of the anterior attachment is then simple.

This technique is effective, but requires some skill with the operating arthroscope. Disadvantages include the risk that excessive traction will be applied to the fragment so that the cut extends more deeply than the original tear, and there is the practical problem that the scissors and basket forceps have a short working life and need frequent replacement. The technique and the disadvantages of the operating arthroscope are well described by Sprague (1982).

Triple puncture technique

If the central approach is used, the arthroscope can be left in situ throughout the procedure and instruments inserted from both antero-medial and antero-lateral approaches. Controlling three instruments is more difficult than two, but the technique allows large instruments to be used to cut the meniscus from the side, instead of relying upon the delicate instruments of the operating arthroscope, which can only be moved parallel with the telescope.

To remove a locked bucket-handle fragment using this technique, the fragment is grasped from the antero-lateral route and its anterior attachment divided with a knife inserted from the antero-medial route (Fig. 10.25). A fragment of meniscus now detached anteriorly and still held with grasping forceps is then divided under tension at its posterior attachment (Figs. 10.26, 10.27). The fragment is easier to divide if it is first twisted with the grasping forceps. The lateral mid-patellar approach can also be used as an alternative to the central approach for the triple puncture technique and avoids violation of the patellar tendon. The techniques for removing bucket-handle fragments are summarised in Figure 10.28.

Powered-instrument technique

The meniscus has a grain of parallel fibres which is easier to follow with hand-operated instruments than

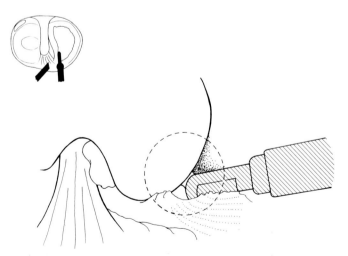

Fig. 10.25 Dividing the anterior attachment of a locked bucket-handle fragment of meniscus using the central approach for the triple puncture technique

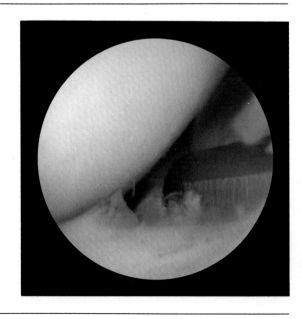

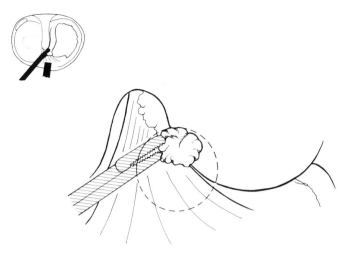

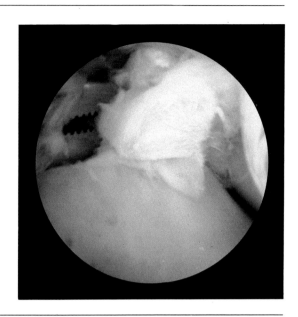

Fig. 10.26   The bucket-handle fragment of meniscus illustrated in Figure 10.25, after division of its anterior attachment. The fragment is grasped with tendon tunnelling forceps

powered cutters. The powered cutter is effective for removing flaps small enough to be sucked into the mouth of the instrument, and for trimming an irregular rim (see Fig. 10.31), but not for cutting across the grain of a bucket-handle fragment. Powered instruments are best used in conjunction with hand instruments and not instead of them.

The meniscal edger cuts meniscus well, but it cuts articular cartilage even better. The ideal instrument for removing menisci would be a wand-like tool 1 or 2 mm in diameter, which would make meniscal tissue melt away on contact with its tip, but would leave articular cartilage unscathed. Such an instrument has not yet been invented, although laser wands may prove to be effective.

Total meniscectomy

The whole of the meniscus can be removed arthroscopically by converting it into a large bucket-handle fragment (Gillquist & Oretorp 1982). The menisco-

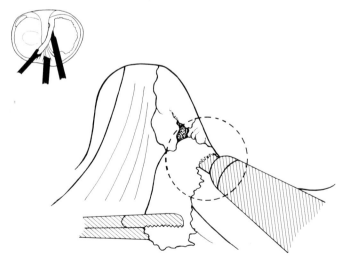

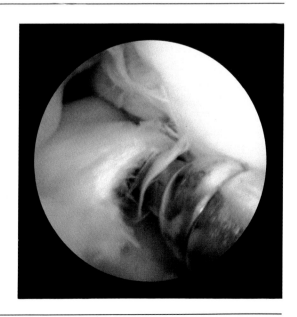

Fig. 10.27   Dividing the posterior attachment of the fragment illustrated in Figures 10.25 and 10.26, while traction is applied

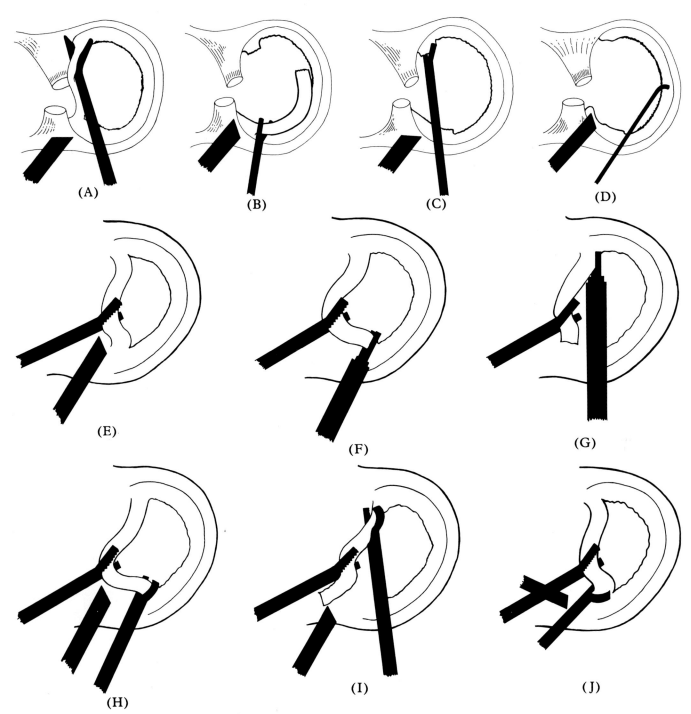

Fig. 10.28 Techniques for removing bucket-handle fragments. Double puncture technique: (A) dividing the posterior attachment; (B) dividing the anterior attachment; (C) trimming the posterior rim; (D) checking the rim with a hook to confirm its integrity. Operating arthroscope technique: (E) the fragment is grasped with forceps inserted from the antero-medial approach, with the arthroscope at the antero-lateral approach; (F) the arthroscope is exchanged for the operating arthroscope and the anterior attachment divided; (G) with the fragment under tension, the posterior attachment is divided. Triple puncture technique: (H) the arthroscope is inserted centrally and the anterior attachment divided with scissors from the antero-lateral approach; (I) the posterior horn is divided under tension with scissors; (J) an alternative triple puncture technique using the arthroscope inserted from the lateral mid-patellar approach

synovial junction is incised, beginning anteriorly, using a knife and carrying the cut as far back in the medial gutter as possible. The arthroscope is then passed through the notch into the postero-medial compartment, and the knife inserted from the postero-medial approach.

The cut is made through intact, healthy meniscal tissue and difficulty can be encountered at several points. First, the junction of the posterior and middle thirds of meniscus, where the superior menisco-synovial junction ends and the popliteus tendon lies in the lateral compartment, is difficult to reach from either the postero-medial or antero-medial approaches with anything except a curved knife passed along the medial gutter and used under control of a 70° arthroscope passed through the intercondylar notch. Damage to the medial collateral ligament can occur, but can be avoided (Gillquist & Boeryd 1982).

The second difficulty is encountered when cutting the posterior third of the meniscus, which tends to slide beneath the knife. Firm downward-cutting movements with a sharp blade are more effective than a sawing action, and a backward-cutting knife is also helpful. Scissors can be used to divide the last few fibres, when the fragment is almost free, but until the space has been created with a knife, there is seldom enough space to admit the blade of a pair of scissors. When the cut has been started, the meniscus is mobilised right up to its posterior attachment, dislocated into the notch and removed in the same way as any other large bucket-handle fragment.

If the principles of conservative meniscal surgery are followed, the indications for this procedure are confined to the removal of shattered menisci, menisci with totally disrupted rims, and cystic degeneration – all conditions in which piecemeal excision is easiest. Despite the narrow indications, the technique is important because it makes arthroscopic meniscectomy available to surgeons who still prefer total to partial meniscectomy, and even to those who consider that removing a normal meniscus is a justifiable procedure rather than a surgical blunder.

Checking the rim

When the fragment has been removed, the rim can be trimmed and checked to make certain that all loose material has gone. To know when the rim has been correctly trimmed requires judgement and can be the most difficult stage of the operation.

The aim of operation should be to remove the offending fragment of meniscus and leave a healthy rim of stable meniscus, rather than paint the lily by removing insignificant scraps and damaging the articular cartilage in the process. The step at the anterior extent of a circumferential tear should be bevelled gently and will round off well with the passage of time (Fig. 10.29), but it cannot be removed completely (Fig. 10.30). The powered cutter can also be used to 'contour' the irregularities of the rim and remove debris (Fig. 10.31), but it is no more effective for this than basket forceps or rongeurs.

When trimming is completed, the rim must again be examined carefully with the hook in the usual way to make certain that it is still stable (Fig. 10.32).

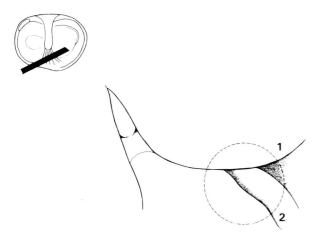

Fig. 10.29 The appearance of a medial meniscus (2) 12 months after removal of an incomplete (type II) tear of the medial meniscus. The step in the meniscus has become smooth, but the posterior part of the meniscus is narrower than the anterior part; medial femoral condyle (1)

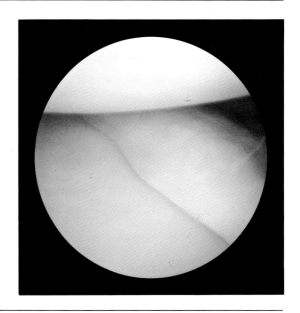

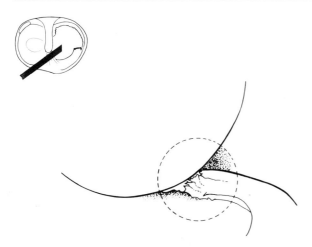

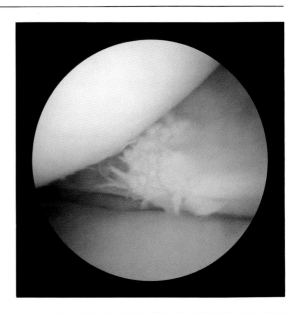

Fig. 10.30 The stump left after division of the anterior attachment of a bucket-handle fragment of medial meniscus involving almost the whole width of the medial meniscus

Special care should be taken not to cut too deeply into the meniscus and cause needless damage to an intact and stable meniscal rim, which can only add to the severity of the original lesion. Although a rim may look irregular, particularly in the posterior third, obsessional attempts to trim it to symmetrical perfection are likely to damage the articular cartilage (Fig. 5.5) and it is better to leave remodelling to nature (Fig. 10.29). As William Shakespeare commented:

There's a divinity that shapes our ends,
Rough-hew them how we will.

(Hamlet, V.ii)

Lost fragments

If the meniscal fragment is divided at both ends and escapes, it must be searched for and removed like any other loose body (p. 86). Sometimes the fragment will escape into the subcutaneous tissues,

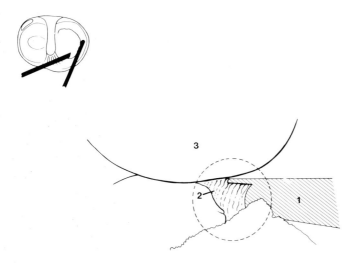

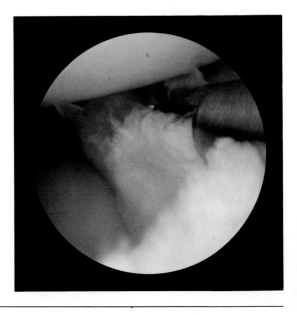

Fig. 10.31 Trimming an irregular meniscal rim (2) using the Stryker shaver (1); medial femoral condyle (3)

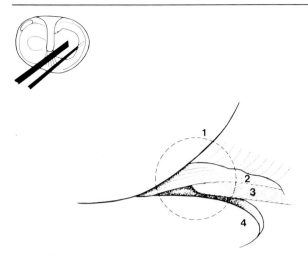

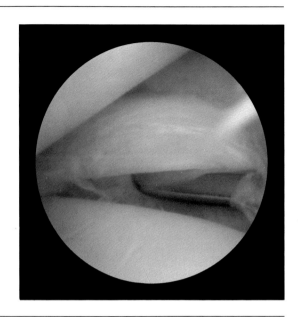

Fig. 10.32 Checking the integrity of the remaining meniscal rim (2) using a blunt hook (3); medial femoral condyle (1), medial tibial plateau (4)

and it has been known to enter the pre-patellar bursa. If the fragment cannot be found after a prolonged search and there is no sign of it in the knee, it is far better to close the wounds and await developments than persevere with the operation. The fragment will usually show itself in the subcutaneous tissues or bursa once the swelling has settled, and can be removed through one of the arthroscopy wounds or a small skin incision under local anaesthetic as an out-patient procedure.

FLAPS

Identifying the anatomy

Flaps can be divided into the following groups:

1. horizontal flaps from the superior surface
2. horizontal flaps from the inferior surface
3. flaps tucked under the body of the meniscus
4. degenerate flaps.

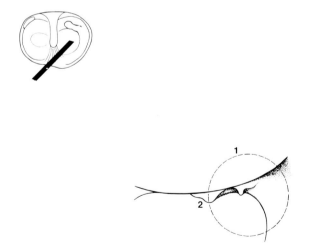

Fig. 10.33 A flap of medial meniscus just visible below the medial femoral condyle (1); medial tibial plateau (2)

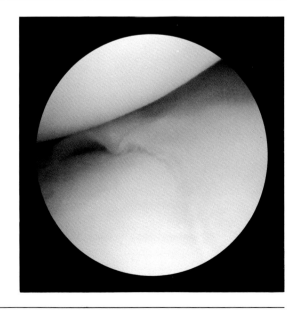

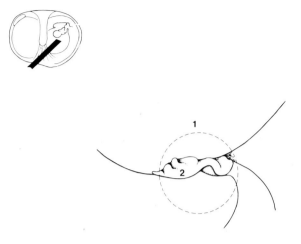

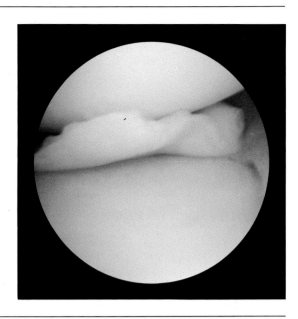

Fig. 10.34 The flap shown in Figure 10.33 (2) is manipulated from beneath the medial femoral condyle (1) by a valgus and external rotation force

Superior flaps

Flaps on the upper surface of the meniscus (Fig. 10.1) and based anteriorly at the junction of the middle and posterior thirds of the meniscus may be inconspicuous at first, but can be exposed with a blunt hook or needle, or simply by a valgus and external rotation force (Figs. 10.33, 10.34). These flaps usually cause a sensation of catching or instability in the postero-medial part of the joint, rather than true locking. The symptoms are relieved by removal of the flap, which is usually the size of a little finger nail (see Fig. 10.42).

Inferior flaps

Flaps arising from the under-surface of the medial meniscus, which are rarer than those arising from the upper surface, are easily missed, but can be found with a percutaneous needle sweeping beneath the meniscus (Fig. 10.35).

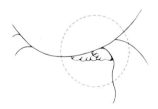

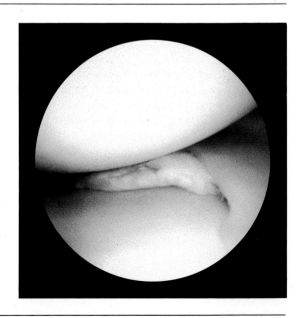

Fig. 10.35 A flap of meniscal tissue arising from the inferior surface of the posterior horn of the medial meniscus

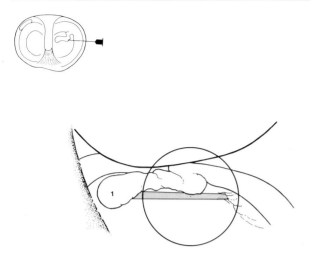

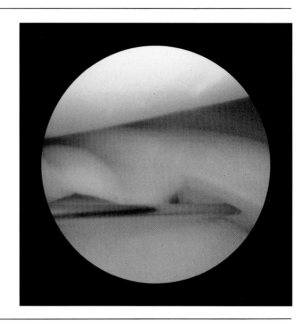

Fig. 10.36   A long fragment of medial meniscus (1) has been dislodged from beneath the meniscal rim

Inverted (tucked-under) flaps

Fragments of medial meniscus can become tucked under the posterior third of the meniscal body to cause a tender nodule on the medial joint-line; this may be so painful that the patient cannot sleep on the side, because of pressure on the joint-line, unless a pillow is placed between the knees. Clinical examination will reveal an extremely tender nodule and, at arthroscopy, the meniscus will appear to have a rounded edge (Dandy 1984). Probing with a needle or hook will reveal a stiff meniscal fragment (Fig. 10.36), turned back beneath the meniscal body and arising either from a superior flap or a type III (concealed) bucket-handle fragment ruptured at its posterior end.

Degenerate flaps

The flaps described above consist of relatively healthy meniscal tissue with one smooth and one

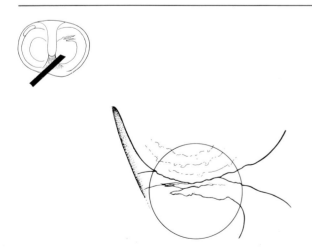

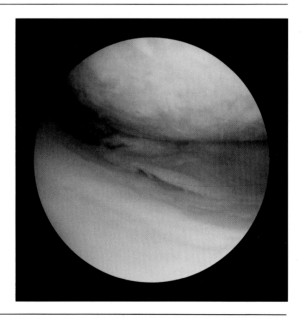

Fig. 10.37   A degenerate flap of medial meniscus. This knee has been distended with gas

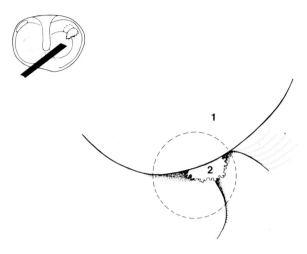

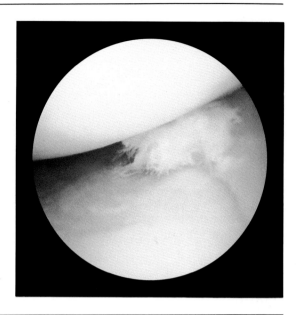

Fig. 10.38   A flap of degenerate meniscal tissue (2) arising from the upper surface of the meniscus has fallen forwards to lie beneath the medial femoral condyle (1)

irregular surface. In older patients with degenerative joint disease, the whole meniscus may be soft and disorganised, and different patterns of flap are seen. Curved oblique tears, a little like the parrot-beak tear of the lateral meniscus (Fig. 10.37), short radial tears and circumferential splits in the margin of the meniscus rather then its body all occur, and the flaps sometimes consist of a mass of fluffy degenerate tissue (Figs. 10.1, 10.38), arising from either the upper or lower surfaces of the meniscus without any specific pattern. The management of these lesions is described below (p. 127).

The shattered meniscus

Some menisci have so many splits and tears that they cannot be assigned to any category and appear as a mass of shredded meniscal tissue (Figs. 10.1, 10.39), all of which must be removed. Shattered menisci are

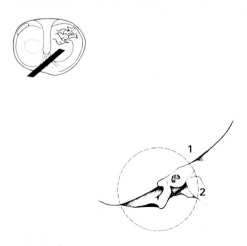

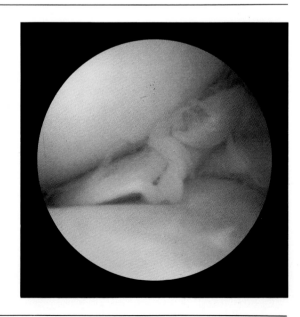

Fig. 10.39   A completely shattered medial meniscus (2) without any intact rim; medial femoral condyle (1)

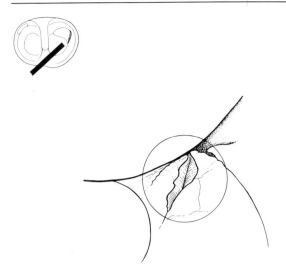

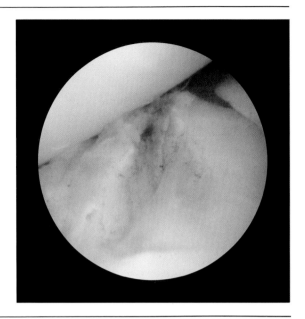

Fig. 10.40   An incision in a degenerate meniscus made with electrocautery

most commonly seen in patients with gross ligamentous instability.

Removing the fragment

Double puncture technique

Superior flaps are best removed with punch forceps, rongeurs or the electrocautery (Figs. 10.40, 10.41). Curved rongeurs, although a little large, can be slipped easily around the medial gutter to the base of the flap. Fine punch forceps are also suitable (Figs. 10.42, 10.43). When the flap has been removed, the base of the lesion can be excised with a knife or side-biting forceps until healthy tissue is reached, taking special care to remove all soft meniscal tissue, if there is any suspicion of cystic change.

Inferior flaps can be removed with basket forceps or rongeurs, but the flaps tend to fall back under the meniscus before they can be grasped. A percutaneous needle can be used to hold the flap forwards, but care must be taken not to amputate the tip of the needle as well as the flap (p. 64).

If an inverted fragment has been removed, intense

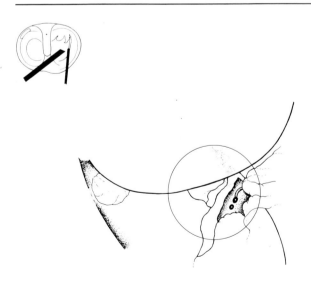

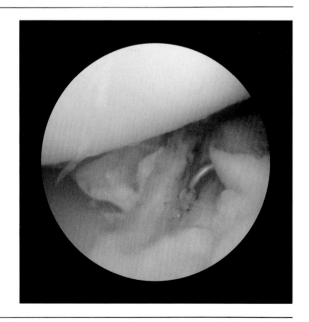

Fig. 10.41   Making the incision shown in Figure 10.40

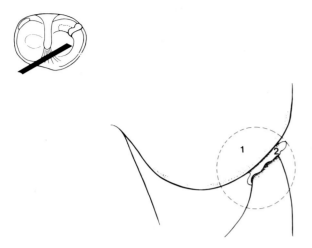

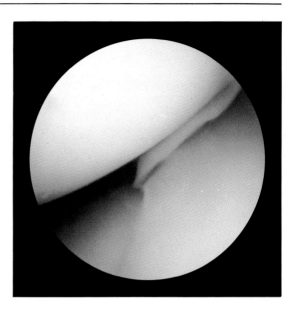

Fig. 10.42 A flap of meniscal tissue involving the upper surface of the meniscus only (2) has come forward beneath the medial femoral condyle (1) to lie in the medial gutter

localised synovitis is often seen beneath the meniscus and may account for the localised pain and tenderness that is so characteristic of this type of tear.

The completely shattered meniscus must either be removed piece by piece with rongeurs and punch forceps until there is an intact and stable rim, or a total meniscectomy performed (p. 133).

Operating arthroscope

The operating arthoscope can be used to remove a flap by applying tension with forceps and cutting its base with the scissors of the operating arthroscope, using basically the same technique as that for a bucket-handle fragment (Figs. 10.44, 10.45). This technique is effective, but requires skill with the operating arthroscope and may damage articular cartilage.

Triple puncture technique

The triple puncture technique is less effective for removing small flaps than bucket-handle fragments, because the medial gutter can be difficult to see from

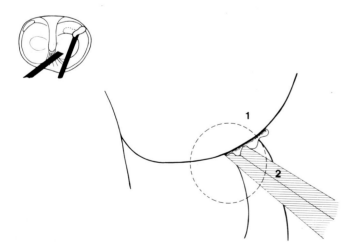

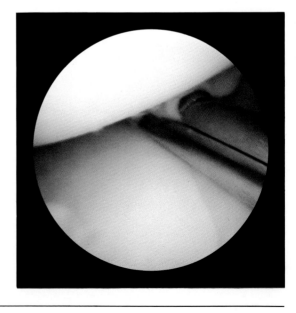

Fig. 10.43 The meniscal flap illustrated in Figure 10.42 is divided at its base with fine punch scissors (2) slipped beneath the meniscus and the medial femoral condyle (1)

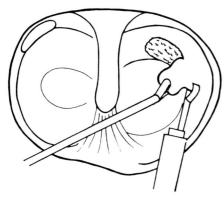

Fig. 10.44 Using the operating arthroscope to remove a flap of tissue while traction is applied with forceps inserted from the antero-lateral route

the central or lateral suprapatellar approach (Fig. 10.46), but it is entirely satisfactory for large flaps.

Checking the rim

Finally, check the rim as described above (p. 135).

OTHER LESIONS

Radial and oblique tears

In the older patient, particularly those with early osteoarthritis, radial and oblique tears of the middle third are sometimes seen which resemble the complex oblique or 'parrot-beak' tear of the lateral meniscus. These lesions do not seem to occur in the younger patient.

The degenerate meniscus

When degenerate osteoarthritis is present, the meniscus shares in the degenerative process and stability of the rim is more important than the smoothness of its surface (Figs. 10.1, 10.47). Fluffy degenerate flaps are too soft to be avulsed neatly and must be picked off carefully with fine basket forceps. Attempts to remove all loose strands of meniscal tissue can be a thankless task; as one small irregularity is removed, two more appear and the surgeon may wish that he had not become involved. By damaging the femoral condyle, attempts to achieve arthroscopic cosmesis may do more harm than good and the surgeon should avoid excessive zeal. Removing only unstable flaps or tags that are in easy reach is quite enough, and the results are most encouraging, with good results in over 80% of patients (Jackson & Rouse 1982, McBride et al 1984).

The debridement of degenerate flaps is often only part of the debridement of a degenerate knee, and may be combined with the excision of osteophytes and loose flaps of articular cartilage (p. 108).

'Cystic' menisci

Although cystic degeneration is much more common in the lateral meniscus than the medial, areas of softening and swelling are sometimes seen at the junction of the middle and posterior thirds of the medial meniscus – just at the point where the

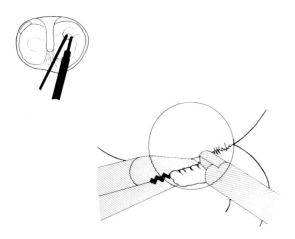

Fig. 10.45 An inferior flap of medial meniscus is grasped with forceps inserted from the antero-lateral route and divided at its base with the scissors of the operating arthroscope

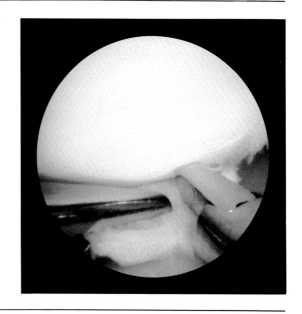

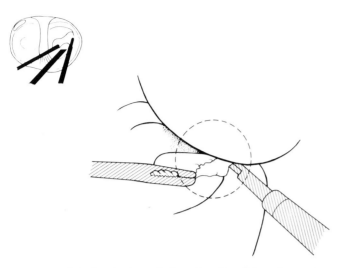

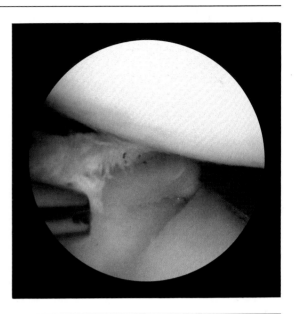

Fig. 10.46 Dividing the base of a long flap of medial meniscus using the triple puncture technique

popliteus tendon would be in the lateral compartment. This type of meniscus is associated with aching, swelling and tenderness on the posteromedial joint-line. At arthroscopy, the meniscus will be torn and the residual rim is soft and mushy. All soft meniscal tissue must be radically removed, or the symptoms will persist.

As in the lateral meniscus (p. 156), the pathology is not cystic at all, but myxoid degeneration (Fig. 10.48).

Retained posterior horn fragments

If symptoms persist after a meniscectomy, it is more likely that meniscectomy was the wrong operation than that insufficient meniscus was removed. A review of patients with persistent symptoms after meniscectomy (Dandy & Jackson 1975) showed that retained fragments were rare, and that the commonest abnormality after meniscectomy was degenerative arthritis. In the days before arthroscopy, the

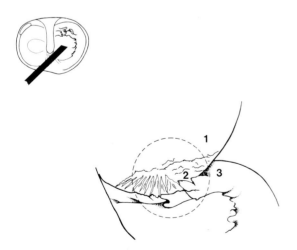

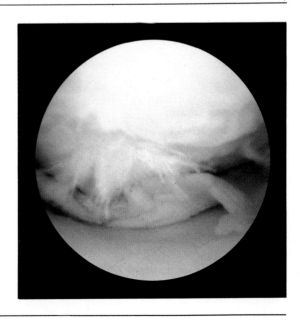

Fig. 10.47 A degenerate tear of the posterior horn of the medial meniscus (3) lying beneath an area of degenerate articular cartilage (2) on the under-surface of the medial femoral condyle (1)

and can easily be removed arthroscopically in the same way as the posterior end of a bucket-handle fragment.

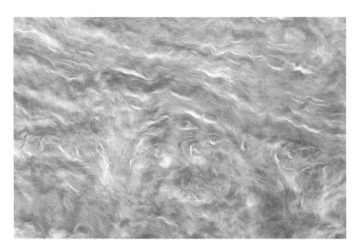

Fig. 10.48 'Cystic' degeneration of the meniscus. The appearances are of myxoid degeneration and no cysts are present

'retained fragment' offered a convenient explanation for the failure of partial meniscectomy, with the result that partial meniscectomy itself often became the scapegoat for a wrong initial diagnosis.

The open removal of retained fragments of posterior horn can be a tedious procedure involving a wide arthrotomy that yields a tatty scrap of tissue so firmly adherent to the bone that excision is difficult and its relationship to the patient's symptoms obscure. It is therefore not surprising that the results of excising retained fragments of posterior horn are unimpressive and that the long-term results have never been reported. Nevertheless, retained fragments of posterior horn do occur occasionally,

References

Barber F A, Stone R G 1985 Meniscal repair: an arthroscopic technique. Journal of Bone and Joint Surgery 67B: 39–41
Dandy D J 1982 The bucket-handle meniscal tear: a technique detaching the posterior segment first. Orthopedic Clinics of North America 13: 369–385
Dandy D J 1984 Arthroscopy of the knee: a diagnostic atlas. Gower–Butterworth, London
Dandy D J, Jackson R W 1975 The diagnosis of problems after meniscectomy. Journal of Bone and Joint Surgery 57B: 346–348
Daniel D, Daniels E, Aronson D 1982 The diagnosis of meniscus pathology. Clinical Orthopaedics and Related Research 163: 218–224
Gillquist J, Boeryd B 1982 Endoscopic total one-piece medial meniscectomy: its effect on the medial collateral ligament. Acta Orthopedica Scandinavica 53: 619–623
Gillquist J, Oretorp N 1982 The technique of endoscopic total meniscectomy. Orthopedic Clinics of North America 13:363–367
Heatley F W 1980 The meniscus – can it be repaired? An experimental investigation in rabbits. Journal of Bone and Joint Surgery 62B: 397–402
Ireland J, Trickey E L, Stoker D J 1980 Arthroscopy and arthrography of the knee: a critical review. Journal of Bone and Joint Surgery 62B: 3–6
Jackson R W, Rouse D W 1982 The results of partial meniscectomy in patients over 40 years of age. Journal of Bone and Joint Surgery 64B: 481–485
McBride G G, Constine R M, Hofmann A A, Carson R W 1984 Arthroscopic partial medial meniscectomy in the older patient. Journal of Bone and Joint Surgery 66A: 547–551
Sprague N F 1982 The bucket-handle meniscal tear. A technique using two incisions. Orthopedic Clinics of North America 13: 337–348
Stone R G 1979 Peripheral detachment of the menisci of the knee: a preliminary report. Orthopedic Clinics of North America 10:643–647
Stone R G, Nolan S E, Ryan P J 1984 Meniscus preservation. In: Grana W A (ed) Update in arthroscopic techniques, pp 53–56. Edward Arnold, London

11

Operations on the lateral meniscus

The lateral compartment differs from the medial in three important respects. First, the anterior edge of the lateral plateau lies a little lower than the medial, and the lateral tibial plateau is arched, whereas the medial plateau is concave. In consequence, instruments inserted immediately above the anterior horn of the lateral meniscus cannot reach the posterior horn, but those inserted from the antero-medial approach will do so if placed approximately 1 cm above the anterior edge of the meniscus and close to the patellar tendon. Secondly, the lateral joint space can be opened more easily than can the medial, and the tibial plateau itself is smaller, so that access to the posterior part of the meniscus is relatively simple if the point of insertion is correct. Finally, the tunnel of the popliteus tendon acts as a localised 'peripheral separation' of the meniscus and influences the pattern of tears and the shape of the meniscal fragments.

The pattern of meniscal lesions in the lateral compartment is also different, with a predominance of complex and oblique flaps involving both surfaces of the meniscus. Myxoid ('cystic') degeneration is more common in the lateral meniscus than the medial, and discoid menisci are, for practical purposes, a lesion of the lateral meniscus only. Because of these differences, lesions in the lateral compartment cannot be approached in the same way as those in the medial.

CIRCUMFERENTIAL TEARS
Identifying the anatomy
Circumferential vertical tears

Circumferential tears are less common in the lateral compartment than in the medial and follow a different pattern. Because the inner margin of the lateral meniscus is shorter than the medial, bucket-handle fragments are shorter and the yield of meniscal tissue from excision of a bucket-handle fragment is smaller.

Although the tear usually extends up to the posterior meniscal attachment or close to it, the anterior limit usually lies either at the anterior edge of the popliteus tunnel (Fig. 11.1) or at the anterior attachment of the meniscus, but not at points in between. The fragment may include the whole width of the meniscus or only part of it.

Fragments which involve the whole width of the meniscus usually affect the posterior half of the meniscus only, and acute tears of this pattern can cause bleeding from a small synovial tear at the anterior edge of the popliteus tunnel. Tears of the posterior third are not always obvious, because, although posterior third tears of the medial meniscus cause an abnormal prominence of the posterior edge in valgus and external rotation, no such prominence occurs in the lateral meniscus, and a needle or hook is needed to demonstrate the tear. The normal mobility of the lateral meniscus varies from person to person and can be difficult to judge, but a meniscus that stays dislocated when the hook is removed must be considered pathological.

Circumferential horizontal tears

Horizontal tears extending from the free edge of the meniscus to its periphery can produce a 'bucket-handle' fragment including only the upper (Fig. 11.1) or, more rarely, the lower half of the meniscus.

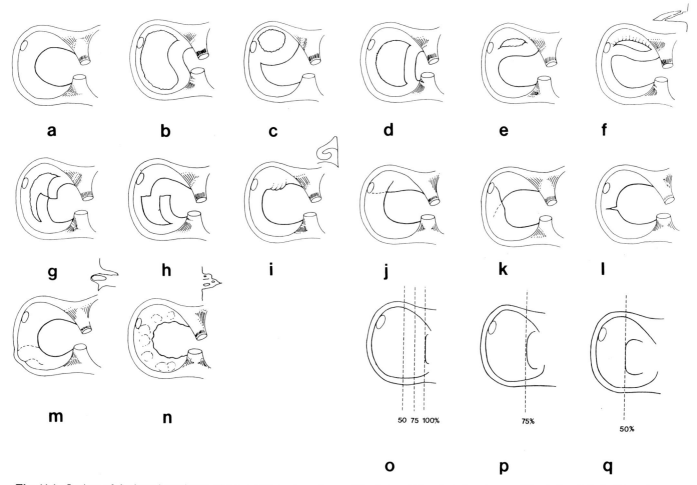

Fig. 11.1   Lesions of the lateral meniscus: (A) normal lateral meniscus; (B) whole-width, whole-length tear; (C) whole-width, half-length tear; (D) whole-length, half-width tear; (E) half-length, half-width tear; (F) half-length, half-width tear with oblique line of cleavage; (G) ruptured bucket-handle fragment; (H) anterior tag; (I) inverted posterior horn tear; (J) complex oblique (parrot-beak) tear involving the posterior portion; (K) complex oblique (parrot-beak) tear involving the mid-portion; (L) radial tear; (M) inferior flap tear of the anterior third, mimicking cyst of lateral meniscus; (N) 'cystic' (myxoid) degeneration; (O) discoid lateral meniscus to show distinction between 50%, 75% and 100% discoid menisci; (P) 75% discoid meniscus; (Q) 50% discoid meniscus

The only sign of the tear, sometimes known as a 'fish-mouth' tear, may be a horizontal fissure on the free edge of the meniscus and a hook or needle is needed to demonstrate the anatomy.

Ruptured bucket-handle tears

Unlike bucket-handle fragments of the medial meniscus, which usually become detached at or near the posterior attachment, in the lateral compartment they can break anywhere (Fig. 11.1). Fragments detached anteriorly can lie in the postero-lateral compartment and should be suspected if the lateral meniscus is unusually narrow. Tags arising from rupture of the fragment at its centre have a characteristic square end (Fig. 11.2) and occur in

pairs, one from the posterior end of the fragment and one from the anterior; both must be removed. Many other patterns, too numerous to mention, are also seen and it is best to regard each tear of this type as unique until its anatomy is clear.

Removing the fragments

Fragments involving the whole length of the meniscus

As with bucket-handle fragments in the medial compartment, the fragment can be divided at each end and removed. This is more difficult in the lateral compartment, because it is smaller than the medial, and a bucket-handle fragment firmly locked in front of the condyle occupies most of the available joint

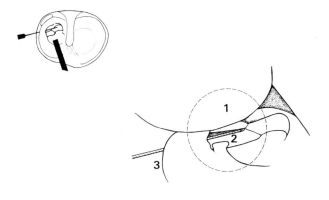

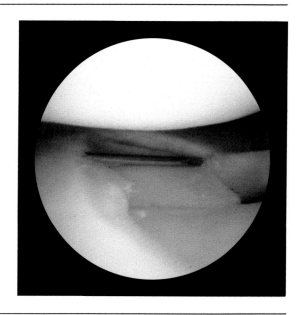

Fig. 11.2 A bucket-handle fragment of the lateral meniscus ruptured at its centre (2) lying beneath the lateral femoral condyle (1) and probed with a percutaneous needle (3)

space (Fig. 11.3). If this is a problem, the fragment can be divided at its centre as if it were a tightly locked fragment of medial meniscus (p. 129).

Narrow fragments involving only part of the meniscal width can be removed by dividing the posterior horn with scissors and avulsing the anterior attachment with rongeurs. Instruments inserted from the antero-medial approach close to the patellar tendon and above the meniscus will reach most parts of the lateral compartment, but the instruments and arthroscope may need to be transposed when the posterior attachment is divided. Full-width fragments not suitable for reattachment can also be removed in this way, but are so tough and thick that they cannot be avulsed and need to be cut at their centre and removed in pieces.

Fragments involving posterior part of meniscus only

Tears that extend only to the popliteus tunnel produce fragments that can become so tightly locked in front of the condyle that it is impossible to slip

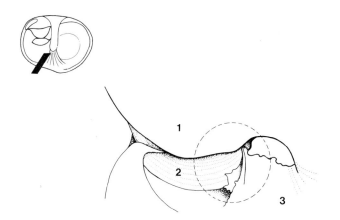

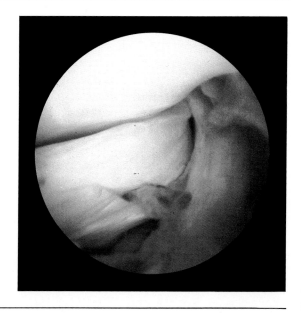

Fig. 11.3 The full thickness of the posterior half of the lateral meniscus (2) has come forward to lie beneath the lateral femoral condyle (1); anterior cruciate ligament (3)

instruments between the condyle and fragment without damaging the articular cartilage (Fig. 5.5). These fragments can be divided at the front first, leaving a long posteriorly based stub which tends to slip back into its normal position under the femoral condyle through the notch into the postero-lateral compartment or into the recess beneath the posterior horn, where they are hard to find. If a large fragment dematerialises in this way, the search must be continued with needle, hook and probe until the fragment is found (Fig. 11.4), when it can be removed like an inverted flap (p. 139) (Fig. 11.9).

Although removal of the loose fragment is still the standard treatment for such lesions, reattachment may be preferable. Even if the meniscus eventually becomes detached and needs to be removed later, the articular cartilage will at least have been protected for a few more years of active life.

Horizontal circumferential tears

Partial-thickness horizontal bucket fragments can be removed in the same way as those involving the whole thickness of the meniscus. The initial division of the fragment is more difficult, however, and care must be taken not to divide the rim completely and produce an unstable rim.

Ruptured bucket-handle fragments

As in the medial compartment, ruptured bucket-handle fragments can be removed by the double puncture technique or the operating arthroscope with the fragment under tension, but it is better to use rongeurs (Fig. 11.5) or punch forceps than fiddle with the tunnel vision and feeble instruments of the operating arthroscope.

Checking the rim

The stability of the rim must be checked carefully, with special attention to the popliteus tunnel. If the tear involves the whole thickness of the meniscus, the popliteus tendon will be exposed without any bridge of tissue crossing it so that the rim of the meniscus is completely functionless.

In these circumstances, the remaining meniscus must be trimmed back to leave a smooth crescent, but it is not necessary to remove every crumb of meniscal tissue. Provided that no unstable tags remain, a firm and even rim is perfectly acceptable and will offer some protection to the underlying articular surface.

If there is a good bridge of intact tissue across the tendon (Fig. 11.6), trimming the rim must be kept to an absolute minimum. It is easy for the bridge to be divided completely by overenthusiastic trimming, and even for the popliteus tendon to be damaged (Fig. 11.7). Irregularities of the rim behind and in front of the popliteus tunnel can be trimmed firmly back to healthy tissue without worry, but a slender popliteus bridge is worth preserving and it is better

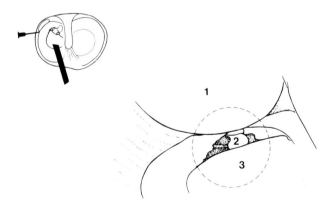

Fig. 11.4 A flap tear of lateral meniscus (2) has slipped backwards beneath the lateral femoral condyle (1) and behind the lateral tibial plateau (3), and is manipulated with a percutaneous needle

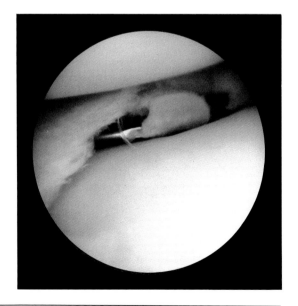

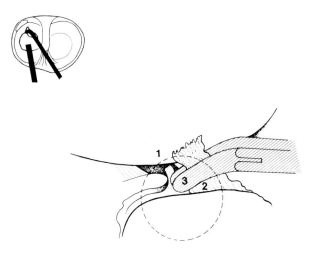

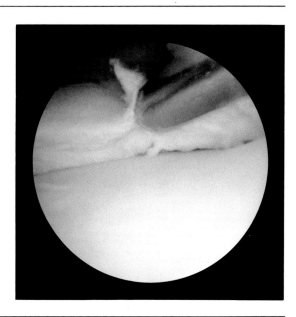

Fig. 11.5 Trimming the fragments of a torn lateral meniscus (2) using curved pituitary rongeurs (3) opposite the popliteus tunnel; lateral femoral condyle (1)

to leave the bridge a little rough than risk dividing it completely.

FLAPS AND TAGS

Identifying the anatomy

Flaps and tags in the lateral compartment differ radically from those in the medial compartment, with a rich profusion of oblique tears based on the popliteus tunnel.

Anterior tags

Anteriorly based tags can arise from a vertical split in the meniscus that runs backwards into a radial tear, creating a fragment that can cause locking and clicking out of all proportion to its size (Fig. 11.1). Exact definition of the anatomy of these lesions can be difficult, because the fragment lies so close to the lens that it may be confused with a bucket-handle tear or even with distended synovium, but it can be defined by passing the arthroscope into the back of

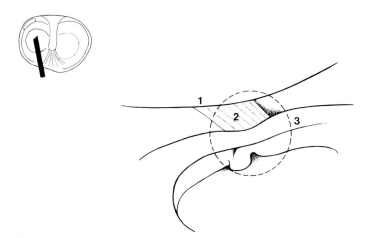

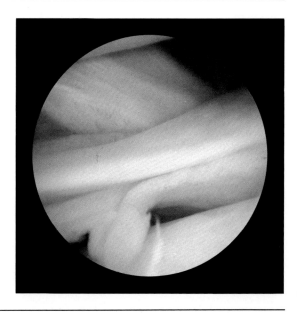

Fig. 11.6 A good bridge of lateral meniscus (3) crossing the popliteus tendon (2); lateral femoral condyle (1). Note the horizontal fissure in the centre of the lateral meniscus

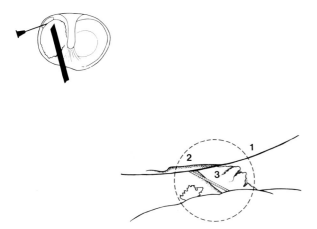

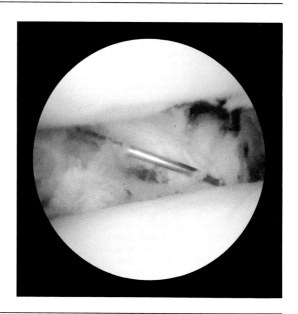

Fig. 11.7 Overenthusiastic trimming of the lateral meniscal rim has damaged the popliteus tendon (3). Longstanding degenerative change (2) is visible on the under-surface of the lateral femoral condyle (1)

the compartment and examining the free margin of the meniscus. If the sharp meniscal edge is lost in the anterior part of the joint and the tissue at the front of the joint corresponds with the defect in the meniscus, there is an anterior meniscal tag.

Posterior flaps

Horizontal or slightly oblique splits in the posterior part of the meniscus can separate a large chunk of tissue (Figs. 11.1, 11.8) attached posteriorly, but not laterally. These fragments may be thicker than the

remaining rim and, because they do not have any lateral attachment, are very mobile. In some patients, the flap becomes inverted and presents a rounded margin (Fig. 11.9), an obvious indication of a concealed flap. The flap is likely to be stiff and will be difficult to extract.

Oblique flap tears and complex oblique tears

Most flaps in the lateral compartment result from tears that run obliquely through the meniscal substance from above and behind to below anter-

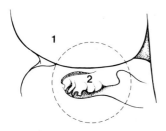

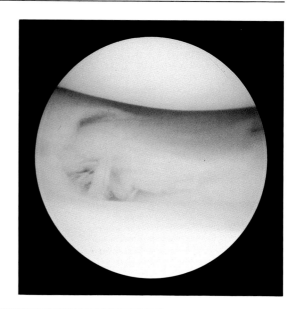

Fig. 11.8 A large flap of lateral meniscus (2) has come forward to lie beneath the lateral femoral condyle (1) as the result of a 'parrot-beak' tear entering the popliteus tunnel

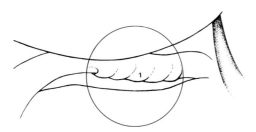

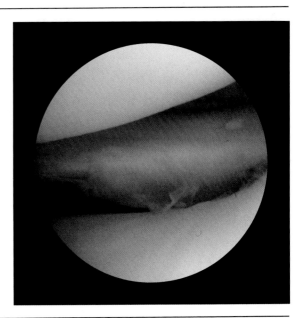

Fig. 11.9   A large flap of lateral meniscus (1) tucked back beneath the posterior horn

iorly. The split appears as a curved radial tear on the upper surface of the meniscus (Fig. 11.10) and an oblique tear on the free margin so that the two sections of meniscus slide over each other to produce the classical 'parrot-beak' appearance (Figs. 11.11, 11.12).

The behaviour of the flap is dictated by the position of the tear and its relationship to the popliteus tunnel. If the lower and anterior end of the tear lies opposite the popliteus tunnel, the flap will be free to move in and out of the joint (Fig. 11.1), but

if the split on the lower surface lies in front of the popliteus tunnel, the flap will be tethered to the lateral side of the knee at its anterior edge (Fig. 11.1) and will not be able to move into the centre of the joint.

Very occasionally, the split on the upper surface of the meniscus lies in front of the popliteus tunnel without extending through to the lower surface, producing a thin sliver of meniscus skived off its upper surface.

Apart from the relationship of the flap to the

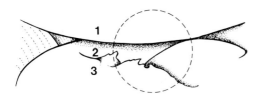

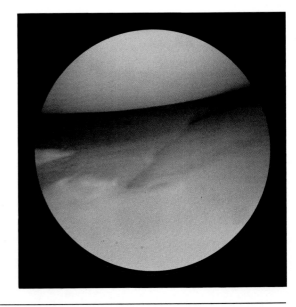

Fig. 11.10   A tear (2) in the lateral meniscus (3) lying anterior to the popliteus tunnel is tethered so that it cannot move into the joint space; lateral femoral condyle (1)

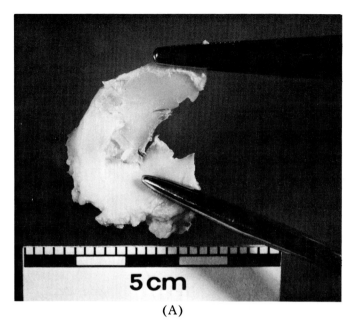

(A)

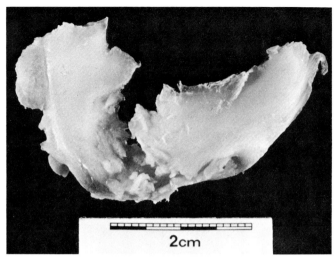

Fig. 11.12   The inferior surface of the meniscus shown in Figure 11.11, demonstrating the complete rupture of the meniscal rim on the inferior surface

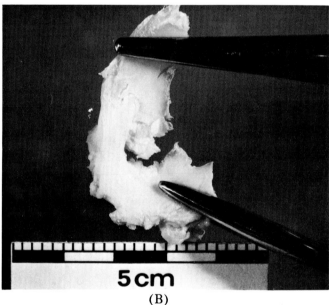

(B)

Fig. 11.11   (A) 'Parrot-beak' tear of the lateral meniscus held in the anatomical position; (B) the meniscus opened to demonstrate the plane of cleavage extending into the popliteus tunnel

popliteus tunnel, these tears also vary according to their lateral extent, some extending right through the rim and some only part of the way. It is important to determine the lateral extent of the tear before operating instruments are inserted.

Radial tears

Small radial splits on the free margin of the lateral meniscus and in its mid-portion are sometimes found unexpectedly and are hard to relate to the patient's symptoms (Fig. 11.1). These lesions may represent the beginnings of a parrot-beak tear. Although there is no evidence that these tears cause symptoms or that cutting them back to their base stops them extending, the procedure is simple and unlikely to cause harm. The tear should be cut with basket forceps or punch forceps until its base is reached, and no further. The edge of the defect is then trimmed to leave a gently curving meniscal margin, taking no more tissue than absolutely necessary and preserving the articular surface.

The 'shattered' lateral meniscus

Apart from the tears described above, multiple splits also occur and leave a tattered fringe of torn meniscal tissue for which the only solution is total meniscectomy. When such a meniscus is found, it can either be removed piecemeal or en bloc by total meniscectomy (p. 133). With either technique, special care must be taken not to damage articular cartilage, while removing the last scrap of degenerate tissue.

Removing the fragment and checking the rim

Tears extending completely through the meniscus into the popliteus tunnel on both upper and lower surfaces sever the rim of the meniscus completely, leaving no alternative to trimming back as much of

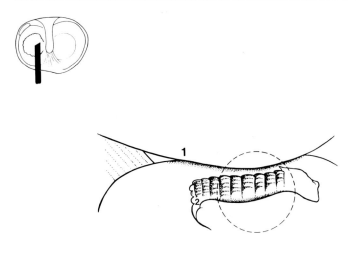

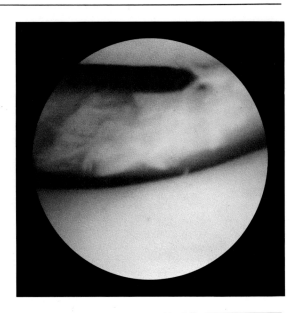

Fig. 11.13 The trimmed rim of a lateral meniscal tear (2) involving part of the meniscal thickness only; lateral femoral condyle (1)

the meniscus as possible both anteriorly and posteriorly. If, however, the tear extends only part of the way through the rim the meniscus can be trimmed back cautiously until the base of the tear is exposed and a gently curving rim is achieved (Fig. 11.13). As with circumferential tears, it is easy to enter the popliteus tunnel and divide the rim completely by misplaced enthusiasm.

Flaps in the posterior third should be dealt with by removing the flap first and then assessing the rim.

If a bridge of healthy tissue is left crossing the popliteus tunnel, the edges can be trimmed lightly, preserving as much of the peripheral rim as possible, but if no such bridge is present, the remaining tissue should be trimmed back firmly to leave a smooth edge.

Partial-thickness flaps raised from the upper surface of the meniscus in its anterior third are best treated by gentle trimming with fine punch forceps or side biters. An alternative is to grasp the free edge

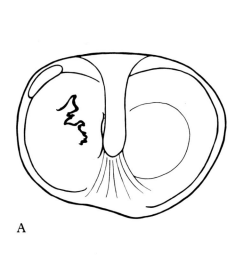

A

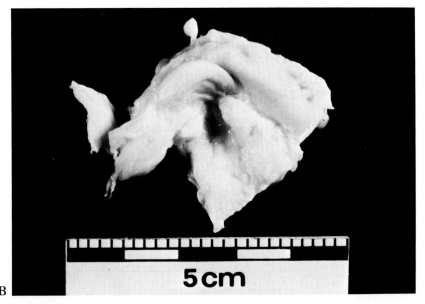

B

Fig. 11.14 (A) A tear of a lateral discoid meniscus involving the upper surface only; (B) a specimen obtained by open meniscectomy

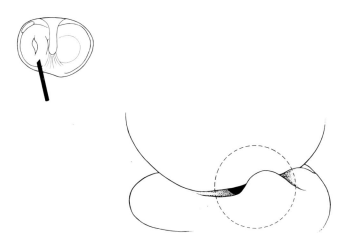

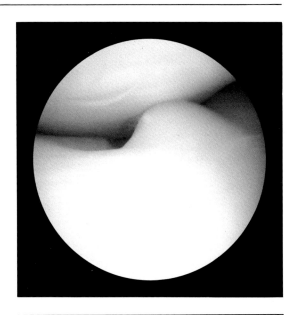

Fig. 11.15 A tear involving the full thickness of a discoid lateral meniscus, with the mobile fragment lying in the intercondylar notch and seen from the antero-lateral approach

of the flap with curved rongeurs and peel the flap back to the anterior meniscal attachment.

OTHER LESIONS

Discoid menisci

It is strange that the incidence of discoid menisci reported in cadaver studies, usually in the region of 7% (Fahmy et al 1983), is less than the incidence found at arthroscopy. Although some discoid menisci may escape notice, this cannot be the whole answer because the absence of a margin to the lateral meniscus is very easy to detect. A more likely explanation is that the incomplete discoid menisci, covering half or three-quarters of the plateau, are recorded as 'broad' menisci at arthroscopy, but 'discoid' at autopsy. This possibility can be investi-

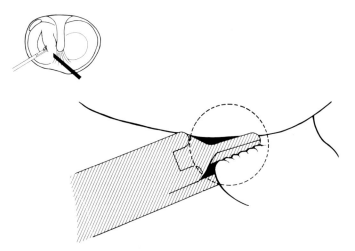

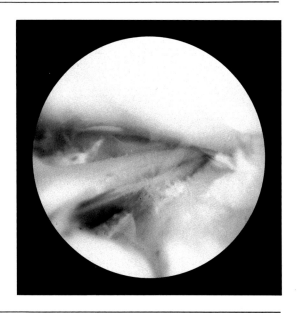

Fig. 11.16 Cutting the anterior attachment of the fragment shown in Figure 11.15, using scissors inserted from the antero-lateral approach, and with the arthroscope inserted from the antero-medial approach

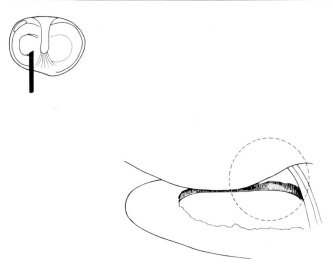

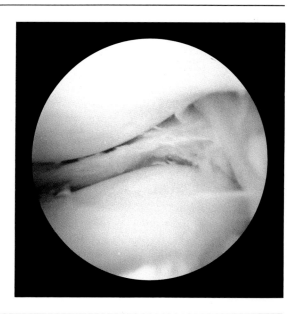

Fig. 11.17   The rim of the meniscus shown in Figure 11.15 after removal of the mobile fragment

gated by recording the approximate percentage of the tibial plateau covered by the meniscus as 50%, 75% or 100% (Fig. 11.1).

An intact discoid meniscus may cause nothing more than asymptomatic loss of extension, but lateral meniscectomy can be followed by osteoarthrosis. The knee with an intact discoid meniscus has a far better future than a knee with no lateral meniscus at all, and a discoid meniscus should not be excised unless the symptoms are bad enough to warrant operation.

Symptoms can be caused by at least three lesions.

In the first, the upper or lower surface of the meniscus tears to produce irregular flaps (Fig. 11.14) and clefts that do not penetrate the full meniscal thickness. In the second, a split develops in the centre of the meniscus to create a fragment that is effectively an enormous locked bucket-handle fragment (Figs. 11.1, 11.15). The third type is a horizontal split in the centre of the meniscus that does not break its surface; this pattern may be a precursor of the other two types of tear.

All three types can be treated by excising the central portion of the meniscus to leave an intact rim, starting in the intercondylar notch and working laterally. Division of the anterior attachment and working outwards from the central defect is an alternative (Fig. 11.16). The aim of excision should be, as always, an intact and stable rim, but with the difference that the resulting rim will be the same width as a normal meniscus (Fig. 11.17). The operation is not difficult, provided that it is done carefully and methodically.

'Cystic' degeneration

'Cystic' degeneration causes pain, tenderness and swelling along the lateral joint-line and a dull toothache-like pain at night, rather than the mechanical symptoms of a meniscal tear (Fig. 11.18).

The arthroscopic appearance of cystic degeneration is often unremarkable. A few small fissures may

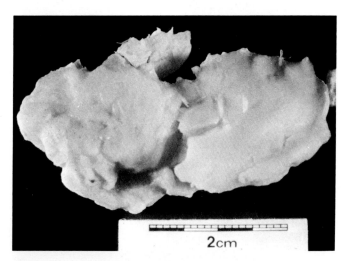

2cm

Fig. 11.18   A lateral meniscus affected by cystic degeneration (removed by open meniscectomy)

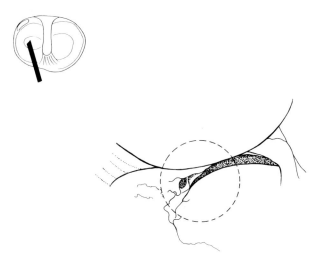

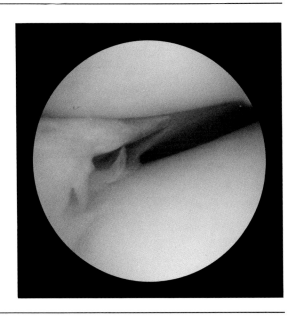

Fig. 11.19   Cystic degeneration of the lateral meniscus

be noted and the usually smooth knife-like edge will be blunted so that the meniscus presents a swollen and somewhat bloated appearance (Fig. 11.19). Although the arthroscopic appearance may be unhelpful, the clinical features of pain, joint-line tenderness and swelling should have suggested the diagnosis long before the patient reached the operating theatre.

Cystic menisci do not split along the grain of their fibres in the same way as healthy menisci with a single tear, and the tissue has a soft and slightly 'springy' feel. Excision is a matter of patient persistence and painstaking piecemeal excision, removing all loose tissue until either a firm rim or the menisco-synovial junction is reached.

Histologically, the appearances are not cystic, but myxoid. The description of 'cystic' is hallowed by time and tradition, but is incorrect and has caused much confusion.

Lateral flap tears

The majority of isolated swellings 1–2 cm in diameter on the lateral joint-line are the result of a tear involving the inferior surface of the meniscus rather than a cyst. These lesions may account for the high incidence of tears associated with cysts (Wroblewski 1973). The fragments are based anteriorly and slip laterally to lie in front of the popliteus tendon, where they can be felt as a swelling on the joint-line

(Fig. 11.20). These swellings, which can be made to disappear by pushing the flap medially with the thumb while the knee is in varus, reappear with a valgus and rotational strain.

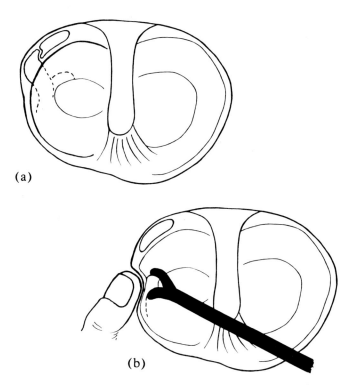

Fig. 11.20   (A) The position of an inferior flap of lateral meniscus mimicking a solitary cyst of the meniscus; (B) the position of the rongeurs for the removal of such a flap

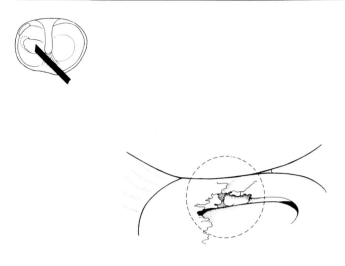

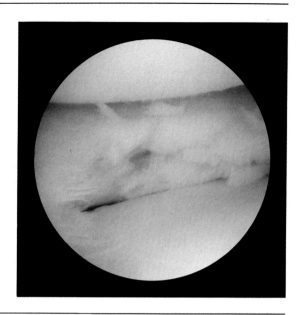

Fig. 11.21 The appearance of the lateral meniscus after excision of an inferior flap simulating a solitary cyst

The fragments can be removed with curved rongeurs inserted from the antero-medial approach, if necessary helping the fragment into the jaws with external finger pressure (Fig. 11.20) to leave a meniscus intact on its upper surface, but with a defect on its inferior surface (Fig. 11.21). An alternative technique is to pass an operating instrument directly beneath the meniscus into the meniscal defect, which is first identified carefully with a percutaneous needle (Fig. 11.22). The arthroscope can be passed through the same incision after the flap has been removed, but it is important to hold the knee quite still after removing the operating instrument so that the incisions in the ilio-tibial tract and joint capsule do not move relative to each other. From this submeniscal approach, there is a clear view of the anterior cruciate ligament and the anterior part of the lateral compartment. This

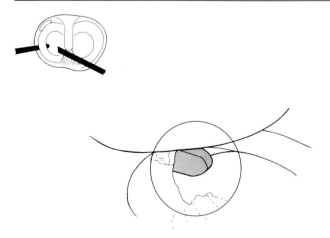

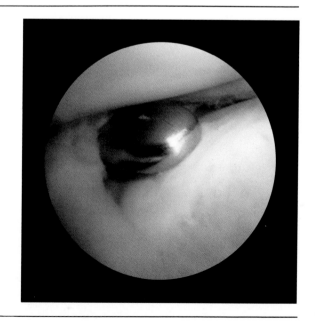

Fig. 11.22 The lateral submeniscal approach. Rongeurs have been passed under the meniscal body to remove an inferior flap tear. The instrument seen is a 70° arthroscope inserted from the antero-medial approach

approach offers an interesting view of the joint from an unusual angle, but is not required for diagnostic arthroscopy.

Both the joint-line swelling and the patient's symptoms disappear after this procedure, but only a long-term study will show if the lesions recur.

Solitary cysts

If the joint-line swelling does not disappear with a little thumb pressure and a varus strain and the meniscus has a clean sharp edge, the swelling is probably a true mucoid cyst of the meniscus, little different from a ganglion. The cyst can be exposed through a short transverse incision splitting the ilio-tibial tract in the direction of its fibres. The cyst can then be excised and its bed curetted without disturbing the intact fibres of the meniscus. Recurrence is unusual (Flynn & Kelly 1976). Rehabilitation after such a limited excision is much simpler and swifter than after a formal arthrotomy, but slower than after arthroscopic meniscectomy.

References

Fahmy N R M, Williams E A, Noble J 1983 Meniscal pathology and osteoarthrosis of the knee. Journal of Bone and Joint Surgery 65B: 24–28

Flynn M, Kelly J P 1976 Local excision of cystic lateral meniscus of the knee without recurrence. Journal of Bone and Joint Surgery 58B: 88–89

Ikeuchi H 1982 Arthroscopic treatment of the discoid lateral meniscus. Technique and long term results. Clinical Orphopaedics and Related Research 167: 19–28

Wroblewski B M 1973 Trauma and the cystic meniscus: review of 500 cases. Injury 4: 319–321

12

Arthroscopy in the management of ligament injuries

A SIMPLIFIED APPROACH TO LIGAMENT LESIONS

Many surgeons find the classification of ligament injuries difficult to understand and unnecessarily complicated, often because of attempts to impose an unnaturally rigid classification upon injuries that are very variable (Dejour et al 1984). A further difficulty is that, once understood, ideas of ligamentous instability change so fast that it is hard to keep pace with either current thinking or the nomenclature (Larson 1983, Lightowler 1983). The result is little short of chaos.

This chapter will offer an uncomplicated – perhaps over-simplified – approach to a difficult problem, emphasising the clinical aspects of the lesions in preference to biomechanical abstractions and replacing rigid classifications with clinical syndromes and 'customised' treatment based on the requirements of the individual patient.

Rotatory instability – a false doctrine?

Rotatory instability began as a wonderfully simple concept (Slocum & Larson 1968) based on excessive forward movement of the medial side of the tibia during the anterior drawer test. The sign was positive in patients with medial ligament injuries and strongly positive in patients with anterior cruciate tears. Undue emphasis was placed on this sign, which was in fact first described by Palmer in 1938. Palmer (1938) saw this sign in its proper perspective:

An increased rotation in flexion is actually one manifestation of the drawer sign, and consequently these two symptoms should be found in parallel. However, scarcely any special clinical significance need be attached to this.

Today, there is general agreement that the symptoms of anterior cruciate insufficiency are due to the 'pivot shift phenomenon' or 'jerk', but the importance of this was not appreciated in 1968 and undue emphasis was placed on tibial rotation. Because of this basic flaw, the concept of rotatory instability did not fit the facts and had to be modified. Antero-medial, antero-lateral, postero-medial and postero-lateral instability were invented, but these instabilities took no account of simple sideways movements and 'straight' instabilities had to be added to the classification. Even this was not enough and 'combined' instabilities were introduced, administering the *coupe de grâce* to Slocum and Larson's original simple idea.

To add to the difficulties, flexion, extension and valgus or varus movements can be seen and measured clinically or radiologically, but this is not possible for rotatory movement about the long axis of the limb which means that the rotational element of the lesion, on which the whole philosophy is based, cannot be quantified and assessment must be largely subjective. The resistance to rotatory forces can, however, be measured in the cadaver (Wang & Walker 1974), but these measurements are no help in the management of the individual patient. The result is a jungle of jargon and biomechanics that helps only those who profess to understand it.

Confusion has been compounded by the term 'lateral pivot shift', which has been misunderstood by many to mean that the axis of rotation (wherever that may be) has shifted laterally. The 'lateral pivot shift' was originally used by Dr David MacIntosh of

Toronto to describe the collapsing of the knee that occurs in patients with anterior cruciate deficiency who report that they feel the bones 'shift' when they pivot on the knee and load the lateral side of the joint (Galway et al 1972, Galway & Macintosh 1980). It is ironic that an attempt to describe a symptom should have added to the misunderstanding that surrounds rotatory instability.

The concept of rotatory instability and the thinking which goes with it has confused and muddled so many surgeons that it deserves to be abandoned. It will not be mentioned again in this chapter.

The ideal knee

As a starting point, it may be helpful to consider how the knee could be redesigned for the greatest convenience of the surgeon. The ideal knee (Fig. 12.1) would have only four types of instability; anterior or posterior displacement of the tibia on the femur and excessive valgus or varus movement. Stability would be maintained by four ligaments constructed of stout tissue that would take and hold a suture well, would have a good blood supply and would always heal soundly. One ligament would be responsible for stability in each direction; the

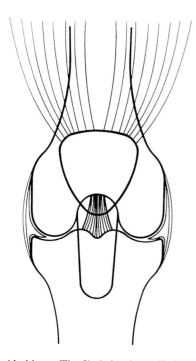

Fig. 12.1 The ideal knee. The fibula has been eliminated and the knee is symmetrical about its midline

anterior ligament would prevent abnormal anterior movement of the tibia, and the posterior ligament abnormal posterior movement. Excessive valgus movement would be prevented by the medial ligament and varus movement by the lateral.

With one ligament ruptured, the function of the others would be unaffected so that excessive anterior movement of the tibia on the femur, for example, would be due to a damaged anterior ligament alone. If two ligaments were damaged, the ideal knee would have anterior and medial instability rather than 'antero-medial' instability, which sounds more like a separate condition instead of the sum of its two component parts. To help further, the correlation between symptoms and signs would be so close that ligament injuries could be correctly diagnosed either from the patient's history or the clinical examination.

As well as the four ligaments responsible for stability, there would be two muscles. The anterior extensor muscle would be the only extensor at the knee and the posterior flexor muscle the only flexor; there would be no medial or lateral muscles. The joint would have a joint capsule, menisci, articular surface and muscles, but damage to these structures would never occur in the presence of a ligament injury. Finally, the convex femoral condyles would sit firmly upon concave tibial plateaux with the menisci deepening the concavity; the joint would be absolutely symmetrical, with the medial and lateral halves mirror images of each other.

The real knee

If we compare the ideal knee with the real knee, there are many similarities, but a few important differences. Although the anterior and posterior cruciate ligament are well placed to act as the anterior and posterior ligament respectively, they also limit valgus and varus movement when medial or lateral stability has been lost. The medial ligament, however, is correctly positioned to act like the medial ligament of the ideal knee, and injuries to it would be easy to detect, if only the anterior and posterior cruciates did not also restrict excessive valgus movement.

In contrast, the lateral ligament bears little resemblance to the ideal. The so-called lateral collateral ligament of the knee runs from the femur to the fibula and not from the femur to the tibia, is tight only when the knee is fully extended or when a varus strain is applied with the knee flexed, and may well have more to do with the stability of the superior tibio-fibular joint than the knee itself. The ilio-tibial band, a much stronger structure, is also under greatest tension when the knee is extended

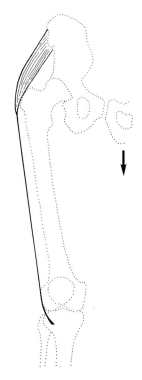

Fig. 12.2   The ilio-tibial tract, linking the tibia and pelvis, is an important stabiliser of the lateral side of the knee

and is probably a more important stabiliser of the lateral side of the knee than the feeble lateral collateral ligament (Evans 1979), even though it runs from the pelvis to the tibia and crosses two joints (Fig. 12.2). This proposition is difficult to test biomechanically in cadavers, because the tract crosses the hip as well as the knee, and because the tensor fasciae latae adds a dynamic component to an otherwise static structure.

When ligaments rupture, the real knee drifts even further from the ideal. Real ligaments do not break cleanly across their centre, but sometimes rupture part of their thickness (Fig. 12.3), or split so that the component parts slide over each other (Fig. 12.4) inside their synovial sheath and unite at a greater length than the original (Fig. 12.5), confusing the physical signs. The comparison is even worse when repair is attempted. Access to the cruciates is difficult, the torn ligament is soft, necrotic (Fig. 12.6), friable, will not hold sutures well, and even if the ends could be accurately apposed, there is no guarantee that a ligament with sutures at its centre would be of the same length or elasticity as the original, considerations which must throw doubt on the wisdom of early repair. As Hey-Groves commented in 1917, 'It is impossible to regard intra-articular suture of the ligaments either by soft sutures or by wire as an efficient procedure or as one free from the risk of leaving loose bodies in the joint.'

The medial ligament presents different problems

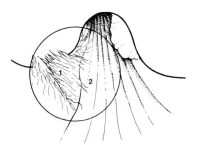

Fig. 12.3   Partial rupture of the anterior cruciate ligament. The postero-lateral band (1) is ruptured, but the antero-medial band (2) is intact

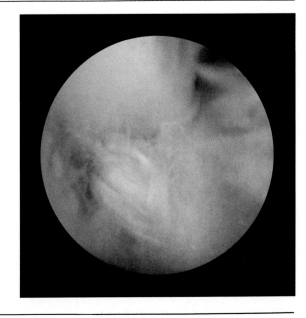

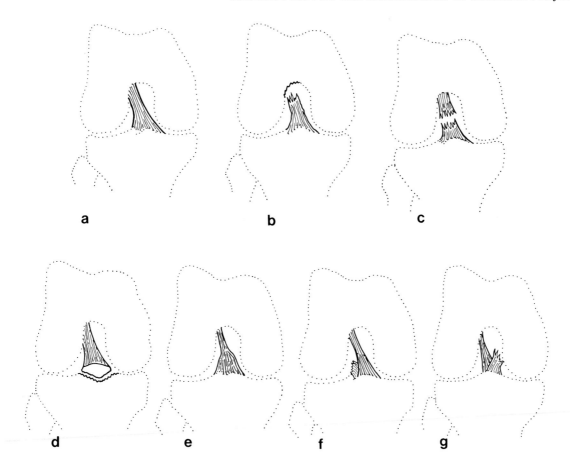

Fig. 12.4 Lesions of the anterior cruciate ligament: (A) normal; (B) avulsion from the femur; (C) mid-portion rupture; (D) avulsion from the tibia with bone block; (E) rupture within the synovial sheath; (F) rupture of the postero-lateral band; (G) rupture of the antero-medial band

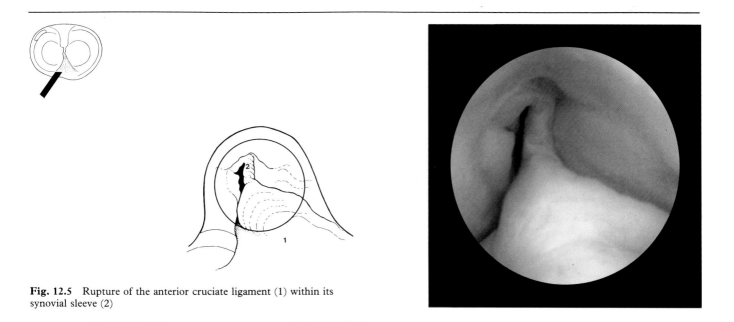

Fig. 12.5 Rupture of the anterior cruciate ligament (1) within its synovial sleeve (2)

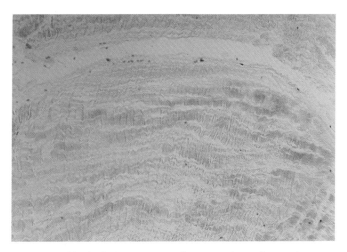

Fig. 12.6 Histological appearance of a ruptured anterior cruciate ligament. Few nuclei are visible. The ligament is dead

from the cruciates. Although exposure is easy, the tissue does not hold sutures well and the problems of restoring precise length and elasticity still apply.

The muscles around the knee are also different. There is only one extensor, but the hamstrings are divided into two groups, one medial and one lateral, and the femoral origins of the gastrocnemius affect the relative positions of the tibia and femur in flexion. On the lateral side, the popliteus muscle is

neither small enough to be ignored nor large enough to be useful when the knee is under stress. The popliteus contracts during internal rotation of the tibia on the femur (Mann & Hagy 1977) and is said to reverse the 'screw-home' movement in full extension to unlock the fully extended knee, but patients with knees locked in extension because of popliteus deficiency are not seen, whereas patients with popliteus ruptures can flex their knees without difficulty. The usefulness of the popliteus – if any – is still obscure and the clincal relevance of the 'screw-home' is open to debate.

Perhaps most important of all, the real knee also differs in the involvement of adjacent structures. Injury to a ligament does not render the patient immune to meniscus lesions or articular cartilage damage, but actually makes them more likely, and the symptoms of these lesions may overshadow those of the ligament lesion.

Finally, the real knee is not symmetrical. The lateral condyle and plateaux are not only smaller than the medial, but the lateral plateau, when covered with articular cartilage, is convex and the femoral condyle slightly concave, the reverse of the medial compartment (Fig. 12.7). Looking critically at the lateral compartment, it seems so intrinsically unsta-

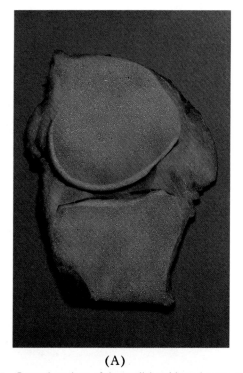

(A)

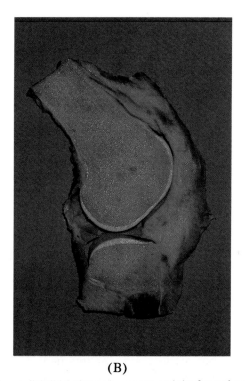

(B)

Fig. 12.7 Coronal sections of the medial and lateral compartments: (A) the medial tibial plateau is concave and the femoral condyle is convex; (B) the lateral compartment has a dome-shaped lateral plateau and the condyle is flat with a concave recess

ble that the tibia and femur can only remain in their correct relationship if the anterior cruciate ligament is both intact and accurately placed.

In short, the ideal knee resembles the real knee in many respects, particularly in the anatomy of the anterior and posterior cruciate and the medial ligaments, the position of the extensor muscles, and the shape of the medial tibial plateau and medial meniscus. The principal differences are the bizarre design of the lateral compartment and lateral ligament, the effect of associated injuries on symptoms, and the impossibility of restoring a ruptured ligament to complete normality by surgical repair.

Despite these differences, the cynic might observe that many reports of cruciate reconstruction and repair seem to have been written about the ideal rather than the real knee; exposure is easy, accurate repair straightforward, and damage to other structures is seldom mentioned. In 1920, Hey-Groves commented on reports of surgical repair of ruptured anterior cruciates as follows: 'I confess that I find it difficult to understand these statements, because in my cases the ligament has been so destroyed, or torn out from their bony attachments, that direct suture would have been impossible.' The quality of the tissue has not improved since 1920, yet accounts of meticulous reconstitution of the ligament still abound.

Clinical patterns of instability

The anatomical classification of instability can be replaced by the recognition of clinical syndromes, but the clinical features of these syndromes must be carefully defined.

Anterior cruciate rupture and the pivot shift phenomenon

History The clinical features of anterior cruciate instability are easily recognised. First, the patient can remember the moment when the ligament ruptured as clearly as if he had broken his leg and will often describe the exact moment of rupture with great clarity, even many years after the event. The injury often occurs during sport with a blow to the lateral side of the tibia, when the knee is slightly flexed and the foot planted, but the ligament can also be ruptured by indirect violence either by landing on the foot while twisting, as in a rugby football line-out

or a game of basketball, or by turning sharply while running at speed, especially in studded boots on a muddy field or rubber-soled shoes on a wooden floor. At the moment of rupture the patient feels something crack in the knee; he may comment that he thought 'he had broken his leg' and other players may report hearing something break. The knee swells and becomes painful, but, paradoxically, this will be less obvious if the joint capsule is also ruptured, because the blood and synovial fluid will escape into the soft tissues of the leg rather than cause tension in the capsule.

When the pain and swelling of the injury has subsided, the patient will find that the knee gives way beneath him when he twists with the weight on the leg and that he can run in straight lines, but cannot turn corners. Collapsing can also occur when walking over rough or uneven ground, stepping off a chair or stool or, in very loose knees, while walking over level ground. The collapsing is accompanied by a sensation of the bones moving, dislocating or shifting, and the patient may describe this with a sudden jerking moving of the hands, often with the two fists held one above the other (Fig. 12.8). It is this clinical syndrome that MacIntosh described as the 'pivot shift' (Galway et al 1972), but Hey-Groves was probably the first to observe this symptom when wrote in 1920: 'In active exercise, when the foot is put forward and the weight of the body pressed upon

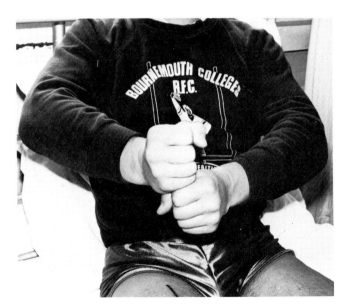

Fig. 12.8 The two fist sign. The patient indicates his sensation of instability with two fists. Note the rugby club jersey

the leg, then the tibia slips forward. Sometimes this forward slipping occurs with a jerk, as in the case shown in Figure 414...'. 'Figure 414' is a photograph of a patient subluxing the upper end of the tibia by applying a valgus strain with the foot planted.

Mechanics The cause of the collapsing episodes is the precarious stability of the lateral compartment, which depends upon the anterior cruciate ligament to hold it together. Without the anterior cruciate ligament, the convex tibial plateau and the femoral condyle slip off each other with the same inevitability as one billiard ball balanced upon another. The ilio-tibial tract is responsible for the sudden jerk; when the knee is extended, the tibial insertion of the ilio-tibial tract lies in front of the axis of flexion, but as the knee is bent, the insertion of the ilio-tibial tract moves back until it crosses the axis of movement and pulls the tibia sharply backwards in the sagittal plane – without any rotational element – into its reduced position (Fig. 12.9). This sudden reduction is the basis of the pivot shift test (Galway et al 1972), Hughston's jerk (Hughston et al 1976), Losee's sign (Losee et al 1978), the flexion rotation draw (Noyes

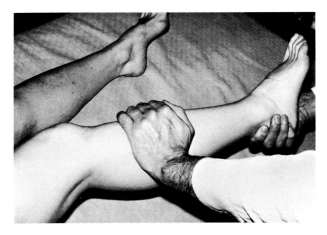

Fig. 12.10 The pivot shift test. The upper end of the tibia is pushed forwards, the foot is internally rotated, a valgus strain is applied and the knee is flexed and extended

et al 1980), the antero-lateral rotatory instability test and other variants.

Examination When examining the knee for the jerk or pivot shift test, the patient should be relaxed and a gentle valgus strain applied to the knee to load the lateral compartment. The tibia is then rotated internally and its upper end pushed forwards to bring the lateral tibial plateau in front of the femur (Fig. 12.10). Maintaining this position, the knee is gently flexed until the tibial plateau jerks backwards into the reduced position. Many patients will recognise this manoeuvre as likely to 'put their knee out' and involuntarily tighten up to prevent it occurring – the pivot shift 'apprehension' sign – just as a patient with recurrent dislocation of the patella is apprehensive when the patella is pushed laterally.

The pivot shift sign or jerk test is positive in every patient with a ruptured postero-lateral band of the anterior cruciate ligament unless there is a block to extension caused by a locked meniscus or other derangement, or a ruptured medial ligament. If there is a block to extension, the tibia cannot be dislocated in front of the femur and therefore cannot be reduced with a jerk. If the medial ligament is ruptured, the valgus strain applied to the joint will open up the medial compartment instead of loading the lateral compartment, so that the jerk will be less obvious.

The anterior draw test with the knee in flexion is the 'traditional' test for cruciate deficiency, but cannot be elicited if the hamstrings are contracted, and is positive only if the antero-medial band of the ligament is ruptured. The Lachman test, however,

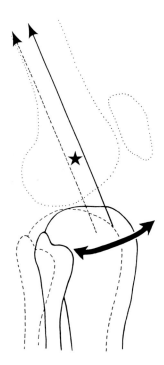

Fig. 12.9 The mechanism of the pivot shift phenomenon. The dome-shaped lateral plateau slips backwards and forwards across the lateral femoral condyle from the dislocated position (solid line) to the reduced position (broken line). The 'flip-flop' effect is provided by the ilio-tibial tract slipping backwards and forwards across the axis of rotation on the femur indicated by ★

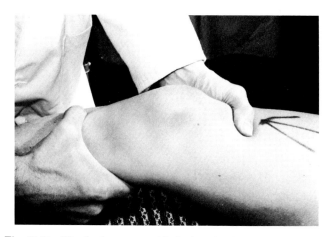

Fig. 12.11 The Lachman test with the knee in almost full extension. The tibia is moved forwards and backwards relative to the femur

can be elicited in even the most apprehensive patient (Fig. 12.11) (Torg et al 1976). The Lachman test is not difficult, and consists only of the anterior draw performed in almost full extension. Rupture of the postero-lateral band of the anterior cruciate ligament is largely responsible for producing the pivot shift and Lachman signs, and the antero-medial for the anterior drawer. If the Lachman sign and pivot shift sign are positive, and the anterior drawer sign is negative, it will generally be found that the antero-medial portion of the anterior cruciate ligament is intact and the postero-lateral band ruptured. If the anterior drawer is positive, and the Lachman and pivot shift signs negative, the reverse will be true (Table 12.1).

Posterior cruciate instability

History Posterior cruciate ligaments are usually ruptured either by a blow to the upper end of the tibia, when the knee is flexed, or by forced hyperextension (Kennedy & Walker 1979) and, as with anterior cruciate ruptures, patients can usually remember the moment of rupture. In some, the posterior cruciate may have been only one of several injuries and may be overlooked. A motorcyclist with a fracture dislocation of the hip, for example, may be unaware of his ligament injury until he has recovered

fully from the dislocation and begins to use his limb normally.

The disparity between the symptoms and physical signs in patients with posterior cruciate rupture is remarkable; many patients may have no evidence of their rupture apart from a massive posterior draw, but others will be disabled (Dandy & Pusey 1982). Some patients can achieve, either by planned conservative treatment or simply by missed diagnosis, a clinical and functional result so good that any surgeon would be proud to take the credit for it had he operated upon it, but other patients with less obvious posterior draw signs may be incapacitated by recurring collapsing of the knee. Accordingly, the indications for reconstruction of the posterior cruciate ligament should be based on symptoms rather than physical signs.

Examination The posterior draw sign is easily detected if it is marked, but minor degrees often escape notice, or may be mistaken for an anterior draw sign. If in doubt, a straight edge can be held against the tibia to aid comparison with the other side (Fig. 12.12).

If the posterior cruciate ligament is torn, the lateral tibial plateau can slip backwards off the

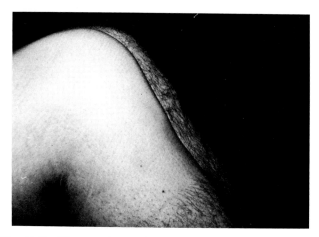

Fig. 12.12 The posterior sag sign. The tibia sags backwards in relationship to the femur. A straight line drawn up the front of the tibia nearer to the camera would pass through the patella, but a similar line drawn on the far tibia would pass just in front of the patella

Table 12.1 Effect of partial rupture on the signs of anterior cruciate deficiency

	Antero-medial band	Postero-lateral band	Both bands
Anterior draw	+	−	+
Lachman and pivot shift	−	+	+

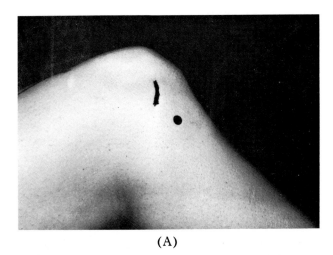

(A)

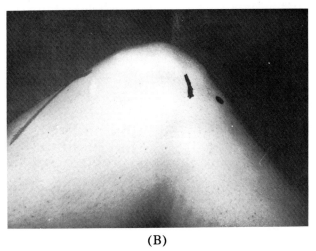

(B)

Fig. 12.13 Postero-lateral instability with the tibia externally rotated: (A) the tibia lies posterior to the femur, but in internal rotation; (B) it is brought into the normal position

ruptured posterior cruciate ligament, even those with a gross posterior draw sign, and the discrepancy between the symptoms and physical signs cannot be completely explained on the basis of postero-lateral instability or the reverse pivot shift sign.

Medial ligament

History Medial ligament ruptures are usually associated with anterior cruciate rupture, but isolated injuries are sometimes seen, following a pure valgus strain caused by a blow to the outer side of the knee. Symptoms from isolated medial ligament ruptures are uncommon, perhaps because valgus strains are more easily avoided than the twisting movements that cause the pivot shift. Although many patients are able to compensate well for a medial ligament deficiency, accidental knocks which push the foot laterally can cause pain and a feeling of discomfort or instability when the medial compartment is loaded. If the anterior cruciate is also ruptured, a pure valgus strain will open the joint widely and cause both pain and instability.

Mechanics Because the medial tibial plateau is larger than the lateral (Fig. 12.7), and is concave at its centre, the medial compartment is much more stable than the lateral (Fig. 12.14). The pivot shift phenomenon cannot occur in the medial compartment, because it is not possible for the femoral

femoral condyle when the tibia is held in external rotation, and relocate as the knee is extended (Fig. 12.13). In some patients, this dislocation and reduction of the tibia on the femur occurs with a jerk and has been called the 'reverse pivot shift sign' by Jakob. The sudden dislocation and reduction of the femur on the tibia is the probable explanation for the collapsing that sometimes follows rupture of the posterior cruciate ligament (Jakob et al 1981). The reverse pivot shift test is performed in much the same way as the test for anterior cruciate insufficiency, except that the tibia begins dislocated in flexion with the foot externally rotated and reduces as the knee is extended, the foot internally rotated and the upper end of the tibia pushed forward. The reverse pivot shift sign is an unusual phenomenon; it is by no means present in every patient with a

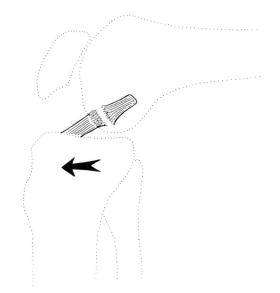

Fig. 12.14 Movement of the medial plateau in anterior cruciate ruptures. Because of the shape of the medial plateau, it cannot sublux in front of the medial femoral condyle if the anterior cruciate is ruptured

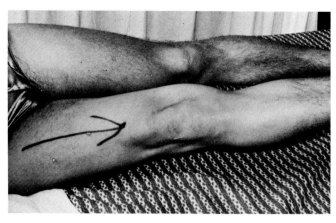

Fig. 12.15 A test for medial ligament instability. Adducting the leg against gravity produces a feeling of insecurity if the medial ligament is ruptured, and may demonstrate abnormal medial laxity

condyle to slide off the medial tibial plateau even, if the patient has abnormally lax ligaments and a very small tibia. Instead of the pivot shift, there is an increased range of backward and forward movement of the femur on the tibia, which the patient experiences as an unpleasant sliding sensation.

Examination On clinical examination, excessive opening of the medial compartment is easily demonstrated by applying a valgus strain with the knee fully extended. It is sometimes helpful to ask the patient to adduct the leg against gravity (Fig. 12.15) so that the weight of the leg applies the valgus strain; patients with an unstable medial ligament will be unable to lift the leg in this way, and the test reproduces their symptoms.

Lateral collateral ligament

The structures responsible for the stability of the lateral side of the knee have already been described (p. 162), and the importance of the ilio-tibial band stressed. The lateral collateral ligament and the ilio-tibial tract can be torn or avulsed from their bony insertions, but problems resulting from isolated injuries of these structures are remarkably rare. Although excessive opening of the lateral compartment can sometimes be demonstrated, few symptoms result from this, unless there is an associated lesion of a cruciate ligament, a meniscus or the articular surface, perhaps because the normal valgus angle of the knee is enough to protect the knee from varus strains. Rupture of the lateral collateral ligament alone probably causes no symptoms at the knee, and the importance of this ligament may have been greatly overestimated.

ACUTE INJURIES

Anterior cruciate

Indications for early repair

In the ideal knee, every ligament would cause symptoms if left unrepaired, and repair would be simple and successful in every patient. Reality is different; we do not even know the proportion of unrepaired ligament ruptures that cause late problems, because there is no prospective study of untreated injuries to act as a control group. Some studies have shown that about 70% or 80% of patients with isolated anterior cruciate injuries are able to resume their normal sporting and social activities after correction of meniscal injuries and other internal derangements (Chick & Jackson 1978, McDaniel & Dameron 1980, Jackson et al 1980, Dandy et al 1982, Paterson & Trickey 1983), particularly if the hamstrings are strengthened (Giove et al 1983). This figure is uncomfortably similar to, if not better than, the results of early surgical repair (Feagin & Curl 1976), and acute repair of ligament injuries around the knee may eventually prove to be one of the greatest uncontrolled studies in the history of surgery.

If we accept that some patients do well with conservative management, it follows that, if every patient with an acute anterior cruciate rupture underwent immediate repair, many unnecessary operations would be performed and this would favour a conservative approach. On the other hand, all patients who needed repair would be treated correctly and promptly, but if the opposite approach were adopted and every acute anterior cruciate ligament were managed conservatively, no unnecessary operations would be performed, but definitive repair would be delayed in every patient who needed it.

Although delaying operation until there is definite instability may seem undesirable, there is no firm evidence that early repair gives a better result than late reconstruction. Late reconstruction is an elective procedure carried out after the synovitis and soft tissue trauma of the acute injury has subsided, and the results may well be better than those of early repair. Moreover, if the ligament is replaced with tissue from elsewhere – the medial third of the patellar ligament, for example – the grafted material may well be stronger than two necrotic stubs of ligament with a foreign body (the suture) lying between them.

If the decision is taken to repair the anterior cruciate at once, there is then a choice of operation. Some surgeons will prefer a direct repair of the ligament, some a primary reconstruction using prosthetic material or natural tissue such as patellar tendon, while others will compromise and perform an augmentation with fascia lata or tendon.

The degree of ligament laxity provides some help in selecting patients for early repair, but it does not supply the complete answer. The grading of ligamentous instability still depends upon the subjective 'feel' of the knee compared with the normal and cannot yet be measured mechanically, although many ligament-stressing devices of varying complexity are now available. To grade ligament instability consistently requires experience, not only to gauge the abnormal movement, but also to encourage the patient to relax enough for the knee to be examined. Anterior cruciate ligament laxity, for example, is completely hidden by contraction of the hamstrings, and some patients find it impossible to relax these muscles and place their unstable knee in the hands of a stranger. For these reasons, it is almost impossible to achieve consistent grading between examiners and it is unwise to place much reliance on the grade of instability reported by a colleague whom one does not know well.

The convention is to regard a separation of 5 mm or less as 1 +, 5–10 mm as 2 +, and 10 mm or more as 3 + (Committee on the Medical Aspects of Sport 1968). This, together with the normal knee as grade 0, means that there are four grades of instability. Some surgeons use five grades, 0 for the normal knee, and grades 1, 2, 3 and 4 for the abnormal knee (Insall et al 1981), but to distinguish five grades of instability on the basis of the subjective assessment of a movement measured in millimetres would seem hard to justify. The author's criteria for distinguishing the three grades of instability are that if the knee feels a little loose, but it is difficult to be certain, there is grade 1 laxity. If the laxity is so gross that it is positively alarming and the leg appears to come apart in the examiner's hand, grade 3 laxity is present. Knees that do not fit into either of these categories have grade 2 laxity.

Until we know which patients are likely to do well with conservative management and which need surgery, and until we have some evidence that the long-term results of early repair are better than those of conservative management, the indications for early ligament repair must rely on clinical judgement, rather than unthinking attempts to abolish abnormal physical signs. In some patients, early operation seems the obvious choice. Young patients, for example, in whom a block of bone has been avulsed from the tibia should probably have the block of bone replaced and fixed either with open surgery or arthroscopically (p. 171), even though its blood supply and strength will have been jeopardised by the violence needed to avulse it from the tibia, and the ligament will probably stretch and become incompetent with time.

Patients with sporting aspirations are also candidates for early repair. A 19-year-old professional sportsman should probably have his anterior cruciate ligament repaired at once, whereas a 40-year-old executive who plays occasional badminton for relaxation will probably prefer to be managed conservatively, reserving the upheaval of cruciate reconstruction until it is clearly unavoidable and adequate preparations have been made to minimise the impact on his livelihood (Table 12.2).

If the medial ligament is ruptured as well as the anterior cruciate, early repair of both ligaments is indicated, because the prognosis for patients with ruptures of the medial ligament and anterior cruciate

Table 12.2 Spectrum of conservative to aggressive management of acute anterior cruciate ruptures

Conservative	No patients ever operated upon acutely
	Young patients with avulsed tibial spine
	Patients under 25 with another lesion, e.g. medial ligament rupture
	Professional athletes under 25
	Patients over 25 with another lesion, e.g. medial ligament rupture
	Professional athletes over 25
	Patients under 30 with isolated anterior cruciate rupture
	Patients over 30 with isolated anterior cruciate rupture
	Every patient with a positive pivot shift, regardless of age
Aggressive	Any patient with a haemarthrosis, even if the pivot shift is negative

ligament is worse than for an isolated anterior cruciate rupture (Jackson et al 1980).

The arthroscopic approach

Although arthroscopy of the acutely injured knee presents special problems (p. 59), it is very helpful in the management of acute injuries. A precise diagnosis can be made, the haemarthrosis evacuated, the joint cleaned thoroughly and torn menisci, loose bodies or stubs of ruptured ligaments removed under arthroscopic control. Correction of the internal derangement alone can produce good results in 70–80% of patients (Chick & Jackson 1978, McDaniel & Dameron 1980, Jackson et al 1980, Dandy et al 1982, Paterson & Trickey 1983).

Correction of internal derangements

Loose bodies and torn menisci may be removed in the usual way, and removal of the acutely torn ligament is straightforward. The aim of operation should be to leave the notch free of swollen and oedematous tissue, and this is most easily done by avulsing the tissue with rongeurs.

Repairing avulsed anterior cruciate ligaments

If the block of bone cannot be reduced by manipulation (Fig. 12.16), it can be accurately replaced under arthroscopic control, but there is no reason to suppose that the viability of the ligament is any better after arthroscopic replacement than after open replacement. Apart from the usual problems of a haemarthrosis and operating in the notch, the operative technique is simple, the principal difficulty being to hold the bone fragment down while it is drilled from below. Once the drill holes are made, monofilament nylon can be used to draw the definitive suture throught the fragment. Wire is stiff and unwieldy, but stout braided nylon or silk is quite satisfactory, although it has a tendency to snag on exposed bone trabeculae. Once introduced, the suture material can be tied subcutaneously and a cast applied.

Arthroscopic repair of ruptured cruciates

It is also possible to suture anterior cruciate ligaments ruptured in their mid-portion, but there is no evidence to suggest that the results are any less disappointing than the same procedure done open.

Management after arthroscopy

When the internal derangements have been corrected arthroscopically, a programme of vigorous physiotherapy and rehabilitation can be instituted in full knowledge of the pathology, but the patient should be reviewed carefully and frequently. The

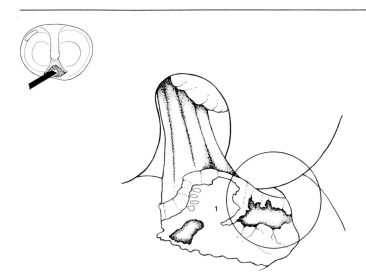

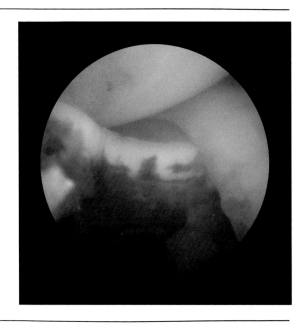

Fig. 12.16 A block of bone (1) from the tibia has been avulsed, leaving the anterior cruciate intact

treatment does not end with removal of the arthroscope; the patient must be watched carefully so that those who are not going to avoid ligament reconstruction can be identified without delay and the reconstruction done at once.

Posterior cruciate

If the posterior cruciate ligament is ruptured in its mid-portion, most patients can expect to achieve a good result without operation (Dandy & Pusey 1982), but if radiographs show that the tibial insertion has been avulsed with a block of bone, open reduction and internal fixation of the bony fragment is probably correct, with the proviso that the strength, length and viability of the ligament will be abnormal. No technique for arthroscopic repair of these lesions has been developed, but there is no reason why the operation should not be straightforward.

Medial ligament

The choice between conservative and operative treatment is less controversial in the management of ruptures of the medial ligament than in ruptures of the cruciate ligaments. If there is grade 1 laxity only on flexion, conservative management in a plaster cylinder is usually sufficient; open repair, however, is indicated, if there is laxity on extension or if the anterior cruciate ligament is also torn. Arthroscopy is useful in dealing with internal derangements and identifying the site of the tear. If the medial ligament or posterior capsule is ruptured, there is often a characterisitic kink in the meniscus (O'Connor 1974). If the meniscus floats high off the tibia, the ligament has been pulled off the tibia, and if the meniscus is in its normal relationship, the lesion is proximal.

LATE RECONSTRUCTION

Anterior cruciate

General considerations

Operations for late reconstruction of the anterior cruciate ligament can be divided into two main groups: those in which the operation is performed outside the joint and those in which something is placed inside the knee to replace the ligament. The extra-articular procedures act by reinforcing the secondary stabilisers of the knee rather than restoring the anatomy to normal. Restoration of the original anatomy by replacing the anterior cruciate ligament in the intercondylar notch is theoretically preferable, but the technical problems of such a procedure are far greater than those of an extra-articular operation. Of the operations performed outside the knee, the pes anserinus transfer has now fallen from popularity and the MacIntosh tenodesis and its variants are more commonly performed.

Extra-articular reconstruction

The pes anserinus transfer was originally recommended for instability on the medial side and postero-medial corner of the knee (Slocum et al 1974), before the importance of the pivot shift was widely recognised and came to be widely used for anterior cruciate instability. The results of pes anserinus transfer for the pivot shift phenomenon are not good (Chick et al 1981, Freeman et al 1982), perhaps because the pes anserinus transfer only alters the action of the dynamic stabilisers of the knee and the anterior cruciate ligament is a static stabiliser. Although the muscles around the joint can help to stabilise it if the stress can be anticipated, they are of little help in protecting the joint against sudden unexpected stresses that do not allow sufficient time for the muscles to contract. For this reason alone, a transposed muscle is a poor substitute for a ligament. Transposition of the pes anserinus can be combined with capsular repair and tightening of the medial ligament (Nicholas 1973).

The MacIntosh operation and its variants, such as the Ellison procedure (Ellison 1979), produce a static stabiliser parallel with the anterior cruciate ligament, but outside the joint, and hold the tibia in external rotation (Fig. 12.17). In performing the pivot shift or jerk test, the tibia must first be rotated internally on the femur so that the lateral tibial plateau lies in front of the femoral condyle. If internal rotation is prevented, this initial subluxation is not possible and the pivot shift test will be negative. In this respect, the operation can be compared with the Putti–Platt operation for recurrent dislocation of the shoulder, because the dislocation is prevented by restricting rotation at the joint.

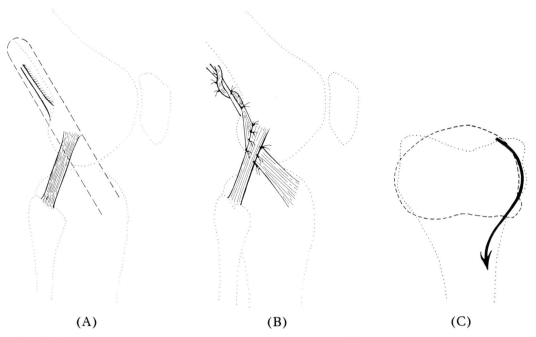

(A)   (B)   (C)

Fig. 12.17 MacIntosh lateral substitution reconstruction. (A) A strip of ilio-tibial band is raised to expose the lateral collateral ligament and lateral intermuscular septum; (B) the strip of ilio-tibial tract is passed beneath the lateral collateral and woven through the lateral intermuscular septum; (C) the strip of ilio-tibial band pulls the tibia into external rotation

The MacIntosh extra-articular tenodesis – technique

The MacIntosh tenodesis is a reliable and simple operation and will abolish the pivot shift sign. The results are good in the short term (Ireland & Trickey 1980), but, like other extra-articular repairs, they tend to deteriorate with time as the transposed slip stretches.

1. After a preliminary arthroscopy, the leg is prepared and placed on a rest (Fig. 12.18), which makes the operation a great deal simpler.
2. With the knee flexed on the rest, a longitudinal incision is made from Gerdy's tubercle to a point 10 cm above the femoral condyle.
3. A strip of ilio-tibial tract about 1–2 cm wide and based distally on Gerdy's tubercle is then raised.
4. The lateral collateral ligament is identified and elevated with a pair of artery forceps, without opening the synovium, and the ilio-tibial is strip passed under it from below upwards.
5. The lateral intermuscular septum is then identified, and a soft-tissue tunnel is created from the lateral collateral to the distal end of the septum, as close to bone as possible.
6. The strip is then passed through the tunnel and

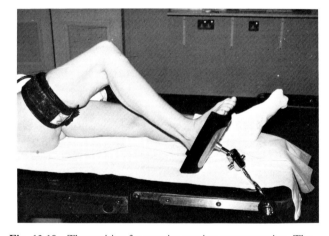

Fig. 12.18 The position for anterior cruciate reconstruction. The foot is resting on a support attached to the operating table which holds the knee flexed to 90° and the foot in external rotation

woven through the septum, keeping the strip next to bone.
7. With the foot in external rotation, the strip is pulled tight and stitched to lateral collateral, soft tissue and intermuscular septum with an absorbable suture such as Vicryl or chromic catgut.
8. The defect in the ilio-tibial tract is then closed as far as the lower limit of vastus lateralis to prevent muscle herniation.

Intra-articular reconstruction

Although correction of the normal anatomy is attractive, there are some practical problems in achieving this. First, the length and tension of the anterior cruciate ligament are critical and difficult to reproduce exactly, because the femoral attachment of the anterior cruciate ligament is placed so far back in the knee that it cannot be seen from an anterior approach. In general, if the attachment of the cruciate substitute to the femoral condyle can be seen from the front of the joint, it has probably been placed too far anteriorly. This criticism applies particularly to procedures involving a drill hole through the femoral condyle; the normal cruciate ligament lies at the very back of the femoral condyle, and any drill hole must be too far forwards.

One third of the patellar tendon is often used as a cruciate substitute (Jones 1970, Clancy et al 1982, Insall 1984), but there is no immutable law of nature to say that the patellar tendon is invariably the same length as the anterior cruciate ligament and, in fact, the ligament is usually too short to reach right to the back of the lateral condyle. To leave the patellar ligament attached distally to the tibia and then attach it to the proximal end as far back on the femur as it will reach is to leave the selection of the site of femoral attachment of the cruciate to chance, while to use the expansion of the tendon over the patella brings weak tissue to the site of femoral attachment.

Fixation of the ligament substitute to bone presents a further problem. While a patellar ligament substitute can be prepared with a bone block at each end, other materials such as the semitendinosus tendon or strips of the ilio-tibial tract do not have such a stout bony attachment and sound fixation to bone is unpredictable and difficult. Vascularity of a ligament substitute is another cause of concern (Arnoczky et al 1982), although Alm et al (1976) showed that revascularisation of the graft occurs quite quickly in dogs. If a strip of ilio-tibial tract, patellar ligament, or semitendinosus tendon is raised, leaving it attached only at one end, the vascularity must be severely impaired and the strip can effectively be regarded as a dead or prosthetic graft. If the graft is indeed avascular and acting only as a prosthesis, it would be more convenient to use a true prosthetic ligament which could be of the correct length and strength, but the problems of fixation to bone would remain (Rushton et al 1983). Many materials have been used as ligament pros-

theses (Trickey 1984), and the least unsuccessful have been those which are porous and allow fibrous tissue to grow into their substance. The technique for replacing the anterior cruciate ligament under arthroscopic control is already available (p. 175), but no suitable prosthetic ligament has yet been developed.

Combined MacIntosh tenodesis and replacement of anterior cruciate using the medial third of the patellar tendon – technique

Because of these uncertainties, a combined intra-and extra-articular procedure is probably the treatment of choice at present. The technique described below is straightforward and reliable (Fig. 12.19).

1.–3. Steps 1–3 are the same as for a MacIntosh tenodesis (p. 173).
4. After raising the lateral collateral ligament, the postero-lateral corner of the knee is identified and opened with a vertical incision long enough to admit a finger.
5. The skin is then reflected far enough medially to reach the patella and tibial tubercle. The patella is reached more easily if the knee is extended and rested on the support.
6. The medial third of the patella tendon is then identified and removed with a block of bone from the tibial tubercle distally and the non-articular portion of the patella proximally, and placed in saline at room temperature. The patellar block should include cancellous bone and measure just less than 1 cm in width.
7. The fat-pad is excised and the femoral attachment of the anterior cruciate identified. A recess is then cut at this site with a reciprocating saw. A finger in the postero-lateral compartment is used to confirm that the recess is correctly placed.
8. A tunnel is made through the tibia to enter precisely at the anterior edge of the tibial insertion of the anterior cruciate.
9. The patellar bone block is then fixed to the femur with 20 gauge wire, using a wire tightener, making sure that the cancellous surfaces are firmly apposed.
10. The tibial bone block is then passed through the tibial tunnel and held with a staple, which 'collapses' the tunnel and holds the plug firmly.

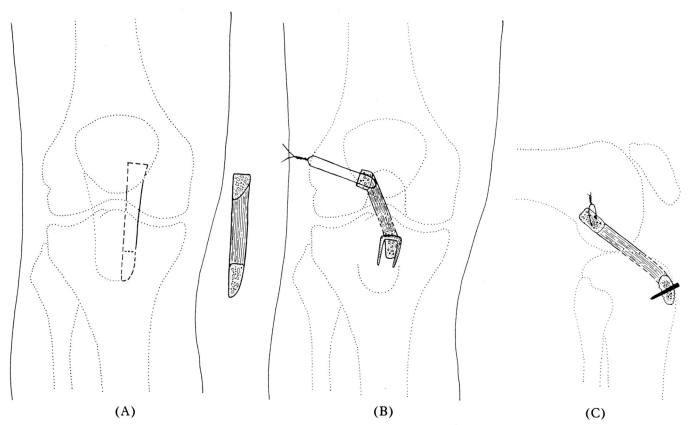

(A)   (B)   (C)

Fig. 12.19 Anterior cruciate reconstruction using the medial third of the patellar ligament: (A) a strip of patellar ligament is removed as a free graft with bone at each end; (B) and (C) the graft is placed in the intercondylar notch and secured proximally with a wire and distally with a staple

11. The postero-lateral capsulotomy is closed with slight overlap and a MacIntosh tenodesis performed in the usual way (p. 155).
12. Cast immobilisation is not required if the fixation has been done correctly.

Arthroscopic replacement of the anterior cruciate with a prosthesis

The main use of the arthroscope in the late management of ligament lesions still lies in assessment (Fig. 4.37) and the correction of internal derangements, but its future role is likely to be more important and the time when a patient's knee can be restrung with a new cruciate ligament as an out-patient procedure may not be too far distant. To insert a ligament prosthesis under arthroscopic control without arthrotomy is not difficult and was described in the first edition of this book (Dandy 1981) (Figs. 12.20, 12.21). The technique awaits only the appropriate prosthetic material, but an extra-articular repair is nevertheless advisable as an

additional procedure, until satisfactory long-term results are available.

The technique described was used with carbon fibre and proved reliable, but the results were not always satisfactory. Synovitis was a common problem and there was little evidence of fibrous ingrowth into the prosthesis, although it quite quickly became covered with a thin layer of flimsy synovium (Rushton et al 1983) (Fig. 12.22).

Technique

1. The arthroscope is inserted from the antero-lateral route and the notch cleared of debris in the usual way from the antero-medial approach.
2. A short incision is made just medial to the tibial tubercle and a bone awl or drill passed through the tibia, preferably with a jig (Fig. 12.23), to enter at the anterior limit of the anterior cruciate insertion onto the tibia. Care must be taken not to damage the arthroscope with the drill.

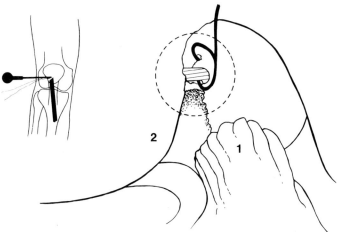

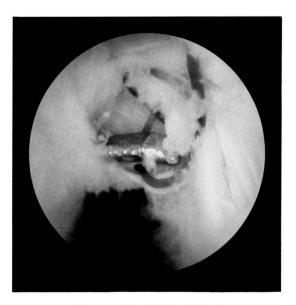

Fig. 12.20 A bone awl carrying a strand of monofilament nylon has been passed through the lateral femoral condyle to the site of attachment of a ruptured anterior cruciate ligament (1). The nylon can then be used to draw a carbon fibre replacement for the anterior cruciate ligament through the lateral condyle (2)

3. A second short incision is made over the back of the lateral femoral condyle, and a bone awl or drill is passed through the condyle to enter the knee at the femoral insertion of the anterior cruciate, with a jig, if available.
4. The two holes are enlarged to the correct size to accommodate the prosthesis.
5. Monofilament nylon is passed through the femoral tunnel, picked up in the notch with forceps and drawn out through the antero-medial approach so that it lies along the roof of the intercondylar notch.
6. The nylon is grasped with fine forceps passed through the tibial tunnel, and withdrawn through the tibia (Fig. 12.24).
7. The nylon is then used to pull the prosthesis through the femur, notch and tibia.
8. The prosthesis is secured to bone. If the fixation ever proves to be adequate, the patient could be left free of immobilisation; when this technique

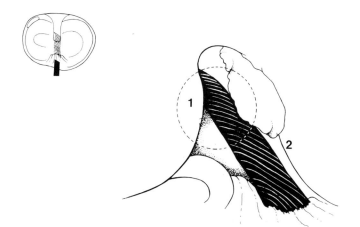

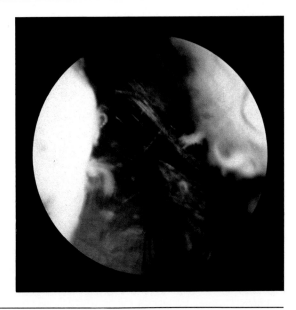

Fig. 12.21 A carbon fibre replacement of the anterior cruciate ligament lying in the intercondylar notch; lateral femoral condyle (1), medial femoral condyle (2). The carbon fibre was inserted under arthroscopic control

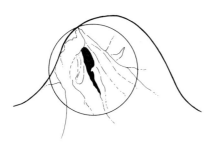
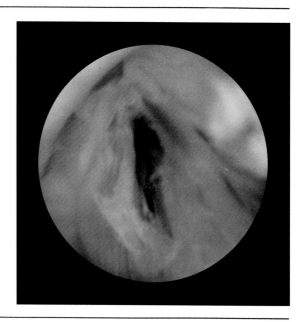

Fig. 12.22 Carbon fibre anterior cruciate replacement two years after insertion. The carbon fibre is visible through a thin fibrous covering

was used with carbon fibre, however, a MacIntosh tenodesis was added to ensure success.

Posterior cruciate

Late reconstruction of the posterior cruciate ligament presents the same problems of anatomical positioning, length, vascularity and bone fixation encountered in reconstructing the anterior cruciate, but with the additional worry that, if the knee is immobilised in flexion, the tibia will hang on the ligament substitute and place great stress upon its fixation. If the knee is immobilised in extension, the ligament substitute will be under tension and

immobilisation in approximately 10–20° of flexion is probably a satisfactory compromise.

If the reverse pivot shift sign is present, the operation should aim to hold the postero-lateral

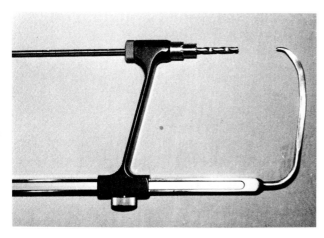

Fig. 12.23 Jig for arthroscopic insertion of anterior cruciate prosthesis

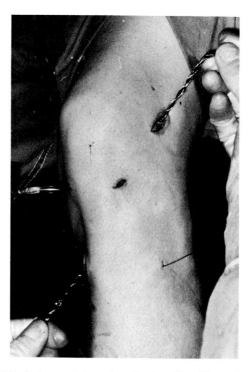

Fig. 12.24 Arthroscopic insertion of carbon fibre. The carbon fibre has been passed through femoral and tibial tunnels under arthroscopic control and will be pulled through a locking tunnel in the tibia, using monofilament nylon, which leaves the skin through a short incision visible at the right of the picture

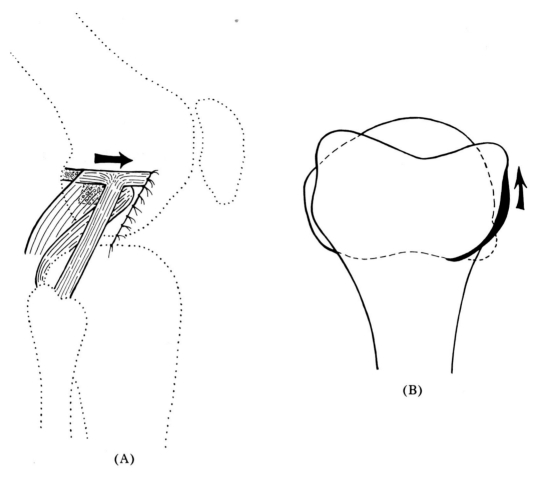

(A)

(B)

Fig. 12.25 Postero-lateral capsular advancement for postero-lateral instability: (A) a block of tissue including the lateral collateral ligament and popliteus tendon is brought forwards in a prepared bed; (B) the tibia is pulled into internal rotation

corner of the tibia forward, but no normal anatomical structure is conveniently placed to perform this function except the popliteus tendon. The popliteus tendon, being attached to the popliteus muscle, is not a true static stabiliser, but its femoral insertion can nevertheless be advanced on the femur so that the tibia is pulled forwards. Advancement of the popliteus, postero-lateral joint capsule and lateral collateral ligament, together with replacement of the posterior cruciate using graft material or the gastrocnemius belly, in addition to popliteus advancement, is probably the treatment of choice at present.

Postero-lateral capsular advancement (after Trillat 1977)

If the patient has disabling collapsing of the knee from posterior cruciate deficiency and a posterolateral sag, advancement of the postero-lateral structures may be effective (Fig. 12.25). The operation is extra-articular and not difficult.

Technique

1. The leg is prepared and placed on a support (Fig. 12.26).
2. A lateral incision is made, splitting the ilio-tibial tract. The synovium is opened just enough to

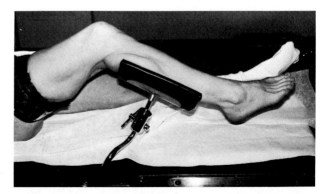

Fig. 12.26 A rest used to support the tibia during posterior cruciate reconstruction. The leg is supported by the rest, which pushes the upper end of the tibia anteriorly

identify the synovial reflection in front of the politeus tendon.

3. The fibular insertion of the fibular collateral ligament and the popliteus tendon are then raised on a single bar of bone about 2.5 cm long and 5 mm wide, and the capsule incised vertically at its ends to create a square flap.

4. The bed from which the bar was lifted is then deepened and extended forwards, and the free edge of the flap pulled forwards and buried to tighten it. The flap is then secured with staples.

5. The overhanging front edge of the flap is sutured to capsule and synovium, but the defect at the back cannot be closed. The ilio-tibial tract is repaired, the wound closed and a cast applied in about 10° of flexion.

Medial ligament

Late reconstruction of the medial ligament and postero-medial corner of the knee present different problems from those of cruciate reconstruction. No intra-articular substitute is required and problems of vascularity or bone fixation are less, but to repair a flat sheet of stretched tissue is not easy. If the ligament has been detached from the tibia, it can be advanced distally by a soft tissue release and secured to the tibia, which is generally effective (Insall 1984). Pes anserinus transfer, which increases the force with which the hamstrings can pull the tibia backwards, is contra-indicated if the postero-medial corner of the knee is lax, because the need then is to pull the tibia forwards rather than backwards.

Lateral ligament

Late instability due to isolated ruptures of the lateral structures of the knee is not a problem encountered in normal clinical practice, but repair of the ilio-tibial band or collateral ligament may be required as an additional procedure when repairing associated ruptures of the joint capsule or the cruciate ligaments.

Correction of secondary derangements

Knees with ligament deficiency are more susceptible to internal derangements than normal knees, and patients with no symptoms of cruciate deficiency may require arthroscopy for a torn meniscus or other lesion (Dandy et al 1982). Long or swollen stubs of ligament can give rise to mechanical symptoms, as can ununited fragments of tibia avulsed with the cruciate. Both can be excised arthroscopically.

Anterior cruciate stubs

If the anterior cruciate ruptures at its proximal femoral attachment, a long stub of tissue will remain.

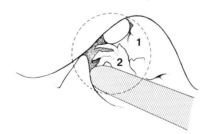

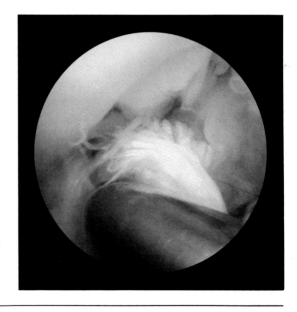

Fig. 12.27 The redundant stub of a ruptured anterior cruciate ligament (2) is removed from the intercondylar notch (1) using pituitary rongeurs inserted from the antero-medial route

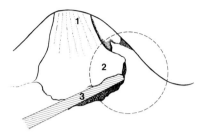

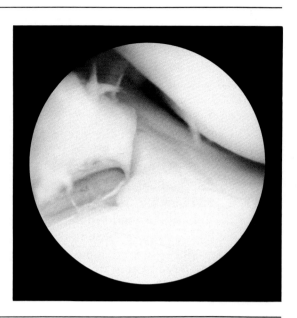

Fig. 12.28 Avulsion of the tibial spine. The anterior cruciate ligament (1) has avulsed a block of bone including the tibial spine (2) from the underlying tibia, and is manipulated with a probing hook (3) inserted from the antero-lateral route with the arthroscope inserted from the antero-medial route

These stubs, which may be over 2 cm in length, are quite long enough to interfere with joint movement, and are sometimes so thick and oedematous that they cause a painful block to extension. Cystic degeneration of the stub is also seen (Dandy 1984). The stub, which is functionally useless, is easily trimmed back to its base from the antero-medial approach with punch forceps or rongeurs (Fig. 12.27). The procedure is simple and well within the grasp of a cautious beginner.

Old avulsed spines

If the lesion is not diagnosed early, either the bed of the fracture can be deepened and the fragment reattached – a difficult procedure with a dubious outcome – or it can be excised arthroscopically. Arthroscopic excision is not difficult if the fragment is first mobilised with a long-handled knife and small osteotome or periosteal elevator, so that it can be removed with rongeurs (Fig. 12.28).

Symptoms following reconstruction

Patients who have undergone cruciate reconstruction also develop mechanical symptoms and require arthroscopy. In these patients, adhesions may restrict flexion, and excessive fibrous tissue can form round the cruciate replacement, obstructing extension and causing crepitus.

Debridement of fibrous tissue from around a cruciate graft is not difficult, apart from the usual problems encountered when working in the notch, but it can sometimes be difficult to know how much tissue can safely be removed. Only experience helps with this decision.

References

Alm A, Lilledahl S O, Stromberg B 1976 Clinical and experimental experience in reconstruction of the anterior cruciate ligament. Orthopedic Clinics of North America 7: 181–189

Arnoczky S P, Tarvin G B, Marshall J L 1982 Anterior cruciate ligament replacement using patellar tendon. An evaluation of graft vascularisation in the dog. Journal of Bone and Joint Surgery 64A: 217–224

Chick R P, Jackson D W 1978 Tears of the anterior cruciate ligament in young athletes. Journal of Bone and Joint Surgery 60A: 970–973

Chick R P et al 1981 The pes anserinus transfer: a long-term follow-up. Journal of Bone and Joint Surgery 63A: 1449–1452

Clancy W G, Nelson D A, Reder B, Narechania R G 1982 Anterior cruciate ligament reconstruction using one third of the patellar ligament, augmented by extra-articular tendon transfers. Journal of Bone and Joint Surgery 64A: 352–359

Committee on the Medical Aspects of Sports 1968 Standardised nomenclature of athletic injuries. American Medical Association, Chicago

Dandy D J 1981 Arthroscopic surgery of the knee. Churchill Livingstone, Edinburgh

Dandy D J 1984 Arthroscopy of the knee: a diagnostic atlas. Gower–Butterworth, London

Dandy D J, Pusey R J 1982 The long term results of untreated ruptures of the posterior cruciate ligament. Journal of Bone and Joint Surgery 64B: 92–94

Dandy D J, Flanagan J P, Steenmeyer V 1982 Arthroscopy of the ruptured anterior cruciate ligament. Clinical Orthopaedics and Related Research 167: 43–49

Dejour H, Chambat P, Aglietti P 1984 Ligamentous surgery of the knee. In: Insall J N (ed) Surgery of the knee. Churchill Livingstone, New York

Ellison A E 1979 Ilio-tibial band transfer for antero-lateral rotatory instability of the knee. Journal of Bone and Joint Surgery 61A: 330–337

Evans P 1979 The postural function of the iliotibial tract. Annals of the Royal College of Surgeons 61: 271–280

Feagin J A, Curl W W 1976 Isolated tears of the anterior cruciate ligament: five year follow-up study. American Journal of Sports Medicine 4: 95–100

Freeman B L, Beaty J H, Haynes D B 1982 The pes anserinus transfer: a long-term follow-up. Journal of Bone and Joint Surgery 64A: 202–207

Galway R D, MacIntosh D L 1980 The lateral pivot shift: a symptom and sign of anterior cruciate insufficiency. Clinical Orthopaedics and Related Research 147: 45–50

Galway R D, Beaupre A, MacIntosh D L 1972 Pivot shift: a clinical sign of symptomatic anterior cruciate deficiency. Journal of Bone and Joint Surgery 54B: 763–764

Giove T P, Miller S J, Kent B E, Sanford T L, Garrick J G 1983 Non-operative treatment of the torn anterior cruciate ligament. Journal of Bone and Joint Surgery 65A: 185–192

Hey-Groves E W 1917 Operation for repair of the crucial ligaments. Lancet 2: 674–675

Hey-Groves E W 1920 The crucial ligaments of the knee joint: their function, rupture and operative treatment of the same. British Journal of Surgery 7: 505–515

Hughston J C, Andrews J R, Cross M J, Moschi A 1976 Classification of knee ligament instability. Part II. The lateral compartment. Journal of Bone and Joint Surgery 58A: 173–179

Insall J N 1984 Chronic instability of the knee. In: Insall J N (ed) Surgery of the knee. Churchill Livingstone, New York

Insall J N, Joseph D M, Aglietti P, Campbell R D 1981 Bone block ilio-tibial band transfer for anterior cruciate insufficiency. Journal of Bone and Joint Surgery 63A: 560–569

Ireland J, Trickey E L 1980 MacIntosh tenodesis for antero-lateral instability of the knee. Journal of Bone and Joint Surgery 62B: 340-345

Jackson R W, Peters R I, Marczyk R L 1980 Late results of untreated anterior cruciate rupture. Journal of Bone and Joint Surgery 62B: 127

Jakob R P, Hassler H, Staeubli H V 1981 Observations on rotatory instability of the lateral compartment of the knee. Acta Orthopedica Scandinavica (suppl 191) vol 52

Jones K G 1970 Reconstruction of the anterior cruciate ligament using the central one-third of the patellar ligament. Journal of Bone and Joint Surgery 52A: 1302–1308

Kennedy J C, Walker D M 1979 The posterior cruciate ligament: a clinical and laboratory study. Journal of Bone and Joint Surgery 61B: 241

Larson R L 1983 The knee – the physiological joint. Journal of Bone and Joint Surgery 65A: 143–144

Lightowler C D R 1983 Difficulties with knees. British Medical Journal 1287: 165

Losee R E, Johnston T R, Southwick W O 1978 Anterior subluxation of the lateral tibial plateau. Journal of Bone and Joint Surgery 60A: 1015–1030

McDaniel W J, Dameron T B 1980 Untreated ruptures of the anterior cruciate ligament: a follow-up study. Journal of Bone and Joint Surgery 62A: 696–705

Mann R A, Hagy J L 1977 The popliteus muscle. Journal of Bone and Joint Surgery 59A: 924–927

Nicholas J A 1973 The five-one reconstruction for antero-medial instability of the knee. Journal of Bone and Joint Surgery 55A: 899–922

Noyes F R, Bassett R W, Grood E S, Butler D L 1980 Arthroscopy in acute traumatic haemarthrosis of the knee. Journal of Bone and Joint Surgery 62A: 687–695

O'Connor R L 1974 Arthrosopy in the diagnosis and treatment of cruciate ligament injuries. Journal of Bone and Joint Surgery 56A: 333–337

Palmer I 1938 On the injuries to the ligaments of the knee joint. A clinical study. Acta Chirurgica Scandinavica suppl 53

Paterson F W N, Trickey E L 1983 Meniscectomy for tears of the meniscus combined with rupture of the anterior cruciate ligament. Journal of Bone and Joint Surgery 65B: 388–390

Rushton N, Dandy D J, Naylor C P E 1983 The clinical, arthroscopic and histological findings after replacement of the anterior cruciate ligament with carbon fibre. Journal of Bone and Joint Surgery 65B: 308–309

Slocum D B, Larson R L 1968 Rotatory instability of the knee. Its pathogenesis and a clinical sign to demonstrate its presence. Journal of Bone and Joint Surgery 50A: 211–225

Slocum D B, Larson R L, James S L 1974 Late reconstruction of ligamentous injuries of the medial compartment of the knee. Clinical Orthopaedics and Related Research 100: 23–55

Torg J S, Conrad W, Kalen V 1976 Clinical diagnosis of anterior cruciate instability in the athlete. American Journal of Sports Medicine 4: 84–93

Trickey E L 1984 Chronic ligamentous injuries. In: Jackson J P, Waugh W (eds) Surgery of the knee. Chapman & Hall, London

Trillat A 1977 Les laxités posteroexternes du genou. Vortrag Knee Workshop, Heidelberg

Wang C J, Walker P S 1974 Rotatory laxity of the human knee joint. Journal of Bone and Joint Surgery 56A: 161–170

13

Arthroscopy in the management of anterior knee pain

Pain around the front of the knee is a formidable problem in clinical practice. The patients most commonly affected are adolescents, usually girls, whose knee prevents them taking a full part in sport or social activities. The condition causes understandable parental anxiety, often to the extent that the accompanying parent – usually the mother – will answer questions on behalf of the patient, and may even give a clear description of symptoms of which the girl herself was unaware.

Many different disorders (Fig. 13.1) can cause anterior knee pain, and each must be managed differently. Separation of one condition from another has been made difficult by the practice of lumping all anterior knee pain together under the diagnosis of chondromalacia patellae, which perhaps reflects the tendency of doctors to translate into

Latin that which they cannot treat effectively. 'Chondromalacia patellae' first appeared in the literature as a pathological diagnosis in 1928 (Aleman 1928) and means only 'softening of the articular cartilage of the patella'. The term places undue emphasis on the articular surface and could usefully be removed from the orthopaedic vocabulary, accompanied, if possible, by 'patello-femoral syndrome'. A syndrome is a collection of symptoms and not a diagnosis; to attribute pain at the front of the knee to 'patello-femoral syndrome' might impress the patient, but indicates that the doctor cannot make a diagnosis. 'Patello-femoral pain' is less mischievous, but can also be criticised because anterior knee pain is often caused by structures other than the patello-femoral joint.

If patients with anterior knee pain are to be treated

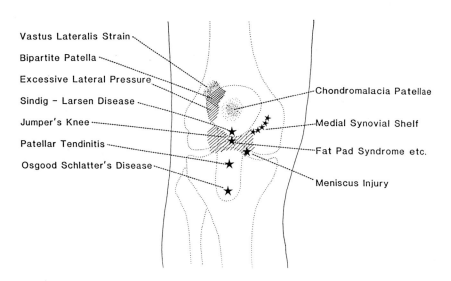

Fig. 13.1 Causes of anterior knee pain.

effectively, as accurate a diagnosis as possible should be made before treatment is started. To separate the many causes of anterior knee pain one from another is difficult and a proper diagnosis cannot be made in every patient; nevertheless there are several clearly recognisable pathological and clinical entities which can be considered according to the structures involved.

PAIN FROM SYNOVIUM

Because inflamed synovium is painful and tender, any generalised synovitis can cause pain in the knee, both at the front of the joint and elsewhere. Generalised synovitis will usually be clinically obvious, but some areas may be so much more tender than the rest that the generalised synovitis passes unnoticed. The areas of synovium which lie in close contact with the femur in full flexion are particularly vulnerable if the knee is flexed for long periods; pain after prolonged sitting, as in a car or cinema, should suggest synovium as the site of pain.

Traumatic synovitis

A blow to the front of the knee can cause a painful, but localised synovitis. The site of the tenderness, the history of trauma and the synovial thickening will usually suggest the diagnosis, but if the patient falls into the habit of walking with a stiff knee, the clinical picture may be confused. Conservative management with rest and anti-inflammatory drugs is usually successful, but patient physiotherapy and continuing optimism may be necessary to correct altered gait patterns.

Synovial shelf syndrome

The synovial shelf (p. 43) is a real structure (Fig. 4.15), but is seldom painful. The synovial shelf syndrome (Fujisawa 1976, Patel 1978, Vaughan-Lane & Dandy 1982) is characterised by pain on flexion of the knee, tenderness of the synovial shelf and an absence of patello-femoral tenderness. A blow to the front of the knee, perhaps on the edge of a desk or a dashboard, is a common precipitating factor. The syndrome should be suspected in patients with localised tenderness when the synovial shelf is rolled against the underlying femoral condyle, particularly if there is a distinct 'painful arc'

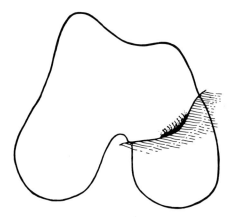

Fig. 13.2   Relationship of the medial synovial shelf and the impingement lesion on the medial femoral condyle. The shelf can catch on the impingement lesion during flexion

between 45° and 60° of flexion. A lesion of the articular cartilage is reported by some, but this is probably nothing more than the impingement lesion (p. 45) (Figs. 4.20, 4.21). This position (Fig. 13.2) corresponds with the movement of the shelf across the condyle, and it is easy to speculate that it is due to contact between an inflamed or scarred shelf and the femoral condyle.

Cynics have observed that many open operations for 'chondromalacia patellae' result in either division of the synovial shelf or relaxation of the medial parapatellar tissues, including the shelf, and they suggest that lateral release, tibial tubercle transposition, arthrotomy, medial meniscectomy and patellectomy may be little more than complicated techniques for dividing the medial synovial shelf. Rival cynics ask why this condition has reached epidemic proportions in the last few years, and find difficulty in understanding why the synovial shelf syndrome did not afflict humanity until the arthroscope was invented.

Whatever the importance of the synovial shelf syndrome, the results of shelf excision (Vaughan-Lane & Dandy 1982) are encouraging. Approximately 85% of patients with pain on flexion of the knee, a history of injury, a broad synovial shelf and tenderness medial to the patella without any other abnormality can expect to be relieved by excision of the shelf (Jackson et al 1982). The technique of shelf excision is described above (p. 76).

Suprapatellar plica

If the suprapatellar membrane is complete and divides the joint into two separate compartments

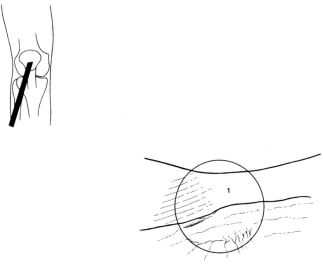

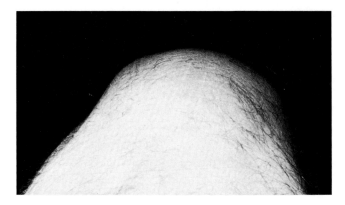

Fig. 13.3   A complete suprapatellar membrane (1)

(13.3), or if it is almost complete and has a split at its centre which acts as a valve, synovial fluid can collect above it to form a tense swelling. Although the condition is very unusual, the symptoms of aching and swelling proximal to the patella after exercise should suggest the diagnosis. Hughston et al (1973) reported symptoms caused by thickening and swelling of the suprapatellar plica, but this has not been reported by others.

If a complete membrane is present, it can be mistaken for the upper limit of the suprapatellar pouch (Dandy 1984), but its presence can be confirmed by probing with the irrigation needle or by looking for the articularis genu muscle (p. 43). If a complete membrane is present, it can easily be divided from either the suprapatellar or antero-medial approach, but the indications for doing so are imprecise. Because a complete membrane can cause symptoms and its division carries little morbidity, there may be some justification for dividing the membrane whenever it is identified.

PAIN FROM THE PATELLA

Mechanical factors

The Q angle, genu valgum, genu varum, the position of the patella (Fig 13.4) and anteversion of the femoral neck have all been proposed as causes of anterior knee pain. Although all of these factors may

Fig. 13.4   A naked-eye skyline view of a normal patella

contribute to some extent, Fairbank et al (1984) found no difference in these measurements between patients with anterior knee pain and normal adolescents. Mechanical factors are more important in patellar instability than anterior knee pain.

Radiological assessment

Radiological assessment of the patello-femoral joint is less helpful than subjective clinical signs, but shows well the effects of overloading the lateral facet (Figs. 13.5, 13.6) and permits lines to be drawn on the radiographs so that angles, distances and the width of joint spaces can be measured, recorded, analysed and compared. Although there are studies which show a relationship between radiological

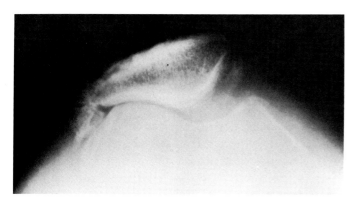

Fig. 13.5   The final result of excessive lateral pressure syndrome. The lateral facet of the patella is worn, the patella tilted laterally, and there is calcification in the lateral retinaculum of the patella

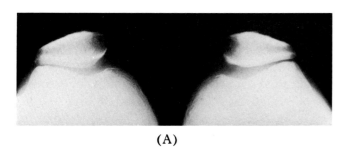

(A)

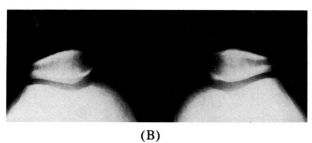

(B)

Fig. 13.6   Tangential (skyline) radiographs (A) in 30° and (B) 60° of flexion in a patient with excessive lateral pressure syndrome. There is erosion on the lateral femoral condyle

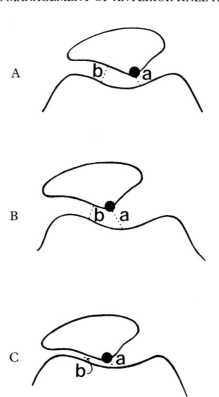

Fig. 13.7   The patello-femoral index, which measures the ratio between the thickness of the medial patello-femoral joint space and the lateral patello-femoral joint space. Measurement 'b' is the narrowest measurement of the lateral patello-femoral space and measurement 'a' is the distance between the median ridge of the patella and the nearest point to the medial femoral condyle. The ratio is abnormal if the patella is displaced laterally (B) or if the lateral joint space is narrowed (C) compared with the normal (A)

measurements and clinical features (Aglietti et al 1983), none has yet been shown to have any correlation with the prognosis or results of operation.

Patello-femoral index

Laurin (Laurin et al 1979) has described a patello-femoral index derived from comparison of the distance between the lateral facet of the patella and the lateral femoral condyle with the distance between the median ridge of the patella and the medial femoral condyle (Fig. 13.7). Although such a measurement is something of a blunt instrument involving many variables, including articular carti-

lage thickness, the position of the patella in relation to the midline of the femur and the amount of patellar tilt (lateral patello-femoral angle) (Fig. 13.8),

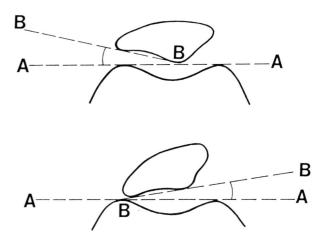

Fig. 13.8   The patello-femoral angle. The angle between the lateral facet of the patella and a transverse line joining the femoral condyles is normally open laterally (A), but is open medially (B) in patients with excessive lateral pressure syndrome

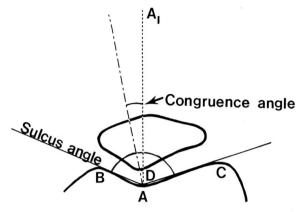

Fig. 13.9 Sulcus angle and congruence angle. The sulcus angle (BAC) measures the depth of the intercondylar groove of the femur. The congruence angle (D) measures the angle between a line bisecting the sulcus angle and a line drawn through the deepest point of the intercondylar groove and the median ridge of the patella. These measurements provide some indication of how well the patella 'fits' the femur

it offers some guide to the load on the lateral facet. The sulcus angle, congruence angle (Fig. 13.9) and other radiological indices are comprehensively described by Insall (1984).

Sulcus angle

The intercondylar groove on the patella is important for stability of the patella, and was exhaustively studied by Brattstrom (1964), who introduced the sulcus angle as a measure of the depth of the groove and found that the angle was normally about 142° (Fig. 13.9). Brattstrom used axial radiographs, which are difficult to obtain, but the angle can also be measured on a 30° tangential view.

Congruence angle

Although the sulcus angle measures the depth of the intercondylar groove, Merchant's congruence angle (Merchant et al 1974) is needed to show how well the patella sits in the groove. The congruence angle is measured by using a line bisecting the sulcus angle as a reference line. The angle between this and a second line drawn from the bottom of the groove through the lowest point of the patella is the congruence angle, angles medial to the reference line being negative, while those lateral to it are positive (Fig. 13.9). Merchant found the normal angle to be about −6° and considered that anything more than +16° was abnormal.

Although it is more often abnormal in patellar instability, the congruence angle is also abnormal in patients with anterior knee pain.

Excessive lateral pressure syndrome

Of all the varieties of anterior knee pain, excessive lateral pressure syndrome (Ficat & Hungerford 1977) is possibly the most common and probably the least understood. The characteristic features of the condition in the early stages are:

1. Pain around the patella when the patello-femoral joint is under load.
2. Tenderness of the lateral facet of the patella when the lateral edge of the patella is pushed against the femur in its normal position, but not when its lateral edge is moved away from the femur.
3. Limited medial mobility of the patella. Although this sign cannot be quantified and is only subjective, it is comparatively easy to identify a patella that is tightly held on its lateral side.
4. If the patella is examined with the naked eye, and the knee flexed to 30° or 60°, the patella often lies tilted like a soldier's beret (Fig. 13.4). This sign is again a subjective assessment, and does not always correspond to the radiological appearances of a 'skyline' view.
5. Patello-femoral crepitus is unusual in the early stages of excessive lateral pressure syndrome, but if the condition persists untreated osteoarthritis of the lateral half of the patello-femoral joint will follow.
6. The patients are commonly adolescents, usually girls near the growth spurt, but adults may suffer from the late effects.

Management

There are no figures to show how many patients with excessive lateral pressure syndrome make a natural and lasting recovery without treatment. Conservative management, including physiotherapy to build up the vastus medialis obliquus is commonly advised, although it is hard to see how selective hypertrophy of one part of the quadriceps – even if this were possible – could produce any permanent stretching of the very tight fibrous attachments of the patella on its lateral side. Even if ineffective, physiotherapy allows time for natural recovery and can do no harm.

Operation

If the symptoms have persisted for more than six months and are interfering seriously with the patient's everyday activities, lateral release of the extensor mechanism can be considered. When the operation has been explained, stressing that the relief of symptoms cannot be guaranteed and that roughly one patient in four is likely to be disappointed with the result, many patients will prefer not to undergo operation. If surgery is undertaken, the best results are in patients with the classical features of excessive lateral pressure syndrome that have already been described, and without any articular cartilage changes. Ogilvie-Harris & Jackson (1984) found that 85% of patients with normal or grade I patellar changes had good results. The operation is least effective in patients who have widespread articular cartilage damage. It is not known whether lateral release works by relieving the load on the lateral edge of the patella, altering its line of movement, changing its blood supply, or by denervating the capsule. The technique of operation is described above (p. 79).

The work of Fulkerson et al (1984), which demonstrated interstitial fibrosis of the nerves in the capsule similar to that seen in Morton's neuroma, may explain the cause of pain in these patients and the success that follows lateral release.

Miserable malalignment

The term 'miserable malalignment' was devised by James (1979) to describe persistent anterior knee pain in adolescents with squinting patella and femoral torsion. The condition can be confused with excessive lateral pressure syndrome, and is not a true patellar instability.

Chondromalacia patellae

Although the term chondromalacia is grossly over-used, articular cartilage softening does occur and the macroscopic appearances and histological features are well known (Ficat & Hungerford 1977). In brief, the pathological process passes through several distinct stages.

1. The 'blister' lesion

The blister lesion (Goodfellow et al 1976) results from degeneration and swelling of the deep layers of the articular surface without disruption of the surface layers (Fig. 13.10). The lesion, which presents a domed blister-like appearance (Fig. 13.11), is probably caused by imbibition of fluid into the disrupted deep layers of articular cartilage, as the long chain proteoglycans break into smaller molecules (Shoji & Granda 1974). The blister lesion can progress in one of two ways.

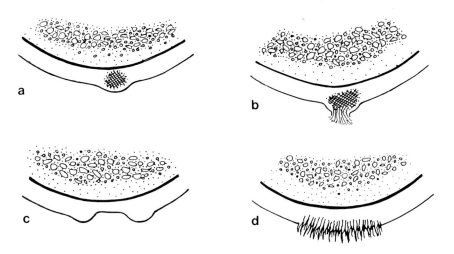

Fig. 13.10 Patterns of chondromalacia patellae: (A) a blister lesion with swelling of the deep layers of articular cartilage; (B) a burst blister with ruptured fibrils protruding through the surface; (C) an umbilicated blister in which an area of softening surrounds a depressed area; (D) generalised fibrillation of the articular cartilage

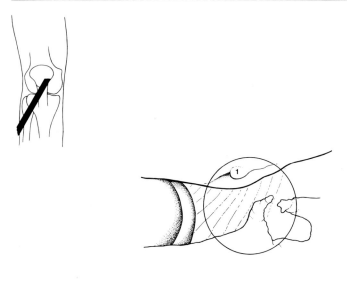

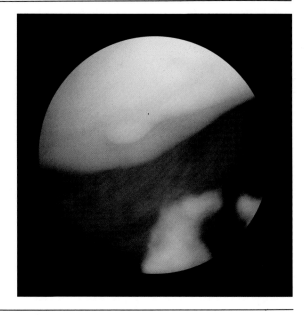

Fig. 13.11 A blister lesion (1) of the patella

2. The 'burst blister'

The blister lesion can rupture at its apex so that a tuft (Fig. 13.10) of damaged deep fibres protrudes (Dandy 1984). Such a lesion weakens the articular surface and provides a starting point for progressive articular cartilage breakdown.

3. The 'umbilicated blister'

A ring-shaped 'blister lesion' is sometimes seen, with a base of firm tissue at its centre consistent with healing or fibrosis (Fig. 13.10), surrounded by a ring of degeneration as the blister process proceeds outwards.

4. Fine fibrillation

Fine fibrillation of the articular cartilage is seen more frequently than the blister lesion, perhaps because it is more easily recognised. Fine fibrillation is also found in elderly patients with degenerative joint disease.

5. Coarse fibrillation

Coarse fibrillation with widespread disruption of the articular surface presents a shaggy 'crab meat' appearance at arthroscopy (Fig. 13.10), and may well result from a more rapid and widespread breakdown of the articular surface than the blister lesion.

6. Late changes

When breakdown occurs faster than repair, the articular cartilage changes proceed to osteoarthritis with exposure of the underlying cortical bone.

Grading

Precise grading of articular cartilage changes is made difficult by the great variation in appearance from one part of the joint to another, and by the indistinct boundary between chondromalacia and degenerative change. The following system, derived from that of Outerbridge (1961), has proved simple and convenient in practice and is based on the worst area of articular change that can be found. The system is similar to that used for the tibio-femoral joint (p. 103).

Grade I. Blister lesions (Fig. 13.11), softening (Fig. 13.12), and all changes up to and including an area of fine fibrillation 1 cm in diameter on the patella surface only (Fig. 13.13).

Grade II. An area of fine fibrillation more than 1 cm in diameter or coarse fibrillation less than 1 cm in diameter, on the patellar surface only (Fig. 13.13).

Grade III. Coarse (Fig. 13.14) or fine fibrillation over an area more than 1 cm in diameter (Fig. 13.13) on one surface, or less than 1 cm on both joint surfaces. Isolated areas of exposed subchondral bone over an area not greater than 2 mm in diameter on

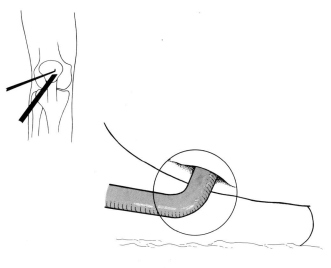

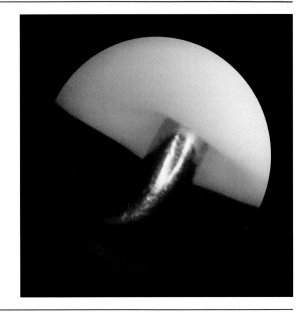

Fig. 13.12   True chondromalacia patellae. The probing hook demonstrates an area of softened, but intact articular cartilage

the patella can also be included as grade III change (Fig. 13.13).

Grade IV.   Exposed subchondral bone over an area more than 2 mm in diameter with surrounding degenerative change (Fig. 13.13). Osteochondral fractures or chondral separations, in which the surrounding articular cartilage is healthy, are classified separately.

Causes of chondromalacia

Traumatic chondromalacia If the patella is struck hard with the knee flexed, the impact is transmitted to the articular cartilage of the patella and femur. Although the patella may appear to recover completely and the patient may remain free of symptoms for as long as two years from the original injury,

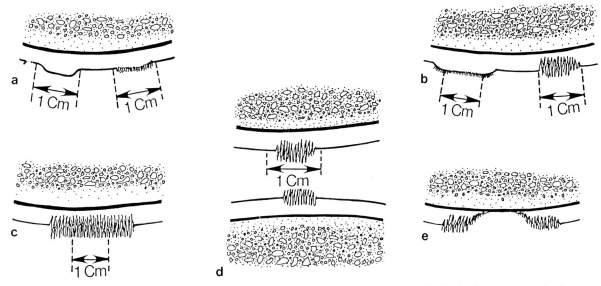

Fig. 13.13   Grading of chondromalacia patellae: (A) grade I change — an area of softening or fine fibrillation less than 1 cm in diameter; (B) grade II change — fine fibrillation more than 1 cm in diameter or coarse fibrillation less than 1 cm in diameter; (C) grade III — coarse fibrillation of more than 1 cm in diameter on one joint surface only; (D) grade III — fibrillation on both joint surfaces less than 1 cm in diameter; (E) grade IV — exposed bone on one or both joint surfaces

degenerative changes can appear later (Chaklin 1939, Soto-Hall 1945); this is an important consideration in the assessment of compensation following road traffic accidents. Because the force required to induce traumatic chondromalacia is less than that required to fracture the patella, a patella that has been fractured by direct injury is very likely to develop the late changes of traumatic chondromalacia, however meticulously it may be repaired (Fig. 13.14).

Idiopathic chondromalacia The pathology of chondromalacia is described by Insall (1984). Idiopathic chondromalacia is similar to traumatic chondromalacia, but lacks the history of definite trauma, and is most commonly seen in adolescents during or after the adolescent growth spurt. No single cause is known, but the articular cartilage of the normal patella is thicker than that of other joints, and the nutrition of its deeper layers may be imperfect. This, with the increased load imposed upon the joint surface by the greater body weight and muscular strength of adolescence, together with the poor nutrition of the joint surface, could tip the balance towards articular cartilage breakdown.

Other causes Any insult to the articular cartilage of the patella such as infection, synovial disease, repeated haemorrhage or prolonged immobilisation can be followed by 'chondromalacia' and progressive articular cartilage breakdown. Malalignment and an increased Q angle (p. 207) may also contribute

(Insall et al 1976), but Fairbank et al (1984) found no such correlation and concluded that overloading was more important.

Subluxation of the patella

Transient subluxation of the patella is most common in patients with lax ligaments and laterally placed patellae; it is often associated with articular cartilage defects, and may present with sudden pain on twisting, rather than a feeling of abnormal patellar movement. Dislocation of the patella is dealt with in Chapter 14.

Operations for chondromalacia patellae

Patellar shaving

Shaving of the patella, a 'traditional' operation, removes loose superficial fibres of degenerate articular cartilage without exposing the underlying subchondral bone. Although shaving undoubtedly produces a better-looking patella and relieves crepitus (Wiles et al 1960), it is hard to see how this alone can bring about permanent healing of the articular surface. When the surgeon has become adept at arthroscopic surgery, there is a temptation to think that any arthroscopic operation must be good. As Dr R.W. Jackson has commented, when you only have a hammer, most things look like nails; this may explain why many surgeons who had discarded open shaving

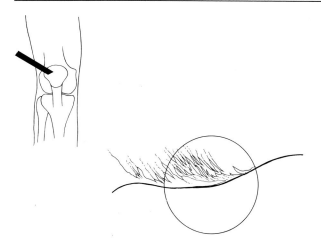

Fig. 13.14 Traumatic chondromalacia. The patient was struck on the patella in a road traffic accident 18 months previously, but had not taken weight on the leg during this period because of lower limb fractures. Note the coarse fibrillation

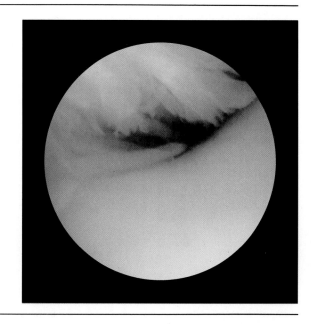

of the patella as ineffective have returned to the operation now that it can be done arthroscopically.

Open shaving, like other operations performed through an arthrotomy, involves many things apart from the procedure itself; these include division and repair of the capsule with an alteration in its tension, and consequently in the patellar alignment; perhaps a haemarthrosis; enforced rest leading to wasting and weakness of the quadriceps, with a consequent reduction in the forces imposed upon the joint; as well as a graded course of physiotherapy to restore function. Arthroscopic shaving of the patella (Fig. 8.16), which involves little more morbidity than simple diagnostic arthroscopy, adds none of these additional insults to the knee, and the long-term results of operation may therefore be different. On the other hand, the long-term results of shaving through an arthrotomy are poor, and there is no reason to suppose that the results will be any better simply because it is done through a smaller hole. Careful and objective assessment of the long-term results of patellar shaving are essential before arthroscopic shaving can become the object of exuberant optimism. The best results of patellar shaving are found in patients with the coarse fibrillation seen in traumatic chondromalacia, of whom 73% of patients with grade II change had good results (Ogilvie-Harris & Jackson 1984). The operative technique is described on p. 104.

Drilling

Drilling subchondral bone to encourage healing is commonly recommended for localised articular cartilage lesions, although it is difficult to see how this can alter the underlying cause of the degenerative change that made the operation necessary in the first instance. Drilling through exposed bone into the underlying cancellous tissue was recommended by Pridie (Pridie 1959, Insall 1967) for osteoarthritis on the grounds that the defects would heal with sound cartilage, but even if new articular cartilage is formed, which some think unlikely (Childers & Ellwood 1979), its spread across the undrilled area would seem improbable (Fig. 8.20).

Drilling through the areas of degenerative articular cartilage rather than exposed subchondral bone is perhaps more likely to be effective, because any healing in the region of the drill holes could provide support for the surrounding articular surface, tipp-

ing the balance in favour of the healing process. Against this must be placed the work of Landells (1957), who has shown that in rabbits the presence of blood in the joint cavity may damage articular cartilage. Decompression of the cancellous core of the patella may also influence the result of operation.

Spongiolisation

Ficat & Hungerford (1977) describe excision of the entire cortex from areas affected by articular cartilage degeneration. Such a procedure is, in effect, a very large Pridie-style drill hole, which creates a cavity at the site of the lesion and may help healing by reducing the mechanical effects of friction and pressure. With the knowledge from Salter's work (Salter et al 1980) that continuous joint motion aids the healing of full-thickness osteochondral lesions, excision of the cortex with early mobilisation would seem a logical treatment and this is supported by the clinical observation that the beds of untreated osteochondral fractures heal well and are often found as incidental asymptomatic findings when loose bodies are removed.

Against spongiolisation, it must be said that the procedure is unusually destructive and places great demands on the healing process in an area where it has demonstrably failed, for if healing had been adequate, the operation would not have been required. Moreover, the edges of the crater may be subjected to particularly heavy loads as healing proceeds at the centre and restriction of weight-bearing with crutches does not solve the problem completely.

Although no figures are available to define the precise indications for drilling or spongiolisation, lesions less than 1 cm in diameter and surrounded by healthy articular cartilage seem particularly suitable for this procedure, whereas the more widespread lesions of osteoarthritis do not. The technique of spongiolisation is described above (p. 106).

At present, it has to be said that we do not know enough about the effects of shaving, drilling, abrasion or spongiolisation to establish the proper indications for these procedures.

Osteoarthritis

Because it is hard to define osteoarthritis as anything more than a progressive and irreversible breakdown of articular cartilage, the point at which chondroma-lacia becomes osteoarthritis is imprecise (p. 102) and any such distinction must be, to some extent, artificial.

Different disorders cause different patterns of osteoarthritis. Excessive lateral pressure syndrome, for example, leads to marked degenerative change on the lateral facet only and these changes may be so marked that there is exposed bone on both the lateral facet of the patella and the lateral condyle, while the medial half of the joint is normal (Fig. 13.6). In theory, a lateral release should be effective in relieving symptoms from this pattern of osteoarthri-tis, but the results are often disappointing and patellectomy offers a more predictable result.

An early lateral release might also avert the onset of osteoarthritis later, but there is no evidence to support the idea of prophylactic lateral release, however sensible this might seem from first prin-ciples.

Fractures of the patella can lead not only to traumatic chondromalacia, but also to a step in the articular surface, which must hasten the onset of frank osteoarthritis. If rapidly progressive osteoar-thritis seems inevitable, the patella should be removed before the femoral surface is involved in the degenerative process.

Operations for osteoarthritis

Tibial tubercle advancement (patello-femoral decompression)

Because the patella bears so strongly against the underlying femur, any procedure that reduces load on the patella is likely to reduce patello-femoral pain and advancement of the tibial tubercle has been widely recommended as a means of reducing patello-femoral load.

Tibial tubercle advancement was originally sug-gested by Maquet (Maquet et al 1967), who described a technique in which the tubercle was advanced 2 cm with a strip of cortex and held with a block of iliac bone under its tip (Fig. 13.15). Secondary skin grafts were needed in 2 of his 49 patients, and the wounds broke down in 2 more (Maquet 1974). Others have encountered similar problems, and one surgeon who practised this procedure made the dismal observation that if the wound could be closed, the tubercle had not been

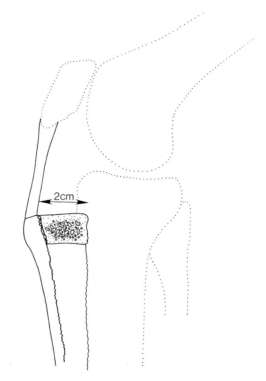

Fig. 13.15 Maquet's operation, in which the tibial tubercle is elevated 2 cm with a block of bone placed under a long tibial strut

advanced far enough. Fracture of the advanced strip of tibial cortex has also occurred (Heatley & Patrick 1979), and most patients, even those with an otherwise successful result, are unable to kneel after operation because the advanced tubercle is sensitive.

Many surgeons who report good results after Maquet's operation are in fact performing Bandi's operation, and this has caused some confusion. Bandi's procedure (Fig. 13.16), in which the tubercle alone is lifted with an osteo-periosteal flap and supported with a 1 cm thick block of cancellous bone, is less drastic than the Maquet procedure and not associated with the same technical problems. Moreover, Nakamura et al (1985) have shown that a 1 cm advancement of the tubercle is mechanically better than a 2 cm advancement, which also distorts the contact areas and interferes seriously with joint function. Bandi also advised that the procedure should include a wide lateral release of the extensor mechanism and debridement of osteophytes, which makes it difficult to identify the results of tibial tubercle advancement alone.

Bandi (1972) has demonstrated mathematically and with a model that advancement of the tibial tubercle by 1 cm produces a substantial reduction in

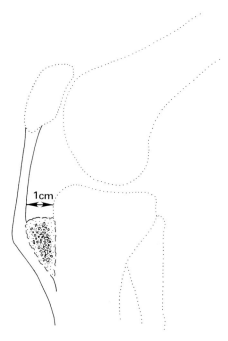

Fig. 13.16 Bandi's operation, in which the tibial tubercle is elevated 1 cm with cancellous bone

Table 13.1 Indications for patellectomy – conservative to aggressive

Conservative	Never
	Gross osteoarthritis confined to the patello-femoral joint
	Comminuted fractures
	Moderate but progressive osteoarthritis
	Recurrence of patellar pain after patellar shaving
	Patellar pain with marked crepitus
	Transverse fracture of the patella
	Painless patellar crepitus
	Undisplaced fractures
	Patellar tenderness, but no crepitus
Aggressive	Mild anterior knee pain with intact articular surface

patello-femoral loading. In effect, advancement of the tubercle produces the same relationship between patella and tibia that is produced by extending the knee a little more and, as the load on the patella increases the more the knee is flexed, this can be helpful. The operation does not, however, produce any absolute reduction in the load on the patella. Tibial tubercle 'advancement' can occur naturally as the result of Osgood–Schlatter's disease, and a similar relationship of tubercle to femur is seen in patients with genu recurvatum. In view of the conflict between the work of Maquet et al (1967) and Nakamura et al (1985) there may be room for a critical review of the biomechanics of tibial tubercle advancement, however good the operation may be in practice, particularly when it is accompanied by a lateral release.

Patellectomy

Indications The indications for patellectomy can be summarised as severe pain in a stable, but irretrievably damaged patello-femoral joint. Conditions which cause irretrievable damage include osteoarthritis, tumours and comminuted fractures, but the point at which the derangement is considered irretrievable varies from one surgeon to the next (Table 13.1).

Bentley (1970, 1977) found that patellectomy was a more reliable operation for chondromalacia patellae than patellar shaving. Some surgeons advise patellectomy for all but the slightest articular cartilage damage, whereas others might treat a comminuted fracture by internal fixation.

Patellectomy has the disadvantage that it is an excision arthroplasty and therefore the last shot in the surgeon's locker; as long as the patella remains, the ultimate salvage operation of patellectomy is still available, but once this has been done, there is little or nothing to offer the patient. Furthermore, patellectomy does not stabilise the patellar mechanism and should not be done unless the patella is stable. Recurrent dislocation of the extensor mechanism following patellectomy may present an insoluble problem.

Against these disadvantages must be set the benefit of replacing a painful joint surface with a smooth tendon so that pain no longer inhibits contraction of the quadriceps. A painless patello-femoral joint with distorted mechanics is better than a painful joint that is dynamically perfect, and patients will often feel that the power of extension is increased after patellectomy, despite the biomechanical disadvantages.

Mechanics At its thickest point, the patella measures 2–3 cm from front to back (Ficat & Hungerford 1977). Removal of the patella allows the extensor mechanism to fall backwards by this amount, bringing the tendon much closer to the axis of rotation and reducing the rotational force on the knee (Kaufer 1971) (Fig. 13.17). At the same time, removal of the patella weakens the power of extension by increasing the functional length of the quadriceps mechanism, and allows the insertions of the vastus medialis and vastus lateralis to migrate proximally.

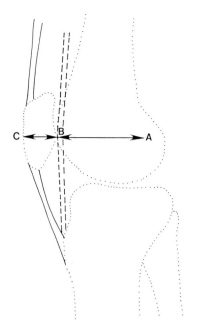

Fig. 13.17 The mechanical effect of patellectomy. Removal of the patella brings the tendon nearer to the axis of rotation (A) by the width of the patella (BC). Shortening the lever arm about the axis of rotation from AC to AB weakens the power of the extensors

Arthroscopy is helpful in selecting patients suitable for patellectomy and excluding surgically correctable derangements, but patellectomy cannot yet be performed arthroscopically.

Many techniques for patellectomy are described, but that of Boyd & Hawkins (1948) is simple, does not disturb the continuity of the extensor mechanism, and permits 'double breasting' of the quadriceps tendon over the defect, which helps to reduce the changes in tendon length and the alignment of the vasti. Because the extensor mechanism remains in continuity, early mobilisation is possible and avoids the disadvantages of cast immobilisation.

Technique

1. After the usual skin preparation, the leg is prepared and draped, and a tourniquet is applied. The line of incision can be in any direction, but a short skin crease incision is entirely satisfactory.
2. The periosteum is incised vertically and cleared from the bone for a few millimetres on either side. The patella is then split vertically in its midline with a broad osteotome (Fig. 13.18).

3. The two halves of the patella are shelled out, preserving the quadriceps expansion over the patella.
4. The soft tissue from each half of the patella is double breasted and sutured with an absorbable suture. Unabsorbable sutures cause painful subcutaneous nodules that do not resolve and should not be used.
5. The tourniquet is released, haemostasis secured, and the skin closed over a suction drain.
6. A firm supportive dressing and a light cast are applied. Quadriceps exercise is instituted at once and flexion commenced as soon as a straight leg raise has been achieved, usually after three or four days, to minimise the risk of adhesion formation.

Osteochondral fractures

Osteochondral fractures of the patella arise from dislocations, direct violence, or sudden twisting movements of the knee, either with or without patella dislocation, and cause pain and haemarthrosis (Rorabeck & Bobechko 1976). Although an osteochondral fracture should always be recognised soon after injury, the fracture often escapes detection (Matthewson & Dandy 1978) until the patient presents with a loose body and pain when the knee is flexed under load. Crepitus is seldom felt under the patello-femoral joint of such knees, but at arthroscopy a healed defect in the articular surface may be seen as a slightly depressed area of articular cartilage that is slightly duller and greyer than normal. Nothing can or need be done about such lesions, and all that is required is arthroscopic removal of the loose body.

If the diagnosis is made early, the joint should be arthroscoped to evacuate blood and assess whether it is technically possible to replace the fragment and fix it internally. The trauma of open reduction and internal fixation is considerable, and this, with the immobilisation needed after operation, may lead to a stiff knee and a worse result than early mobilisation. An osteochondral fracture is functionally the same as the spongiolisation operation of Ficat, so that good results from immediate removal of the fragment and early mobilisation should not be altogether surprising. There is much to be said for immediate arthroscopic removal of the fragment and early movement to encourage healing of the joint surface (Salter et al 1980), but the patello-femoral joint should be protected from load-bearing in flexion for at least eight weeks, and preferably longer.

Chondral separations

Articular cartilage fragments can separate from the patella without detachment of the underlying cortex, leaving exposed subchondral cortical bone. These injuries, like their counterpart in the tibio-femoral joint (p. 98), do not cause any radiological abnormality, and lead to the formation of a loose body of articular cartilage which either remains as a loose body or is converted to fine particulate debris. Arthroscopy may be required to investigate the persistent synovial effusion or diffuse anterior knee pain that may follow a chondral separation.

Once identified, chondral separations can either be left alone or the base can be abraded or drilled to convert them, in effect, into osteochondral fractures. There is no evidence yet to suggest that one

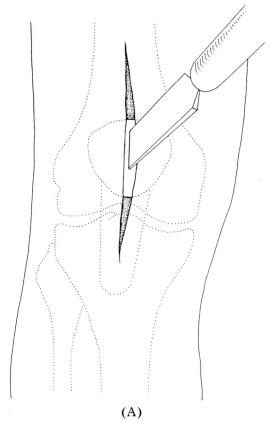

(A)

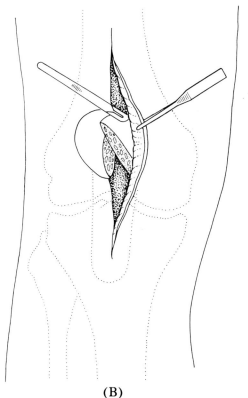

(B)

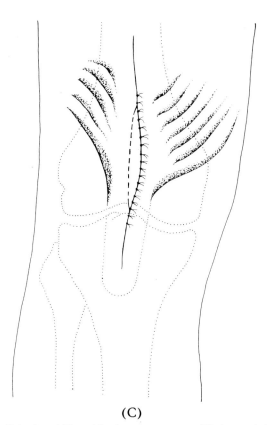

(C)

Fig. 13.18 Patellectomy by the method of Boyd and Hawkins: (A) the patella is split in the midline with a broad osteotome; (B) the two halves are shelled out leaving the extensor tendon intact; (C) the defect is closed and the soft tissues overlapped

treatment is better than another, but it would seem sensible to encourage movement and avoid flexion of the knee under load for several weeks until the lesion has had a chance to heal.

Chondral flaps

Partial-thickness flaps of articular cartilage are sometimes seen after direct violence, such as a kick. The flap may cause mechanical catching or clicking on flexion, and the symptoms can be relieved by removing the flap under arthroscopic control (p. 99). If this is done, it is important to be as gentle as possible with the articular cartilage and not to extend the lesion any more than is absolutely necessary.

Osteochondritis dissecans of the patella

Patients with painful patello-femoral joints sometimes have the radiological appearance of osteochondritis dissecans of the patella (Fig. 13.19) (Edwards & Bentley 1977), which looks more like an ossification defect than the true dissecting lesion of femoral osteochondritis. If a loose body is present, as Edwards and Bentley found in five of their six cases, it should be removed and the bed drilled if it is uneven. More often, arthroscopy shows that the articular surface is intact, with a softened area only detectable with a probing hook, and the lesion should then be left to resolve spontaneously. The natural history of osteochondritis dissecans of the patella with a normal articular surface, and its role as a cause of anterior knee pain, remain uncertain.

Bipartite patellae

Bipartite and multipartite patellae come in many shapes and sizes (Ficat & Hungerford 1977), often without any symptoms attributable to the patello-femoral joint. Some are the result of a fatigue fracture (Devas 1960), and others may be a manifes-

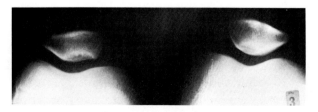

Fig. 13.19 Osteochondritis dissecans of the patella

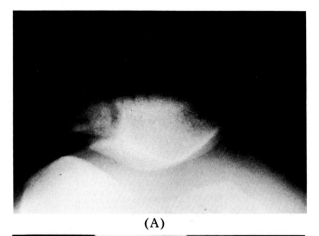

(A)

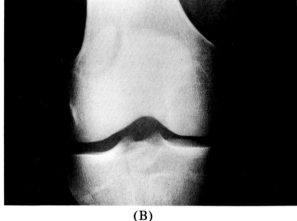

(B)

Fig. 13.20 Bipartite patella: (A) 30° tangential view; (B) antero-posterior view

tation of the excessive lateral pressure syndrome (Fig. 13.20). Most bipartite patellae are asymptomatic, but when they do give rise to symptoms, they cause pain and tenderness at the supero-lateral corner of the patella. At arthroscopy, the articular surface is usually normal, but if there is crepitus under the abnormal area of patella, arthroscopy may show fibrillation over the separated fragment.

If patience, anti-inflammatory drugs and rest do not relieve symptoms, operation must be considered. Excision of the abnormal fragment is usually effective, but this may be nothing more than a needlessly traumatic lateral release. Osborne & Fulford (1982) reported good results after lateral release alone, and Rohlederer (1951) has reported spontaneous union of the separated fragments following lateral release. If the articular cartilage of the separated fragment is degenerate, excision of the loose fragment will be necessary. Excision of the fragment, combined with a lateral release, is therefore a logical procedure, with the proviso that if the articular cartilage of the fragment is entirely normal at arthroscopy, lateral release alone may be sufficient.

PAIN FROM TENDONS

Vastus lateralis strain

Some patients have pain and tenderness localised to the supero-lateral corner of the patella, but no true tenderness of the patella. If the tenderness is confined to the soft tissues and the lateral facet of the patella is not painful, a strain of the vastus lateralis insertion, analagous to tennis elbow, is likely. Natural recovery can be hastened with anti-inflammatory drugs and avoiding unnecessary strain on the joint, but if symptoms persist, steroid injection into the painful area (but not into the joint) can be effective. If all else fails, a lateral release may be required. It is possible that this condition is a 'forme fruste' of bipartite patella. Apart from excluding an internal derangement and performing a lateral release, arthroscopy is not helpful in the management of these lesions.

Patellar tendinitis (jumper's knee)

In adults, pain localised precisely to the centre of the patellar tendon at its insertion on the patella is usually due to a partial rupture of the fibres at their insertion. The condition is known as 'jumper's knee' because of its alleged occurrence in high jumpers, but in practice the condition is no more common in jumpers than tennis elbow is in tennis players. Jumper's knee is probably the result of any unexpected contraction of the quadriceps (James 1979), rather than some movement specific to jumping.

Jumper's knee can be persistent and troublesome, and may not respond to conservative management. Injection of hydrocortisone around the tender spot is often effective, but because of the real risk of tendon rupture following steroid injection, the steroid should be placed around the bone-ligament junction and not into the tendon itself. If steroid injection is ineffective – as it often is – operation may be needed to raise the central fibres of the tendon from the lower pole of the patella, after a preliminary arthroscopy to exclude internal derangements. The underlying bone can then be scarified or drilled, in the belief that, as the surgically created lesion heals,

the original site of pain will be obliterated by sound scar tissue. The operation is comparable to that for release of tennis elbow and carries a similarly uncertain prognosis.

PAIN FROM BONE

Reflex sympathetic dystrophy (algodystrophy)

Sudeck's atrophy following Colles' fracture at the wrist or Pott's fracture at the ankle are well recognised (Schutzler & Gossling 1984), but the same condition at the knee can escape recognition. Although it is rare, the condition must be borne in mind when a persistently painful knee fails to respond to treatment and should always be considered before a patient is labelled as a hysteric or a malingerer.

The clinical features of reflex sympathetic dystrophy are pain, tenderness, warmth, sensitivity to temperature change, and stiffness. The precipitating factor is usually trauma, often nothing more severe than a minor knock on the front of the knee, but perhaps the most common overall cause is haemarthrosis following arthrotomy. This presents a special problem to arthroscopists, who are often referred patients who have undergone unsuccessful arthrotomy elsewhere.

The patella is more often involved in reflex sympathetic dystrophy than the tibia or femur, perhaps because it is more exposed and less well covered by soft tissues. Radiological examination will show osteoporosis (Fig. 13.21) and the knee will be normal on thermography. Radio-nuclide scintigraphy may show increased uptake in the early stages, but uptake may be normal or even reduced in the later stages. The investigations and pathology are described by Ficat & Hungerford (1977), who also found an increase in interosseus pressure and venous stasis in the patella and the lower end of the femur on phlebography.

The natural history of reflex sympathetic dystrophy is of gradual spontaneous recovery over a period of up to two years. The condition follows the usual three stages seen in Sudeck's atrophy with (1) an early period of pain, followed by (2) stiffness with relief of pain, and later by (3) a gradual return of movement. As with Sudeck's atrophy, additional trauma – including arthrotomy or forced manipula-

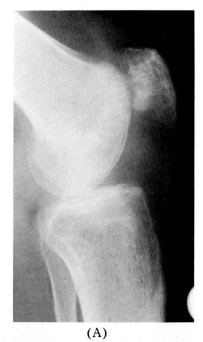

(A)

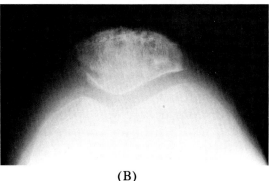

(B)

Fig. 13.21 Reflex sympathetic dystrophy involving the patella and femur: (A) lateral view; (B) 60° tangential view

tion – should be avoided in the first painful phase, but arthroscopy will exclude an internal derangement and does not seem to delay recovery. Gradual mobilisation should be instituted once the acute phase has passed and a diminishing course of steroids may be helpful. Ficat & Hungerford (1977) report good results from administration of Valium, Hydrargine and a non-steroidal anti-inflammatory drug in the early stages, and have also found that sympathectomy can be helpful in the later stages (Hungerford 1980). Continued encouragement and applied optimism may be just as effective.

Osgood–Schlatter's disease

Osgood–Schlatter's disease, or apophysitis of the tibial tubercle (Osgood 1903, Schlatter 1903, Mital et al 1980), can be distinguished from patellar pain without difficulty, but is sometimes seen in an orthopaedic clinic with the initial diagnosis of 'chondromalacia'. Osgood–Schlatter's disease occurs at the start of the adolescent growth spurt, is most common in athletic youngsters, and results from the new-found strength of the quadriceps mechanism being too powerful for its attachment to the apophysis of the tubercle. Partial separation of the apophysis from the tibia leads to pain when the quadriceps is contracted, tenderness and a prominent tibial tubercle.

Spontaneous resolution with growth is the rule. Most patients make a steady, but slow recovery over a period of twelve to eighteen months, if they avoid cross-country running, jumping and other activities which produce pain. Complete restriction of all sporting activities is not necessary, and injection of hydrocortisone into the apophysis is indicated only if the pain is severe and does not resolve within six months of onset. Immobilisation in a plaster cylinder always results in wasting of the quadriceps and very occasionally in relief of symptoms.

A few patients develop an isolated bony spicule at the attachment of the tendon to the tibial shaft, sometimes with the formation of a pseudarthrosis between the spicule and the tibia. The pseudarthrosis may become inflamed, and exuberant synovial proliferation or even granulation tissue may form around the spicule. It is in these patients that injection of steroid is more effective. If the pain persists, excision of the bony spicule may be needed, but the patient should be warned that the pain will persist long after the operation, and that the prominence on the tibial tubercle will not be completely removed. Arthroscopy has no part to play in the management of this condition, except as a preliminary to excision of the spicule, should this be necessary, to exclude an internal derangement.

Sindig-Larsen disease

Sindig-Larsen disease (Sindig-Larsen 1921, Katz 1981) is comparable to Osgood–Schlatter's disease, but involves the lower pole of the patella (Fig. 13.22) and is much more common in patients under the age of 10 than those entering the adolescent growth spurt, a reflection of the earlier fusion of the growth centre for the lower pole of the patella. A prolonga-

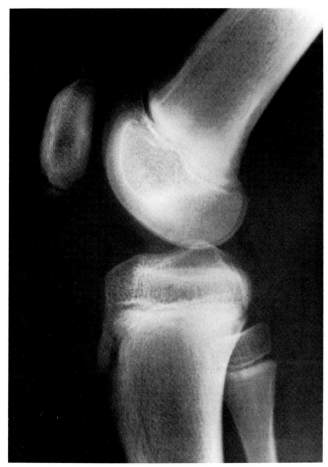

Fig. 13.22 Sindig-Larsen disease

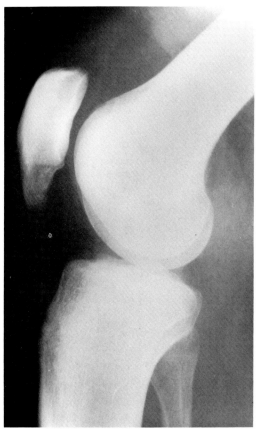

Fig. 13.23 Prolongation of the lower pole of the patella, perhaps the late result of Sindig-Larsen disease

tion of the lower pole of the patella (Fig. 13.23), occasionally seen as an incidental finding in adults, may perhaps be the end result of Sindig-Larsen disease. Sindig-Larsen disease is more easily confused with chondromalacia patellae than Osgood--Schlatter's disease, but can easily be distinguished by the localised tenderness at the lower pole of the patella, the radiological appearance of the slight separation of the lower pole, and the patient's age. In an adult, the same symptoms and signs would suggest jumper's knee.

Miscellaneous lesions

There is probably no limit to the number of lesions which can cause anterior knee pain. An osteoid osteoma of the tibia was found and removed arthroscopically in one patient and many equally bizarre lesions are likely to occur.

PAIN FROM INTERNAL DERANGEMENTS

Ruptured anterior cruciate ligaments

Most surgeons will be able to recall patients with a small effusion and a painless block to extension, who were thought on clinical grounds to have a torn meniscus, but had a full range of extension under general anaesthesia. These patients may have a swollen and oedematous anterior cruciate stub which can be removed under arthroscopic control. There is good evidence that the anterior cruciate ligament is crammed with proprioceptive nerves, and these may somehow be responsible for inhibiting extension. With time, the stub retracts down on to its tibial attachment and forms a nubbin of tissue in the notch, which limits full extension mechanically, and can be painful as well.

Meniscus lesions

Although lesions of the menisci are often associated with pain at the front of the knee, it is unusual for

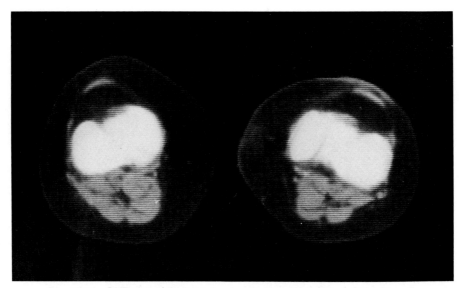

Fig. 13.24   CAT scan of the knee showing the size and position of the fat-pad

pain to be the only symptom, or for tenderness at the front of the joint to be the only abnormal sign. Despite this, meniscus lesions can present with nothing more than tenderness over the medial or lateral side of the patellar tendon, and the possibility of a meniscus lesion should not be forgotten in a patient with pain over the anterior horn of meniscus in the absence of any other symptom or physical sign.

Fat-pad

Inflammation of pads of fat and synovial fronds have been incriminated as a cause of anterior knee pain since at least 1904 (Hoffa 1904), but the condition has sometimes been considered a diagnosis of desperation. The fat-pad is a normal structure, but it is so large and in such a vulnerable position (Fig. 13.24) that it is remarkable that it seldom causes symptoms. The characteristic features of the 'fat-pad syndrome', which have been well described by Smillie (1978), include pain on hyperextension with tenderness of the fat-pad on firm palpation. The condition is most often seen in adolescent girls, who find that the pain is worse when walking barefoot or in low-heeled shoes than in high heels.

If the symptoms persist and the fat-pad is explored (p. 81), it will usually appear normal, although haemorrhagic lesions are sometimes seen in its substance or along its free margin. Excision of the fat-pad is effective, but Smillie has advocated the

alternative procedure of tethering the prominent synovial fronds with a suture to stop them intruding into the joint.

It is entirely possible that some of the good results of fat-pad excision occur in patients who have had pedunculated lipomata, ganglia or the synovial shelf syndrome. The medial synovial shelf runs into the infrapatellar fat-pad and excision of the fat-pad may alter the tension in this structure, even if it is not completely divided.

Ganglia

Ganglia in the knee are uncommon, but are sometimes seen beneath the synovium at the base of the anterior cruciate ligament. The ganglia can be either sessile or pedunculated, and cause a deep-seated aching pain on full extension. Arthroscopic excision is simple (p. 82).

Lipomata

Small pedunculated lipomata can cause pain at the front of the knee, particularly if the pedicle is twisted at its base and the tumour becomes necrotic. The lesions are so rare that it is impossible to make the diagnosis clinically. At arthroscopy, the lesion will be seen as a purplish mass resembling a haemorrhoid and arthroscopic excision of the lesion is straightforward (p. 82).

References

Aglietti P, Insall J N, Cerulli G 1983 Patellar pain and incongruence. I Measurements of incongruence. Clinical Orthopaedics and Related Research 176: 217–224

Aleman O 1928 Chondromalacia posttraumatica patellae. Acta Chirurgica Scandinavica 63: 149–190

Bandi W 1972 Chondromalacia Patellae und Femoro-Patellare Arthrose. Helvetica Chirurgica Acta suppl II: 3–70

Bentley G 1970 Chondromalacia patellae. Journal of Bone and Joint Surgery 52A: 221–232

Bentley G 1977 Surgical treatment of chondromalacia patellae. Journal of Bone and Joint Surgery 59B: 107–108

Boyd H B, Hawkins B L 1948 Patellectomy – a simplified technique. Surgery, Gynecology and Obstetrics 86: 357–358

Brattstrom H 1964 Shape of the intercondylar groove normally and in recurrent dislocation of the patella. Acta Orthopedica Scandinavica suppl 68: 134–148

Chaklin V D 1939 Injuries to the cartilages of the patella and the femoral condyle. Journal of Bone and Joint Surgery 21: 133–140

Childers J C, Ellwood B C 1979 Partial chondrectomy and subchondral bone drilling for chondromalacia. Clinical Orthopaedics and Related Research 144: 110–113

Dandy D J 1984 Arthroscopy of the knee: a diagnostic atlas. Gower–Butterworth, London

Devas M B 1960 Stress fractures of the patella. Journal of Bone and Joint Surgery 42B: 71–74

Edwards D H, Bentley G 1977 Osteochondritis dissecans patellae. Journal of Bone and Joint Surgery 59B: 58–63

Fairbank J C T, Pynsent P B, van Poortvliet, Phillips H 1984 Mechanical factors in the incidence of knee pain in adolescents and young adults. Journal of Bone and Joint Surgery 66B: 685–693

Ficat R P, Hungerford D S 1977 Disorders of the patello-femoral joint. Williams & Wilkins, Baltimore, Md

Fujisawa Y 1976 Problems caused by the medial and lateral synovial folds of the patella. Kansetsukyo 1: 40–44

Fulkerson J P, Tennant R, Grunnet M 1984 Evidence of nerve damage the retinaculum of patello–femoral pain patients. Proceedings of the Fifth Triennial Meeting of the International Arthroscopy Association, London

Goodfellow J W, Hungerford D S, Zindel M 1976 Patello–femoral mechanics and pathology. 2 Chondromalacia patellae. Journal of Bone and Joint Surgery 58B: 291–299

Heatley F W, Patrick J H 1979 A three–year prospective study of the tibial tubercle advancement operation. Journal of Bone and Joint Surgery 61B: 518

Hoffa A 1904 The influence of the adipose tissue with regard to the pathology of the knee joint. Journal of the American Medical Association 43: 795–796

Hughston J C, Stone M, Andrews J R 1973 The suprapatellar plica: its role in internal derangement of the knee. Journal of Bone and Joint Surgery 55A: 1318

Hungerford D S 1980 Dystrophie sympathique reflexe et chondromalacie de la rotule. Revue Chirurgie Orthopédique 66: 259–261

Insall J N 1967 Intra–articular surgery for degenerative arthritis of the knee; a report on the work of the late K H Pridie. Journal of Bone and Joint Surgery 49B: 211–228

Insall J N 1984 Disorders of the patella. In: Insall J N (ed) Surgery of the knee. Churchill Livingstone, New York

Insall J N, Falvo K, Wise D W 1976 Chondromalacia patellae: a prospective study. Journal of Bone and Joint Surgery 58A: 1–8

Jackson R W, Marshall D J, Fujisawa Y 1982 The pathological medial shelf. Orthopedic Clinics of North America 13: 307–312

James S L 1979 Chondromalacia of the patella in the adolescent. In: Kennedy J C (ed) The Injured adolescent knee. Williams & Wilkins, Baltimore, Md

Katz J F 1981 Non-articular osteochondroses. Clinical Orthopaedics and Related Research 158: 70–76

Kaufer H 1971 Mechanical function of the patella. Journal of Bone and Joint Surgery 53A: 1551–1560

Landells J W 1957 The reactions of injured human articular cartilage. Journal of Bone and Joint Surgery 62A: 1232

Laurin C A, Dussault R, Levesque H P 1979 The tangential X-ray investigation of the patello-femoral joint: X-ray technique, diagnostic criteria and their interpretation. Clinical Orthopaedics and Related Research 144: 16–26

Maquet P 1974 Advancement of the tibial tuberosity. Clinical Orthopaedics and Related Research 115: 225–227

Matthewson M H, Dandy D J 1978 Osteochondral fractures of the lateral femoral condyle: a result of indirect violence to the knee. Journal of Bone and Joint Surgery 60B: 199–202

Mital M A, Matza R A, Cohen J 1980 So-called unresolved Osgood–Schlatter lesions. A concept based on fifteen surgically treated lesions. Journal of Bone and Joint Surgery 62A: 732–739

Ogilvie-Harris D J, Jackson R W 1984 The arthroscopic treatment of chondromalacia patellae. Journal of Bone and Joint Surgery 66B: 660–665

Osborne A H, Fulford P C 1982 Lateral release for chondromalacia patellae. Journal of Bone and Joint Surgery 64B: 202–206

Osgood R B 1903 Lesions of the tibial tubercle occurring during adolescence. Boston Medical and Surgical Journal 148: 114–117

Outerbridge R E 1961 The aetiology of chondromalacia patellae. Journal of Bone and Joint Surgery 43B: 752–757

Patel D 1978 Arthroscopy of the plicae-synovial folds and their significance. Americal Journal of Sports Medicine 6: 217–225

Pridie K H 1959 A method of resurfacing osteoarthritic knee joints. Journal of Bone and Joint Surgery 46B: 618

Rohlederer O 1951 Atiologie und Symptomatologie der Praeluxio Patellae. Zentralblatt fur Chirurgie 76: 103–115

Rorabeck C H, Bobechko W P 1976 Acute dislocation of the patella with osteochondral fracture. A review of eighteen cases. Journal of Bone and Joint Surgery 58B: 237–240

Salter R B, Simmonds D F, Malcolm B W, Rumble E J, Macmichael D, Clements N B 1980 The biological effect of continuous passive movement on the healing of full-thickness defects in articular cartilage. Journal of Bone and Joint Surgery 62A: 1232–1251

Schlatter C 1903 Verletzungen des Schnabel Formigen Fortsatzes der Oberen Tibiaepiphysis. Beitrage zur Klinische Chirurgie 38: 874–887

Schutzler S F, Gossling H R 1984 The treatment of reflex sympathetic dystrophy syndrome. Journal of Bone and Joint Surgery 66A: 625–629

Shoji H, Granda J L 1974 Acid hydrolases in the articular cartilage of the patella. Clinical Orthopaedics and Related Research 99: 293–297

Sindig-Larsen C M F 1921 A hitherto unknown affection of the patella in children. Acta Radiologica 1: 171

Smillie I S 1978 Diseases of the knee joint. Churchill Livingstone, London

Soto-Hall R 1945 Traumatic degeneration of the articular cartilage of the patella. Journal of Bone and Joint Surgery 27: 426–431

Vaughan-Lane T, Dandy D J 1982 The synovial shelf syndrome. Journal of Bone and Joint Surgery 64B: 475–476

Wiles P, Andrews P S, Bremner R A 1960 Chondromalacia of the patella. A study of the late results of excision of articular cartilage. Journal of Bone and Joint Surgery 42B: 65–70

14

Arthroscopy in the management of patellar instability

Although there are many different types of patellar instability, there is a tendency for recurrent dislocation of the patella – rather like 'chondromalacia patellae' – to be regarded as a single disorder and for one operation to be applied to every case. This chapter will try to separate the various patterns of instability and show how the arthroscope can help, an approach first used by Wiberg in 1941.

TYPES OF DISLOCATION

Recurrent dislocation of the patella

In patients with recurrent dislocation, the patella dislocates suddenly and completely to the lateral side and the dislocations are separated by periods of weeks or months. The patients, usually adolescents or young adults, often describe these episodes as 'dislocations of the knee', which may direct the attention of the unwary away from the patella. The first dislocation is often caused by a sharp twisting movement of the knee on the sports field or the dance floor, but with time the patella will dislocate more and more frequently and with diminishing trauma.

Clinical examination will usually demonstrate abnormal mobility of the patella when it is pushed laterally, and the patient may feel that the patella is about to dislocate. The patient's apprehension may be so great that she may grab the examiner's hand to stop him dislocating the patella, but a feeling of mild agitation or misgiving is more usual. If the knee is examined shortly after a dislocation, there is usually an effusion and medial parapatellar tenderness.

Radiographs often show small ossicles of bone on the medial side of the patella, the result of acute osteochondral fractures from contact between the lateral femoral condyle and the medial edge of the patella at the moment of dislocation. These fractures were first described by Coleman in 1948 and are sometimes called 'Coleman's fractures' (Fig. 14.1).

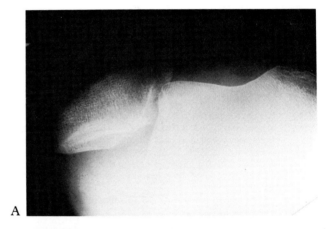

A

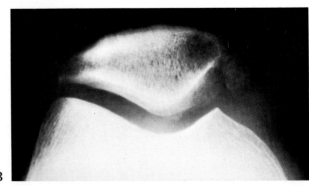

B

Fig. 14.1 Coleman's fractures: (A) a fracture of the medial margin of the patella at the time of dislocation; (B) the late result of such a fracture

Arthroscopy is useful in assessing the stability of the patella, the state of the articular surface, and checking that there is no other internal derangement but it has little, if anything, to offer in identifying the cause of patellar instability, which is usually determined by clinical and radiological examination. If the arthroscope is placed in the lateral gutter with the lens directed upwards, the median ridge of a dislocatable patella will easily be seen as it is pushed laterally, but in the normal knee it is unusual to see much more than a third of the patella, however hard it is pushed laterally. The lateral suprapatellar approach can also be used, but the insertion of the arthroscope distorts the anatomy and the antero-lateral approach is preferable.

Characteristic vertical fissuring of the articular surface of the medial facet may be present, presumably from repeated contact with the femoral condyle, and osteochondral fractures or chondral separations can sometimes be recognised. Subsynovial haemorrhage is often seen medial to the patella after a recent dislocation and ectopic ossicles may be identified beneath the synovium (Fig. 14.2).

Habitual dislocation of the patella

In patients with habitual dislocation, the patella dislocates every time the knee is flexed, in contrast to the patient with recurrent dislocation, where months may pass between dislocations. The clinical features include pain and unsteadiness of the knee, with obvious dislocation of the patella when the knee is flexed, and radiographs show patello-femoral incongruity.

The greater frequency of dislocation causes more extensive damage to the articular surface than in recurrent dislocation, even though the dislocations are less dramatic. Arthroscopy is useful in determining the full extent of the damage to the patella.

The lateral part of the extensor mechanism is often abnormally short in these patients and must be lengthened to achieve stability. The patella may also be abnormal in shape, and operation is therefore a formidable undertaking, requiring extensive lateral release and perhaps elongation of the quadriceps mechanism in a joint which already has degenerative changes and bony incongruity.

Permanent dislocation

If the patella is irreducible and never returns to its correct anatomical position, the dislocation is described as permanent, or persistent (Insall 1984). Arthroscopic release of tight structures may be helpful, but open operation is usually required. Arthroscopy is difficult in these knees.

Congenital dislocation

Congenital dislocation is an uncommon condition first reported by Conn (1925), and differs from permanent dislocation only in being present from

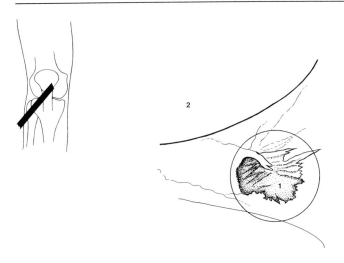
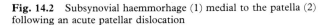

Fig. 14.2 Subsynovial haemmorhage (1) medial to the patella (2) following an acute patellar dislocation

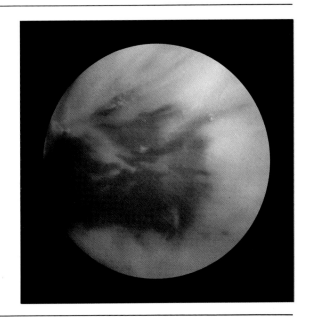

birth. The patella lies on the lateral side of the femur (Fig. 14.3) rather than in the intercondylar groove, and never comes into the correct position at any point of joint movement (Green & Waugh 1968). The condition is present at or shortly after birth, but is often identified later because the subcutaneous fat and valgus deformity of early childhood may delay diagnosis.

Because the dislocated patella lies on the lateral side of the femur, the quadriceps tendon acts as an abductor of the knee as well as an extensor, and the patient may find it easier to walk with a rather stiff-legged sideways shuffle than a normal gait. The extensor mechanism is even shorter than in patients with habitual dislocation, the patella is abnormal in shape, and articular cartilage changes are the rule. Operation is difficult and uncertain, but efforts should be made to elongate the extensor mechanism, release the capsule laterally and, if necessary, stabilise the patella in its correct position with a bone graft under the lateral condylar ridge of the femur (Albee 1919).

Subluxation on extension

The patella will sometimes flick laterally as the knee is actively extended, and reduce when the knee is flexed (Dandy 1971). The patella is usually small and high, and the lateral margin of the lateral femoral condyle deficient. Subluxation on extension usually presents between the ages of 5 and 10 years, and can progress to recurrent frank dislocation before skeletal maturity.

On examination, the patella dislocates laterally when the knee is actively extended by the quadriceps, but not when extended passively, and reduces on flexion. Some patients progress to recurrent frank dislocation of the patella, but natural recovery

without operation can occur as the ligaments become tighter and the bones enlarge through normal growth.

If the patients present before skeletal maturity, it is important to avoid damage to the tibial apophysis (Fig. 14.4) (Fielding et al 1960, Crosby & Insall 1976, Pappas et al 1984), and management should be as conservative as possible. Physiotherapy to build up the vastus medialis may be helpful, and arthroscopy is useful in assessment and to confirm that there is no other abnormality, but any reconstructive operation should, if possible, be delayed until all growth at the knee has ceased.

If operation cannot be delayed until growth is complete, a semitendinosus tenodesis, which does not involve the growth plates or the apophysis of the tibial tubercle, may be sufficient, but lateral release alone is usually unsuccessful. If operation can be delayed until growth has ended, elevation of the lateral condyle and advancement of the vastus medialis obliquus is often helpful.

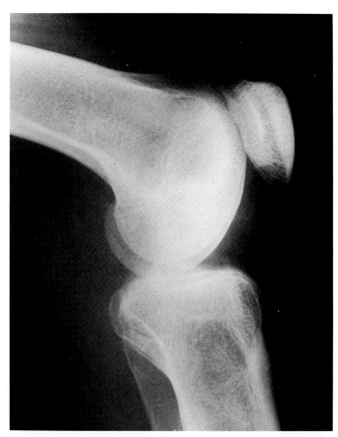

Fig. 14.4 Growth arrest of the anterior margin of the tibia following injury to the tibial tubercle in childhood. Note the abnormal relationship of the tibial plateau and the anterior margin of the tibia

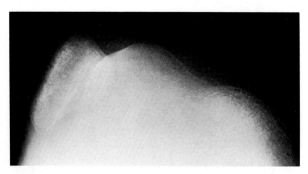

Fig. 14.3 Habitual dislocation of the patella with dysplastic femoral condyles

Excessive lateral pressure syndrome

The excessive lateral pressure syndrome has already been described in Chapter 13 and is mentioned here only because the patella lies in an abnormal position and because some authors refer to the condition as 'subluxation of the patella' (Metcalf 1982). The fact that the patella is placed incorrectly does not necessarily mean that it is unstable. In this condition, the patella is bound more tightly to the femur than normal and the patello-femoral joint has an excess of stability. The condition does not progress to dislocation, and the term 'subluxation' should not really be applied to such a joint.

CAUSES OF INSTABILITY

Ligamentous laxity

Recurrent dislocation of the patella is common in patients with generalised ligamentous laxity (Carter & Sweetnam 1958), voluntary posterior subluxation of the shoulder or clicking of the temporo-mandibular joint. Apart from providing an explanation for the dislocation, to diagnose generalised ligamentous laxity is no help, except as a warning that it will be difficult to achieve stability and that the opposite patella might dislocate also.

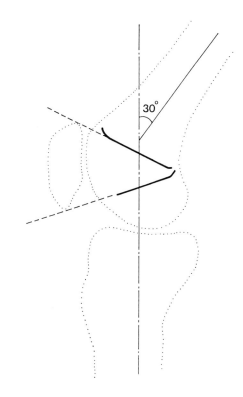

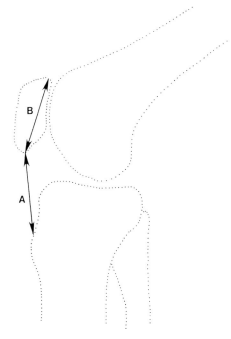

Fig. 14.5   The index of Insall and Salvati, which compares the length of the patella with the distance between its lower pole and the tibial tubercle

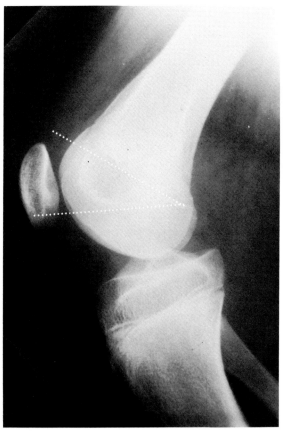

Fig. 14.6   Blumensaat's lines. Lines drawn along the lower femoral epiphysis or its scar and the roof of the intercondylar notch should bracket the patella in 30° of flexion

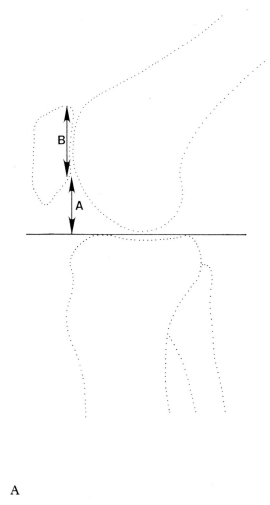

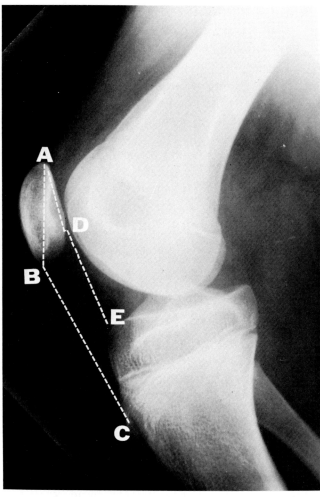

A   B

Fig. 14.7 (A) The index of Blackburne and Peel, which measures the length of the articular surface of the patella with the distance between the lower edge of the articular surface and a horizontal line drawn through the centre of the tibio-femoral joint. (B) compares the index of Blackburne and Peel (AD/DE) with the index of Insall and Salvati (AB/BC) in a patient with a small patella

Proximal realignment with a fascial sling or plication of the medial capsule, either with or without a vastus medialis obliquus advancement, may be effective in these patients, but the repair may stretch. Lateral transposition of the tibial tubercle is unlikely to be helpful if the basic pathology is ligamentous laxity and the tubercle is already in its normal position; in these patients, medial transposition of the tubercle with medial plication can be followed by medial dislocation.

Patella alta

The normal patella depends for stability upon its central 'keel' sitting in the intercondylar groove of the femur, the alignment of the extensor mechanism and its insertion on to the tibia, the action of the vasti medialis and lateralis, and the tension in the medial and lateral retinacula. In patients with patella alta, the patella rides higher than usual, the patella itself and the median ridge are often smaller than usual, and the mechanical stability of the patella in its groove is therefore greatly reduced.

With the help of radiographs, it is not difficult to define which patellae are abnormally high. Insall & Salvati (1971) defined the normal relationship of the patella and femur by comparing the lengths of the patella and patellar ligament (Fig. 14.5). Blumensaat (1938) defined the normal height of the patella by relating its position to the epiphyseal scar and the roof of the intercondylar notch on the lateral radiograph taken at exactly 30° of flexion (Fig. 14.6). The method of Blackburne & Peel (1977), which compares the length of the articular surface of the patella with its height above the tibial plateau (Fig. 14.7), is probably the simplest and most reliable of these measurements, but none replaces clinical examination and the height, shape and mobility of a patella can best be assessed with the fingers. To base clinical decisions on lines drawn on radiographs is an unsound principle; clinical decisions should be made at the bedside, not at the viewing box.

Genu recurvatum

If the knee hyperextends, the patella is not tightly applied to the intercondylar groove in full extension and, at the instant flexion begins, the patella is particularly unstable. If the genu recurvatum is itself the result of generalised ligamentous laxity, the patient will have two conditions contributing to patella instability, both affecting the proximal stability of the joint, and stabilisation will be difficult.

Q angle

The extensor mechanism does not run in a straight line from origin to insertion, but makes a gentle turn laterally at the patella. As a result, the quadriceps pulls the patella laterally as well as upwards, the lateral force being resisted by the lateral condyle and the tension in the medial structures.

The amount by which the line of the extensor mechanism deviates is known as the 'Q' (for quadriceps) angle; it lies between a line drawn from the anterior superior iliac spine to the centre of the patella and another line from the centre of the patella to the tibial tubercle (Fig. 14.8). The hip should be in neutral rotation at the time of measurement, with the muscles relaxed, because either incorrect positioning of the leg or contraction of the quadriceps can alter the Q angle. The normal Q angle is 15° and anything over 20° is probably abnormal (Insall 1984).

Although the Q angle is easy to measure, it is only one of many factors contributing to patellar stability and cannot be taken in isolation. There is a regrettable tendency to place undue importance upon the Q angle, perhaps because it appears so simple and requires such little expertise in its measurement. The Q angle is influenced by anything that affects the position of the fixed points from which it is measured, and therefore depends on the width of the pelvis and the position of the tibial tubercle relative to the tibial crest. The position of the tibial tubercle, however, is affected not only by

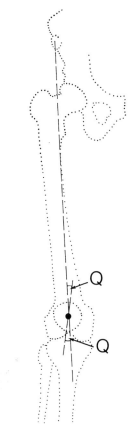

Fig. 14.8 The Q angle between a line drawn from the anterior superior iliac spine and the centre of the patella, and another line drawn from the centre of the patella to the tibial tubercle

its relation to the crest, but also by the relationship of the tibia to the femur. A short patient with genu valgum and a broad pelvis, for example, will have a larger Q angle than a tall slim patient with a narrow pelvis and genu varum.

Femoral or tibial osteotomy will correct a valgus deformity at the knee and reduce the Q angle, but it is so drastic that it should not be considered as a routine procedure for recurrent dislocation of the patella. On the other hand, if a patient has enough genu valgum to merit correction in its own right and also has a dislocating patella, stabilisation of the patella can be deferred until the result of the tibial osteotomy is known.

Congruence angle

The congruence angle (Merchant et al 1974) indicates how well the patella 'fits' the femur. This angle, like so many radiological parameters, is something of a blunt instrument and is abnormal both in the unstable patella-femoral joint and the joint with chondromalacia patellae (Insall 1984). The congruence and sulcus angles have been described above (p. 186).

Quadriceps contracture

If the quadriceps mechanism is abnormally short or there is an abnormal attachment of the patella to the ilio-tibial tract (Jeffreys 1963), its tension will be increased as the patella moves around the front of the femur and the patella will tend to take the shortest possible route from origin to insertion, which is along the lateral side of the femoral condyle and not the long way around the front of the condyle. This is an uncommon cause of patellar dislocation, but it is sometimes seen in patients who have received many intra-muscular injections in the lateral side of the thigh in the neonatal period, or scarring in this area for any other reason (Lloyd-Roberts & Thomas 1964).

Quadriceps contracture can cause habitual dislocation of the patella or a permanent dislocation that may be confused with congenital dislocation. Because the quadriceps mechanism is shorter than normal, attempts at stabilisation will restrict flexion, unless the extensor mechanism is also lengthened.

Dysplastic condyles

The lateral pull of the quadriceps on the patella is resisted by the lateral lip of the intercondylar groove (Brattstrom 1964) as well as the shape of the patella. The height of the condylar ridges and their proximal extent can only be measured accurately by CAT scans (Figs. 14.9, 14.10), but arthroscopy can give a fair estimate of their height and relationship to the patella. Deficiency of the lateral femoral condyle contributes to subluxation of the patella on extension of the knee and perhaps to other patterns of patellar instability, and can be corrected by Albee's operation (Albee 1919).

OPERATIONS FOR PATELLAR INSTABILITY

Proximal realignment procedures

Vastus medialis obliquus advancement

Advancement of the lowermost part of the vastus medialis, the vastus medialis obliquus (VMO),

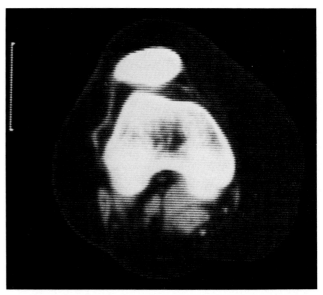

Fig. 14.9 A CAT scan showing the relationship of patella and femur in full extension in a normal knee

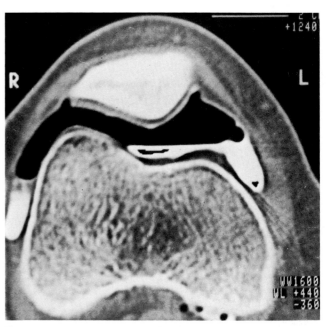

Fig. 14.10 A double-contrast arthrogram of the patello-femoral joint in full extension

increases the pull of the vastus medialis relative to the vastus lateralis (Fig. 14.11) (Madigan et al 1975). The operation is simple, does not produce any irreversible alterations in the anatomy of the knee and, because growth areas around the knee are not affected, the operation can be performed before growth has ceased. The operation is also useful in generalised ligamentous laxity and patella alta.

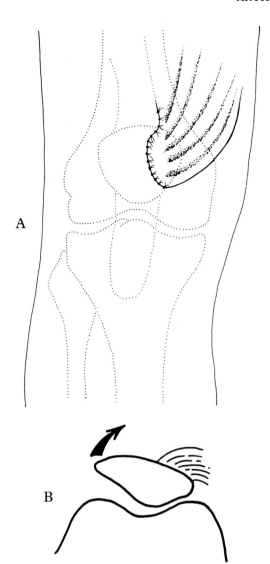

Fig. 14.11 Vastus medialis advancement: (A) the muscle belly is transposed distally and laterally on the patella; (B) the altered action of vastus medialis can tilt the patella

Disadvantages are that the power of the vastus medialis, like other transposed muscles, may be reduced by changing its position, and that moving its insertion nearer to the centre of the patella tilts the lower pole of the patella upwards and the upper pole downwards. It is also possible that the transposed tissue will stretch so that the muscle gradually migrates back to its proper insertion. Finally, if non-absorbable sutures are used, tender nodules form between the skin and the patella, making kneeling impossible. Unabsorbable subcutaneous sutures give rise to long-term problems and should not be used in front of the patella or tibial tubercle.

Lateral release

If the action of the quadriceps is to be modified so that the patella is pulled more medially than lateral, either the vastus lateralis can be weakened or the vastus medialis strengthened. On the principle that it is easier to break something than to make something, a lateral release of the extensor mechanism with division of the vastus lateralis tendon (Fig. 14.12) is even simpler and less complicated than vastus medialis obliquus advancement. The technique of operation is described above (p. 79).

When a lateral release is performed for recurrent dislocation of the patella, the whole of the vastus lateralis tendon must be divided, which means that the incision should be carried well above the upper pole of the patella so that the vastus medialis will act unopposed, pulling the patella medially. As well as pulling the patella medially, the unopposed action of the vastus medialis also pulls the median edge of the patella upwards, but it is unclear if this has any unfortunate consequences.

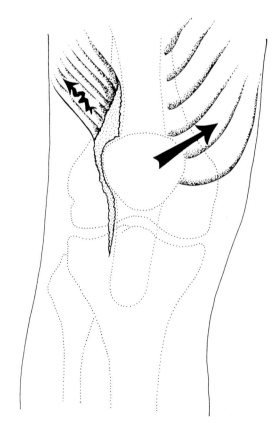

Fig. 14.12 Lateral release. Division of the vastus lateralis weakens it and makes the vastus medialis relatively stronger

Semitendinosus tenodesis

Semitendinosus tenodesis can be either a proximal or a distal realignment. The distal realignment is preferred (p. 212).

Distal realignment procedures

Goldthwait's procedure

Goldthwait described two operations. In 1895, he reported on a patient with bilateral patellar dislocation present for twenty years in whom he successfully stabilised one patella by detaching the patellar tedon with a sliver of bone and suturing it into a prepared subperiosteal bed beneath the pes anserinus. The result was so good that operation was undertaken on the other knee, this time transposing the tendon with a block of bone which was secured in a prepared bed with a nail. The bone block became infected, the wound was slow to heal and Goldthwait discarded the bone-block technique (Goldthwait 1899). We shall never know whether the procedure now known as Goldthwait's operation would ever have been invented, if this wound had not become infected.

In the operation usually associated with Goldthwait, the lateral half of the patella tendon is transposed medially (Goldthwait 1904). It is geometrically impossible to move the insertion of the patella tendon on the tibia by much more than its width, and the action of transposing the lateral slip of the patella tendon also tilts the lateral edge of the patella backwards (Fig. 14.13). This change in position may have a more far-reaching effect upon the patella alignment and dynamics than simply moving the patella tendon medially. Goldthwait's procedure is simple and leaves the patellar mechanism intact so that the rehabilitation is rapid, but it does not correct the proximal part of the patellar mechanism.

Tibial tubercle transposition

Transposition of the entire tibial tubercle with a block of bone (Hauser 1938) makes it possible to reposition the tibial tubercle and reduce the Q angle considerably. In patients with lax ligaments, the tubercle can be moved distally as well as medially but distal transposition of the tubercle may also restrict flexion, increase pressure on the patella surface, and thus accelerate degenerative change.

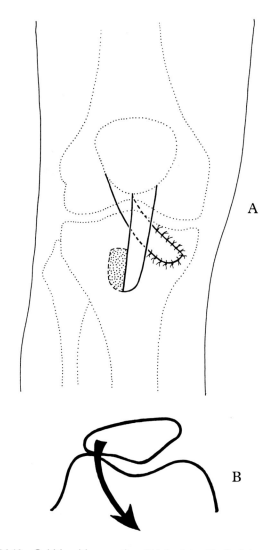

Fig. 14.13 Goldthwait's operation: (A) the lateral half of the patellar tendon is passed behind the medial and sutured to the tibia; (B) this transposition can increase the pressure on the lateral margin of the patella

Smillie described a technique for tibial tubercle transposition in which the tubercle is excised with a rectangle of bone, set into a diamond-shaped recess and rotated to lock it under the tibial cortex, making external immobilisation and internal fixation unnecessary (Smillie 1974) (Fig. 14.14). Although this is an absorbing exercise in surgical technique, the operation has two disadvantages. First, the medullary cavity of the tibia must be extensively excavated to make enough room to insert and then rotate a block of bone. Secondly, the tubercle must be recessed beneath the tibial cortex by at least the thickness of the cortex itself – perhaps 5 mm – so that the operation is effectively a 'reverse Maquet' or

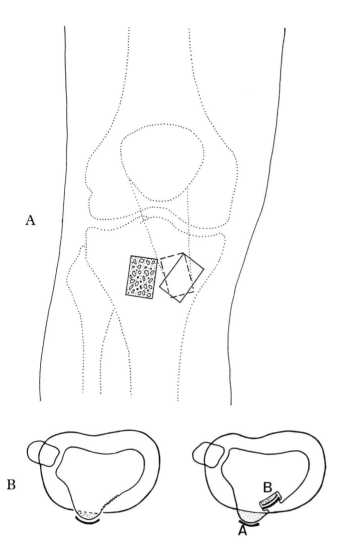

Fig. 14.14 Hauser's operation with recession of the tibial tubercle: (A) to show the change in position; (B) to show how the tibial tubercle is recessed

recessing it (Fig. 14.15). A wide lateral release is necessary for the Hauser, Elmslie–Trillat and most other procedures, which makes it difficult to separate the effect of a lateral release alone from that of a tubercle transposition.

There are many other types of tibial tubercle transposition apart from these, but all disturb the tubercle and must be avoided while growth is continuing, if genu recurvatum is to be avoided (Fielding et al 1960, Crosby & Insall 1976, Pappas et al 1984). As well as the effect on growth, median transposition of the quadriceps insertion causes the muscle to act as an external rotator of the tibia and, if the ligaments are lax, external rotation of the tibia about its long axis will bring the tubercle back to the same relationship with the patella as before operation.

tubercle recession. Such a procedure must alter the stresses upon the patellar surface, and if Maquet's operation to advance the tibial tubercle really does reduce the pressures on the articular surface, recessing the tubercle is likely to increase them by a corresponding amount.

Alternatively, the tubercle can be lifted on a flake of tibial cortex as an osteo-periosteal flap, moved distally, and swung medially to be secured on a prepared bed by a screw. This operation, which was first used by Elmslie (1978), but not formally described by him, was made popular by Trillat (Trillat et al 1964) and is now commonly called the Elmslie–Trillat procedure. The operation actually advances the tibial tubercle slightly, rather than

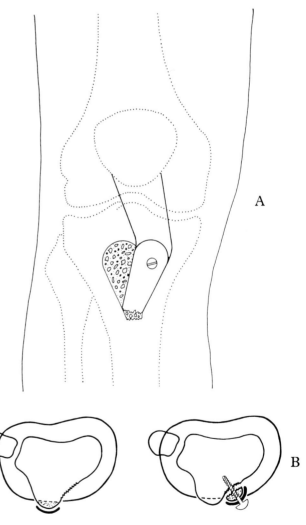

Fig. 14.15 Elmslie–Trillat transposition. The tibial tubercle is swung on an osteo-periosteal flap (A), which advances the tibial tubercle slightly (B)

Semitendinosus tenodesis

Semitendinosus tenodesis (Fig. 14.16), which uses the semitendinosus tendon as an additional ligament to limit lateral motion of the patella, does not disturb the growing areas of the knee, and can be performed before growth has ceased. The operation can be done in one of two ways. Either the tendon can be detached above and the distal part passed through the patella from below upwards (Baker et al 1972, Hall et al 1979), or the tendon can be detached at its tibial insertion and attached to the patella from above – which is a proximal realignment. The first version is the more useful and is simple once the semitendinosus tendon has been identified proximally in the thigh. The operation should be accompanied by a lateral release.

Although the operation is effective in correcting dislocation or subluxation of the patella in younger patients, as the patient grows and the shape of the knee changes, the semitendinosus tendon may then become too tight when the knee is flexed, producing a 'medial compression syndrome'. This is easily relieved, however, by dividing or lengthening the transposed tendon.

Fascial slings

Fascial slings placed under the quadriceps tendon to hold it medially (Fig. 14.17) will produce a stable

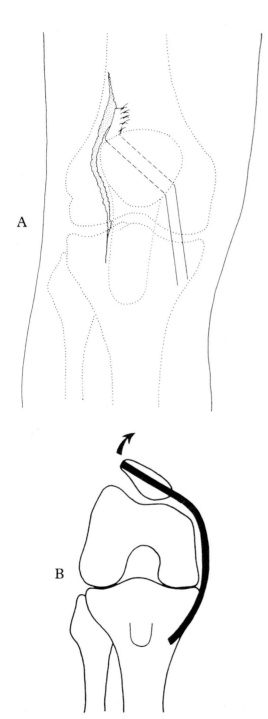

Fig. 14.16 Semitendinosus tenodesis. The tendon is passed through the patella from below upwards after a wide lateral release (A), and can tilt the patella upwards (B)

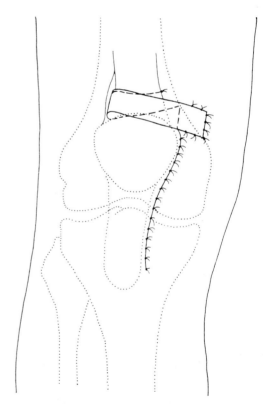

Fig. 14.17 Fascial sling. A strip of fascia from the medial side of the knee is used to pull the patellar tendon medially and the defect closed to pull the patella medially

extensor mechanism at the end of the operation, but slings are less satisfactory in the longer term, because instability may return as the graft stretches. A lateral release is not always advised as part of this procedure, but it is strongly recommended, because to excise a slip of capsule medially and close the defect without an accompanying lateral release must increase the load on the patella. Because the fascial sling pulls the quadriceps tendon medially, it increases the Q angle and is therefore unsuitable for patients in whom this angle is already excessive. However, the fascial sling is useful in patients with lax ligaments.

Tibial osteotomy

Tibial or femoral osteotomy are too extensive and destructive to be considered as a primary operation for recurrent dislocation of the patella alone. Despite this, osteotomy may be considered, if the patient has genu valgum severe enough to warrant osteotomy in its own right as well as patellar instability.

Albee's operation

Albee's operation increases the height of the lateral femoral condyle at the upper end of the intercondylar groove (Fig. 14.18). Although simple in conception, the operation is more difficult than Albee's original description (Albee 1919), in which the elevated condyle was supported by a tibial graft held in position with bone pegs and kangaroo tendon, might suggest. To lift the lateral condyle with an osteotome and hold it up with a bone graft sounds straightforward, but in practice it is impossible to do this without creating a split in the articular surface of

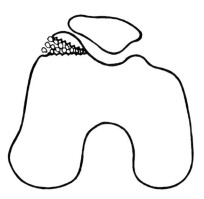

Fig. 14.18 Albee's operation. Bone graft is packed under the lateral condylar ridge to increase its height

the femur. The lateral condyle is convex at its upper end, raising a wedge leaves an articular cartilage defect at the lateral margin, and packing bone graft under the elevated segment creates a raw bone surface inside the synovial cavity, which can lead to intra-articular bleeding and joint stiffness. These problems can be overcome in part by elevating the lateral condyle at its very upper limit and by stripping the synovium from the lateral condyle before entering the bone, so that the synovium can be laid over the defect. The operation is more destructive than a soft tissue procedure alone, but it is useful both for subluxation of the patella on extension and for dysplasia of the lateral femoral condyle in the adult patient.

Selection of operation

In the management of the unstable patella, it is important to select the operation appropriate to the pathology. If the Q angle is larger than normal, it is not sensible to perform a medial plication and vastus medialis obliquus advancement to increase it still further; nor is it sensible to reduce the Q angle, if it is already normal.

Arthroscopy is helpful in assessing the joint surfaces and the patellar position, as well as in the correction of associated internal derangements such as loose bodies and chondral separations, but the choice of operation is based largely on clinical and radiological examination. Selection of operation is often difficult, and it may be necessary to combine one or more of the techniques.

References

Albee F H 1919 Orthopaedic and reconstructive surgery, p 627. W B Saunders, Philadelphia, Pa
Baker R H, Carrol N, Dewar P, Hall J E, 1972 Semitendinosus tenodesis for recurrent dislocation of the patella. Journal of Bone and Joint Surgery 54B: 103–109
Blackburne J S, Peel T E 1977 A new method of measuring patellar height. Journal of Bone and Joint Surgery 59B: 241–242
Blumensaat C 1938 Die Lageabuweichungen und Verrenkurigan der Kniescheibe. Ergebnisse der Chirurgie und Orthopaedie 31: 149–223
Brattstrom H 1964 Shape of the intercondylar groove normally and in recurrent dislocation of the patella. Acta Orthopedica Scandinavica suppl 68: 134–148
Carter C, Sweetnam R 1958 Familial joint laxity and recurrent dislocation of the patella. Journal of Bone and Joint Surgery 40B: 664–667
Coleman H M 1948 Recurrent steochondral fracture of the patella. Journal of Bone and Joint Surgery 30B: 153–157
Conn H R 1925 A new method for operative reduction of congenital luxation of the patella. Journal of Bone and Joint Surgery 7: 370–383

Crosby E B, Insall J N 1976 Recurrent dislocation of the patella. Journal of Bone and Joint Surgery 58A: 9–13

Dandy D J 1971 Recurrent subluxation of the patella on extension of the knee. Journal of Bone and Joint Surgery 53B: 483–487

Elmslie R C 1978 Unpublished work, St Bartholomew's Hospital, London 1912–1932. In: Smillie I S Diseases of the knee joint. Churchill Livingstone, London

Fielding J W, Liebler W A, Tambakis A 1960 The effect of a tibial tubercle transplant in children on the growth of the upper tibial epiphysis. Journal of Bone and Joint Surgery 42A: 1426–1434

Goldthwait J E 1899 Permanent dislocation of the patella. Annals of Surgery 29: 62–68

Goldthwait J E 1904 Slipping or recurrent dislocation of the patella with a report of eleven cases. Boston Medical and Surgical Journal 150: 169–174

Green J P, Waugh W 1968 Congenital lateral dislocation of the patella. Journal of Bone and Joint Surgery 50B: 285–289

Hall J E, Micheli L J, McManama G B 1979 Semitendinosus tenodesis for recurrent subluxation or dislocation of the patella. Clinical Orthopaedics and Related Research 144: 31–35

Hauser E D W 1938 Total tendon transplant for slipping patella. Surgery Gynecology and Obstetrics 66: 199–214

Insall J N 1984 Disorders of the patella. In: Insall J N (ed) Surgery of the knee. Churchill Livingstone, New York

Insall J N, Salvati E 1971 Patella position in the normal knee joint. Radiology 101: 101–104

Jeffreys T E 1963 Recurrent dislocation of the patella due to abnormal attachment of the ilio-tibial tract. Journal of Bone and Joint Surgery 45B: 740–743

Lloyd-Roberts G C, Thomas T G 1964 The etiology of quadriceps contracture in children. Journal of Bone and Joint Surgery 46B: 498–502

Madigan R, Wissinger H A, Donaldson W F 1975 Preliminary experience with a method of quadricepsplasty in recurrent subluxation of the patella. Journal of Bone and Joint Surgery 57A: 600–607

Merchant A C, Mercer R L, Jacobsen R H, Cool C R 1974 Roentgenographic analysis of patellofemoral congruence. Journal of Bone and Joint Surgery 56A: 1391–1396

Metcalf R W 1982 An arthroscopic method for lateral release of the subluxating and dislocating patella. Clinical Orthopaedics and Related Research 167: 11–18

Pappas A M, Anas P, Toczylowski H M 1984 Asymmetrical arrest of the proximal tibial epiphysis and genu recurvatum deformity. Journal of Bone and Joint Surgery 66A: 575–581

Smillie I S 1974

Trillat A, Dejour H, Couette A 1964 Diagnosis et traitement des subluxations recidivantes de la rotule. Revue de Chirurgie Orthop4édique et Reparatrice de l'appareil Moteur 50: 13–24

Wiberg G 1941 Roentgenographic and anatomic studies of the femoro-patellar joint. Acta Orthopaedica Scandinavica 12: 319–410

15

Learning arthroscopic surgery

Skill with a hammer and osteotome is not transferable to the arthroscope, and many otherwise competent surgeons find arthroscopic surgery exceedingly difficult. Triangulation is a particular problem and demands such fine co-ordination of hand and eye that it has even been suggested that some people are physically incapable of this kind of work. This is probably incorrect, but it is certainly true that different surgeons learn at different rates and that some surgeons skilled in conventional techniques find triangulation virtually impossible. For an experienced surgeon to go back to learning basic manual skills requires a self-discipline not possessed by everyone, and the teaching of arthroscopic surgery therefore presents special problems.

SELF-TEACHING

Learning arthroscopic surgery is a lonely business. Most arthroscopists learn by repeating the mistakes of their predecessors so that the trainee becomes his own trainer, critic and examiner. There are many powerful arguments against such a haphazard system of learning, but there is also the advantage that because surgeons share the same experience as they learn, they can chart their progress with some accuracy, so that the learning process can be conducted in a safe and orderly progression from the simplest operations to the most difficult. Although the rate of learning will vary from one individual to the next, the following general outline should be helpful as a guide to the order in which new techniques should be attempted, and when.

Arthroscopic honeymoon

The first five or ten arthroscopies are associated with the excitement and enthusiasm that come with the first experience of any new procedure. The underwater scenery of the knee is spectacular and the beauty of the first clear glimpse down the arthroscope is so exciting that the inevitable early failures are easy to bear. This stage is short-lived.

Depression

In contrast to the previous period, the next 20 or 30 examinations are attended by gloom and disillusion. Early successes prove unrepeatable, the encroachment on available operating time becomes apparent, and the patience of the operating theatre staff begins to wear thin. No clinical benefit from the procedure can be seen, and there is a great temptation to abandon arthroscopy and return to the old ways that once served so well. The decision to abandon arthroscopy is seldom made consciously at this stage, but the intervals between arthroscopic attempts gradually become longer and longer until the arthroscope is packed away for ever. This temptation must be recognised and overcome.

Success

Once the period of depression has passed – usually after some 30 or so attempts – the examination becomes predictable and most of the knee will be seen in most of the patients. The findings of arthroscopy will generally be confirmed at arthrotomy, and the surgeon will begin to have as much confidence in his arthroscopic findings as in his clinical judgement. During this period, anaesthetists and other colleagues come to accept arthroscopy as an inevitable time-wasting prelude to arthrotomy, and there is some justification for this belief, because preliminary arthroscopy can only add to the theatre time required for open meniscectomy. Despite this criticism, some positive benefits can at last be seen when the findings of arthroscopy lead to a smaller and more precise arthrotomy.

The next great landmark comes when the decision is made not to proceed to arthrotomy and to accept that the arthroscopic findings are more likely to be correct than clinical and radiological investigations. When this step has been taken, usually after some 30 or 40 examinations, even the theatre staff will begin to see the real advantages of arthroscopy. Patients will be returned to the wards with their knees intact, and knowledge of the exact pathology will allow the arthrotomies that are still necessary to be done more swiftly and neatly than was previously possible.

Triangulation

With the nursery slopes behind him, the surgeon can turn his attention to advanced diagnostic techniques. It must be emphasised yet again that no attempt at meniscectomy or any other surgical procedure should be made until the surgeon is utterly confident in his arthroscopic findings and in the basic techniques of arthroscopic surgery.

The first and simplest 'exercise' in triangulation is to identify the tip of the irrigation needle in the suprapatellar pouch. When the needle tip can be found without conscious effort, it can be used to probe or manipulate the medial suprapatellar plica, the under-surface of the patella and the synovial shelf. Attempts to grasp and remove a loose body at this stage are permissible, but unlikely to succeed (p. 88). Triangulation is difficult for everyone at first, and it may be helpful to revert to the straightahead 0° telescope instead of the 30° fore-oblique telescope.

Percutaneous probing needles along the joint-line can also be tried at this stage. The point of insertion is most easily found by looking at the desired point of entry through the arthroscope and placing the needle just below the point of transilluminated skin (p. 55). The needle should be slipped either above or below the meniscus, rather than into its substance, but insertion directly into the body of the meniscus

itself may be needed to dislodge a flap or expose a lesion in the posterior horn. More than one meniscus must be felt before an accurate assessment can be made, but this should not be taken as a licence to poke needles into healthy menisci at will.

Synovial biopsy

Synovial biopsy from the lateral suprapatellar approach is simple and yields excellent specimens for histological study, as well as an opportunity to become familiar with the insertion and handling of the instruments. It is sensible to send specimens of unexpectedly inflamed synovium to the laboratory for histological study, and the opportunity therefore arises frequently.

Probing hooks

A probing hook can be used both to improve triangulation and to 'rehearse' operations. If the diagnostic arthroscopy shows a torn medial meniscus, it is entirely reasonable to insert a hook from the antero-medial approach to assess its mobility, even if the joint is then opened. Bucket-handle tears of the medial meniscus can be manipulated with a blunt hook (Fig. 10.7) placed just above the anterior horn of the medial meniscus and about 1 cm from the medial edge of the patellar tendon – a little lower and more medial than the ideal point of insertion for the excision of a meniscal fragment. Care should be taken not to prang the end of the arthroscope with the tip of the trocar, by taking the precautions described in Chapter 4.

Once inserted, the hook can be passed slowly, gently and under direct arthroscopic vision at all times to the medial meniscus, which may be picked up and manipulated as described in Chapter 4. When the medial meniscus can be manipulated easily, it is safe to try the higher and more lateral insertion of the hook needed for examination of the lateral meniscus. When fully confident in all aspects of the probing hook, and not a moment sooner, it is safe to insert cutting instruments in place of the hook and excise simple lesions.

Removing flap and tags

Stubs of anterior cruciate ligament long enough to cause mechanical symptoms (Fig. 12.27) and detached bucket-handle fragments of medial meniscus are ideal lesions for the first attempt at arthroscopic surgery (Fig. 10.13).

When a suitable lesion has been found, it should be grasped firmly at its base with rongeurs and removed, weakening the base first with knife or scissors if necessary. Although removal of these lesions is quick, simple and satisfactory, the surgeon must still restrain himself from attacking large bucket-handle fragments or complex oblique tears, and must be prepared to accept defeat and open the knee if he runs into difficulty.

Bucket-handle tears

When flaps and tags at the front of the joint can be removed simply, the removal of a bucket-handle fragment can be considered. The easiest bucket-handle fragments are type 1 tears of the medial meniscus that are less than 5 mm wide (Fig. 10.2), and the procedure will be easier if the anterior cruciate ligament is ruptured. Thicker fragments are more difficult and placement of the instruments must be exact, if there is a normal anterior cruciate ligament as well as a thick bucket-handle fragment in the notch. The different techniques for meniscectomy are described in Chapters 10 and 11.

Complex meniscal tears

Having successfully dealt with a type 1 bucket-handle tear, it is safe to proceed to type 2 and type 3 peripheral tears, thick bucket-handle fragments and loose bodies, but it is sensible to wait a little longer before tackling an extensive parrot-beak tear or a partial-thickness posterior third tear of the medial meniscus. When these lesions can be handled simply, it is safe to move on to other procedures.

TEACHING AIDS AND COURSES

Before attempting arthroscopic surgery in the operating theatre, it is helpful to read a book on the subject to understand both the problems and the philosophy of arthroscopic surgery, which sometimes differ radically from 'traditional' teaching. Courses on arthroscopic surgery are also valuable, but can only supplement the teaching obtainable from books, while video tapes help with the recognition of structures and pathology, but not with practical skills. A visit to a centre where knee surgery is practised regularly may be useful so that the problems can be seen at first hand.

Knee models

Knee models (Fig. 15.1) are useful for learning practical skills such as depth perception and triangulation, and may accelerate the development of visuospatial skills (Fig. 15.2) (Sweeney 1982). There is no need for the models to be lifelike; triangulation can be practised just as well with the skin of the model

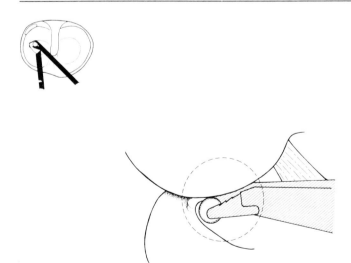
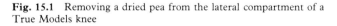

Fig. 15.1 Removing a dried pea from the lateral compartment of a True Models knee

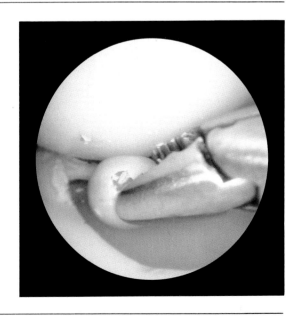

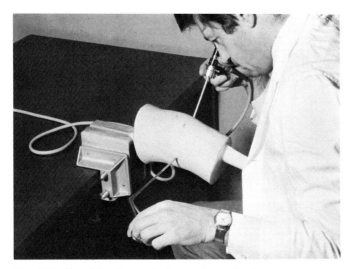

Fig. 15.2 Practising the manipulation of operating instruments inserted from the postero-medial approach using the True Models knee

connecting the irrigation and drainage systems used with powered instruments, and to use the powered instruments themselves. These models are ingenious, but do not produce the operating conditions accurately, and have several disadvantages. First, even though great care has been taken to keep leakage and overflow to a minimum, they are messy. Secondly, many are fixed at their lower end like a plant in a pot; thus they cannot be manipulated like a normal leg attached to a patient at the upper end. Thirdly, most wet models are much stiffer than the normal knee, which makes the trainee concentrate more on the instruments he is using than on important points of technique such as the correct site of insertion or proper manipulation of the leg.

removed (Fig. 15.3) as with it in place. Models also provide the opportunity to recognise different patterns of meniscal tear (Fig. 15.4) and to rehearse the various stages of an arthroscopic operation outside the operating theatre, but, however realistic they may be, there is no substitute for the live, bleeding, human knee, and operating on knee models must always remain an artificial exercise.

Cadavers

The cadaver knee or amputation specimen, while having a certain macabre appeal, is less satisfactory than a model knee. The inevitable mess associated with any cadaveric specimen is made worse by distending the synovial cavity. The cell membranes lose their function after death, and distension with saline results in exudation of fluid from the joint and a large extra-articular collection of saline, which tracks to the point of insertion of the instrument, where it leaks out and dribbles down the arthroscope to the trainee's hand, elbow, and sometimes his eye. To add to these formidable difficulties, the cadaveric knee is stiff, unless it is warmed before use, whole-

Wet models

'Wet' knee models allow the surgeon to become fully familiar with the correct sequence for setting up and

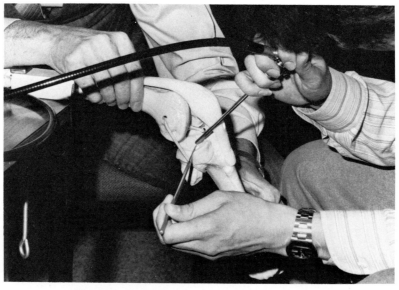

Fig. 15.3 Using a knee model with the skin removed

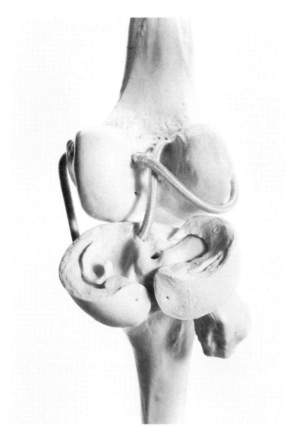

Fig. 15.4 A knee model opened to show the removable menisci and the meniscal lesions

leg amputation specimens are difficult to hold steady, and the view inside the cadaveric knee is quickly obscured by debris. Arthroscopy is therefore more difficult and less realistic in the cadaver than in a live bleeding human knee or a model, but if a cadaver must be used, the article by Fullerton et al (1981) describes a practical method of mounting and preparing the limb.

Other aids

A simple aid to develop the visuo-spatial skills can be made by placing a variety of everyday objects in a box with holes drilled in the side, through which the arthroscope or instruments can be passed. These devices offer nothing more than familiarity with the instruments and do not reproduce the cramped field of vision found within the knee, but they are inexpensive, easy to produce and may help with triangulation.

A hollowed-out grapefruit also makes a simple, but useful model. The grapefruit is sliced in two, the segments removed to leave the fibrous septa with a few pips, and the grapefruit reassembled with adhesive tape to make a worthwhile – though sticky – model for practising depth perception and triangulation. Cabbage, lettuce and Starfire Fuji mums can also be pressed into service (Sweeney 1982).

Television is the ultimate teaching aid and has been described in Chapter 3. It is interesting to note that television was first described as a teaching aid (Poehling 1978) and not as an adjunct to the operation itself. If television is not available, a dual viewing aid alone is an excellent substitute (Figs. 2.21, 2.22).

All these aids shorten the learning period and increase the confidence of the surgeon. Even if none is available, the learning process will be safe for the patient provided that the surgeon only attempts procedures that he knows to be within his competence, and observes the four basic rules of arthroscopic surgery which are:

1. identify the pathology precisely
2. plan the approach carefully
3. keep the tip of the operating instrument in view at all times
4. always rehearse the operation with a hook before inserting cutting instruments.

References

Fullerton L R, Protzman R W, Wincheski J 1981 Arthroscopy training. American Journal of Sports Medicine 9: 38–39
Poehling G G 1978 Arthroscopic teaching technics. Southern Medical Journal 71: 1067–1069
Sweeney H J 1982 Teaching arthroscopic surgery at the residency level. Orthopedic Clinics of North America 13: 255–261

Index